OBSTETRICS AND GYNECOLOGY:
A Competency-Based Companion

Michael Belden MD

Clinical Assistant Professor
Jefferson Medical College
Philadelphia, Pennsylvania
Department of Obstetrics and Gynecology
Lankenau Hospital
Wynnewood, Pennsylvania

Series Editor: Barry D. Mann MD, FACS

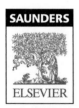

SAUNDERS

ELSEVIER

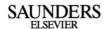

SAUNDERS
ELSEVIER

1600 John F. Kennedy Blvd.
Ste 1800
Philadelphia, PA 19103-2899

OBSTETRICS AND GYNECOLOGY: ISBN: 978-1-4160-4896-1
A COMPETENCY-BASED COMPANION

Notices

Knowledge and best practice in this field are constantly changing. As new research and experience broaden our understanding, changes in research methods, professional practices, or medical treatment may become necessary.

Practitioners and researchers must always rely on their own experience and knowledge in evaluating and using any information, methods, compounds, or experiments described herein. In using such information or methods they should be mindful of their own safety and the safety of others, including parties for whom they have a professional responsibility.

With respect to any drug or pharmaceutical products identified, readers are advised to check the most current information provided (i) on procedures featured or (ii) by the manufacturer of each product to be administered, to verify the recommended dose or formula, the method and duration of administration, and contraindications. It is the responsibility of practitioners, relying on their own experience and knowledge of their patients, to make diagnoses, to determine dosages and the best treatment for each individual patient, and to take all appropriate safety precautions.

To the fullest extent of the law, neither the Publisher nor the authors, contributors, or editors, assume any liability for any injury and/or damage to persons or property as a matter of products liability, negligence or otherwise, or from any use or operation of any methods, products, instructions, or ideas contained in the material herein.

Library of Congress Cataloging-in-Publication Data
Obstetrics and gynecology : a competency-based companion / [edited by] Michael Belden.
   p. ; cm.—(Competency-based companion)
   Includes bibliographical references.
   ISBN 978-1-4160-4896-1
   1. Obstetrics—Case studies.   2. Gynecology—Case studies.   3. Clinical
clerkship.   I. Belden, Michael.   II. Series: Competency-based companion.
   [DNLM: 1. Diagnostic Techniques, Obstetrical and Gynecological—Problems and
Exercises.   2. Diagnosis, Differential—Problems and Exercises.   3. Gynecologic Surgical
Procedures—Problems and Exercises. WQ 18.2 01425 2010]
   RG106.027 2010
   618—dc22
                                                              2009015330

Acquisitions Editor: Jim Merritt
Developmental Editor: Christine Abshire
Design Direction: Lou Forgione
Marketing Manager: Jason Oberacker

Printed in the United States of America
Last digit is the print number: 9   8   7   6   5   4   3   2   1

Working together to grow
libraries in developing countries

www.elsevier.com | www.bookaid.org | www.sabre.org

ELSEVIER   BOOK AID International   Sabre Foundation

for Katherine
Michael, Erica, Daniel

Foreword

Mastery is not a destination. It is a path upon which a physician, from the beginning of his or her training, travels for the length of his or her medical career. For a medical student, the first steps on this arduous journey begin the transformative process toward wisdom, meaning, and service. However, learning the art and science of medicine, much less treading the path of mastery, is no easy task. It takes levels of dedication, practice, motivation, mental discipline, and relational acumen that few in our society are willing to muster and even fewer understand. It is, however, not a solo journey; the young trainee should not and cannot travel this road alone. Wise and learned guides and role models must light the way, encouraging students to stay on the path, guiding them back on the path when they stray, and encouraging them when the way grows long and dark. In a practicing physician's life these guides and role models are often peers and colleagues; in the lives of medical students and residents they are their seniors: faculty and residents who have traveled the road before them. The best teachers have almost a mystical ability to provide the right instruction, at the right moment, for the right reason, and in the right domain.

In order to guide teachers and learners on the path to mastery, the ACGME identified six core competencies essential to the development of a physician and the effective practice of medicine. These six competencies—(1) medical knowledge, (2) patient care, (3) interpersonal and communication skills, (4) professionalism, (5) practice-based learning and improvement, and (6) systems-based practice are the educational lanterns that light the road of mastery in clinical practice. There is, however, a paucity of educational tools in obstetrics and gynecology linking the competencies to the teaching and learning needs of faculty, students, and residents. This textbook, *Obstetrics and Gynecology: A Competency-Based Companion,* by Michael Belden, fills this critical educational need.

Building on the successful format of the first book in this series, *Surgery: A Competency-Based Companion* by Barry D. Mann, this text on obstetrics and gynecology is both useful and profound. In Section I, Dr. Belden demystifies the competencies through an effective, dynamic, and readable overview and introduction to the six competencies along with useful tips to help students, residents, and faculty thrive in the clinical educational environment. The book then provides case presentations in a logical, progressive, organized fashion integrating and illustrating the six competencies with scenarios students are likely to encounter during their obstetrics and gynecology clerkship experience. The book also utilizes learning and teaching methodologies that will provide learners with a wide variety of learning styles (visual, auditory, kinesthetic, etc.) to engage with the material in a deep and meaningful way.

This text will prove an invaluable tool to assist students, whether they ultimately pursue obstetrics and gynecology as a specialty or not, on their journey toward mastery in medicine in general and obstetrics and gynecology in particular. Similarly, faculty and residents will find this book a welcome tool on their journey of mastery in teaching: guiding students of all levels and interests as they acquire the knowledge, skills, and attitudes needed by a practicing physician as she or he continues on the road to mastery.

With this book every student can walk an illuminated path and every teacher can become a Master Teacher. Dr Belden and his team deserve high praise and admiration for this effort. Their contribution to obstetrics and gynecology education is also their gift to you as a teacher, learner, and/or, practicing physician. Read it and enjoy.

Timothy P. Brigham MDiv, PhD
Senior Vice-President, Department of Education, ACGME

Series Preface

In the beginning of this decade when the Accreditation Council for Graduate Medical Education (ACGME) brought forth the idea of competency categories, it was essentially left to the discretion of individual program directors to define and develop competency content, and then teach and evaluate accordingly.

Elsevier's Competency-Based Companion Series is the first publisher's attempt to demonstrate that the ACGME competencies are indeed the real components of what makes the art and science of doctoring a multidimensional profession.

Surgery: A Competency-Based Companion, the first volume of the competency-based series, was an initial effort to call the question, "What do we actually mean by each competency?" For the surgery volume, I personally called upon more than one hundred surgical educators to flesh out each of the six ACGME competencies in the various chapters of that volume. Early in the process it became clear that the authors had different understandings of what might be meant by each of the six competencies. Actualizing such a six-pronged curriculum was not destined to be a simple task for surgical educators, but proved to be an enriching educational journey.

Dr. Michael Belden's *Obstetrics and Gynecology: A Competency-Based Companion* is the second effort to offer competency content within the expanse of a clinical curriculum. Following the paradigm set forth in the surgery volume, Dr. Belden's book aims to teach students and residents to begin their clinical thinking with differential diagnosis and to use their tools of medical history, physical examination, laboratory tests, and imaging to work through the sorting process in a logical, systematic, expeditious, and cost-effective manner.

Reflecting on the Competency-Based Companion Series, the question arises: "Why crowd a book addressed to students and residents who are hungry for *clinical science* with the 'fluffy' issues of Interpersonal and Communication Skills, Professionalism, or issues of how best to use the system?" The woman's health curriculum inherent in Dr. Belden's OB-GYN volume speaks clearly to this issue: these harder-to-measure competencies are actually quite **integral** to clinical science and should not be separated from it. Indeed the competencies of interpersonal skills and professionalism are frequently called upon when dealing with both obstetrical issues and gynecologic care! In almost all aspects of both fields, personal intimacy and social issues hover at the core of the patient–doctor interaction. The practitioner discussing sexually transmitted infections (STIs), as one of many examples, must possess not only up-to-date medical knowledge of causative organisms and antibiotic sensitivities but also the appropriate interpersonal skills and professionalism to negotiate delicate patient–partner issues, to offer counseling when appropriate, and even to help navigate system-based financial considerations.

I salute Dr. Belden for his excellent work in assembling and editing *Obstetrics and Gynecology: A Competency-Based Companion* and for having ensured that it is a convincing demonstration of how competency components merge in educating quality practitioners in his field. And I salute Elsevier for the courage and persistence to believe that this series will ultimately have an impact on the quality of medical education.

Barry D. Mann MD

Preface

When the ACGME introduced the six clinical competencies into the language of medical education in 1999, many approached the concept with some skepticism. It is now more than ten years later, and it is clear that the clinical competencies do indeed bring value to medical education. The competencies enable us to more effectively describe and delineate the characteristics of being a "good doctor," those qualities our predecessors presumed we would ultimately incorporate into our professional lives by example, hard work, and rigorous study. By better defining the underlying principles of sound medical practice into six straightforward categories, it is now easier (and to some degree more acceptable) to identify an individual trainee's deficiencies so that these deficiencies can be directly addressed and appropriately remediated.

How can the ACGME competencies best be applied to help train the next generation of obstetrician/gynecologists? *Obstetrics and Gynecology: A Competency-Based Companion* provides a framework. The chapter contributors as well as the competency and section editors have identified the most commonly encountered obstetric and gynecologic disease processes and have outlined the approach to and management of each with full integration of the competencies. Medical Knowledge and Patient Care are heavily emphasized. In addition, the competency editors, as well as the Series Editor, Barry Mann, MD, have done their best to identify particular issues of Professionalism, Interpersonal and Communication Skills, Practice-Based Learning and Improvement, and Systems-Based Practice that are relevant to the topics addressed in each chapter. These competency paragraphs (color-coded "boxes") can be sorted by competency and can be downloaded separately from www.studentconsult.com. This "vertical read" format helps students better understand the breadth of definition of each competency and facilitate its discussion and mastery. Program directors, clerkship coordinators, and students should feel free to pursue these competency-specific curricula as a way to better incorporate the competencies into their clinical training. The Competency Self-Assessment Forms found on pages 41 and 42 may also be helpful. These forms can be downloaded or photocopied in order to enable students and residents to compile a portfolio which, we hope, will help with their mastery of the topics and will assist their instructors with documentation of growing competence.

This book also contains five "Teaching Visuals" that address important clinical topics we face in obstetrics and gynecology. In theory, there could be a teaching visual for every chapter. Nonetheless, we have elected to focus on five of the most commonly encountered problems that will benefit most from a more "visual" approach. These chapters should help the student or resident who is a visual learner obtain a better grasp of the subject matter. These visuals may also serve as templates to help trainees explain complex medical concepts to patients, colleagues, and their own future students.

Section IX is devoted to Operations and Procedures. This section addresses the most commonly encountered obstetric and gynecologic surgeries arranged in a competency-based format. This section has been devised to help the student/resident prepare for the cases on which she or he will be asked to assist in the operating room.

Finally, I feel compelled to add a few words about obstetrics and gynecology as a specialty. Within the field of medicine, obstetrics and gynecology is unique. I say this because, as a father and husband, I can find no greater joy than in my own family. Obstetricians are integral in allowing the concept of "family" to happen by providing competent, compassionate care. As an obstetrician your primary job will be, to the very best of your ability, to "get it right" every time. Your patients will expect nothing less. While every pregnant woman cannot be guaranteed a perfect baby, as an obstetrician you will guide your patients from the earliest stages of their pregnancy through delivery with the vigilance and oversight needed to provide the best possible outcome for each family. Learning to be a competent and confident obstetrician and gynecologist takes time and a true commitment to the care of women. I hope that in some small way this textbook can act as a framework to allow this process to begin.

Michael Belden MD
February, 2010

Acknowledgments

Obstetrics and Gynecology: A Competency-Based Companion is being published as the second book in the Competency-Based Companion series, which was originally conceived by Barry Mann. I owe Dr. Mann my deepest gratitude for offering me the opportunity to edit this book. Barry was one of my surgical instructors during my third-year surgical clerkship at the Medical College of Pennsylvania, and we have been friends and colleagues for many years. He has served as a mentor, sounding-board, inspiration, and friend. I thank him for entrusting me with the development and editing of this work.

I must also acknowledge the great help and insight provided to me by my Developmental Editor at Elsevier, Christine Abshire. She has been a great help to me and an advocate for this project. James Merritt, Acquisitions Editor at Elsevier, was instrumental from the outset in helping Dr. Mann conceive this series, and his support for this project has been unwavering.

I cannot emphasize enough my deepest thanks to the many contributors who have made this book possible, including the Section Editors, Competency Editors, and my editorial assistant, Mehdi Parva, MD. Special thanks also to Jordan Bloom, Ian Hayden, Matthew Weber, and Reuben Abraham. These hardworking third-year students performed the painstaking task of checking the many Elsevier references that are cited throughout the book. Their speed and accuracy has been much appreciated.

I have been impressed with the quality of the clinical expertise manifested in the fluid medical writing found in this text. In this regard, my job as editor has been easy. I offer my deepest appreciation and respect to the many members of the Department of Obstetrics and Gynecology at Lankenau Hospital, my home institution. This book contains numerous chapters that were conceived and written by our largely volunteer faculty. In particular, Drs. Andrew Gerson and Nancy Roberts have been especially supportive and helpful. Having first served as my teachers, they are now my highly valued colleagues. My residents from the Lankenau Hospital Obstetrics and Gynecology program and my students from Jefferson Medical College have been a great inspiration to me over the years and have helped me refine my teaching skills. Furthermore, they have helped me understand how the clinical competencies can best be incorporated into medical teaching.

Special thanks, indeed, are due to my three partners in practice, Patricia McConnell, MD; Maggie Peden, MD; and Mark Finnegan, MD. Patty, Maggie, and Mark have been profoundly supportive of my work on this project even when, at times, it increased their share of the work that sustains our practice. They are all very gifted teachers in their own right, and they are great proponents of the volunteer-faculty teaching model. Having these three physicians as partners has been a true joy for me throughout my years of practice. They make the day-in, day-out, work of being an obstetrician truly enjoyable. I am lucky and privileged to have these three doctors as my partners and as my friends.

Finally, I offer my greatest thanks to my wife, Katherine Belden, MD, who has been kind enough to contribute greatly to this project as chapter author and as section co-editor. Katherine has given me much advice and unfailing encouragement, and for this I will always be truly grateful.

Contributors

Emily Abramson-Chen MD
Resident in Family Medicine, Department of Family and Community Medicine, Christiana Care Health System, Wilmington, Delaware

Jennifer E. Agrusa
Medical Student, Obstetrics and Gynecology, New York University School of Medicine, New York, New York

Jennifer L. Aldrich MD
Clinical Specialist, Infectious Diseases, Department of Medicine, Lankenau Hospital, Wynnewood, Pennsylvania

Asma Ali MD
Resident, Obstetrics and Gynecology, Lankenau Hosptial, Wynnewood, Pennsylvania

Kelly C. Allison PhD
Assistant Professor of Psychology in Psychiatry, Center for Weight and Eating Disorders, Department of Psychiatry, University of Pennsylvania School of Medicine, Philadelphia, Pennsylvania

Lucinda S. Antosh DO
Resident, Obstetrics and Gynecology, Lankenau Hospital, Wynnewood, Pennsylvania

Janine M. Barsoum DO
Staff Physician, Teaching Faculty, Department of Obstetrics and Gynecology, Lankenau Hospital, Wynnewood, Pennsylvania

Maureen E. Basha PhD
Assistant Professor, Pharmacology and Physiology, Drexel University College of Medicine, Philadelphia, Pennsylvania

Renee M. Bassaly DO
Fellow, Female Pelvic Medicine and Reconstructive Surgery, Department of Urogynecology, University of South Florida; Department of Obstetrics and Gynecology-Urogynecology, Tampa General Hospital, Tampa, Florida

Katherine A. Belden MD
Instructor of Medicine, Division of Infectious Diseases, Department of Medicine, Jefferson Medical College, Thomas Jefferson University Hospital, Philadelphia, Pennsylvania

Michael Belden MD
Clinical Assistant Professor, Jefferson Medical College, Philadelphia, Pennsylvania; Department of Obstetrics and Gynecology, Lankenau Hospital, Wynnewood, Pennsylvania

Dale Berg MD
Professor of Medicine, Jefferson Medical College; Co-Director, University Clinical Skills and Simulation Center, Thomas Jefferson University, Philadelphia, Pennsylvania

Katherine Berg MD, MPH
Associate Professor of Medicine, Jefferson Medical College; Co-Director, University Clinical Skills and Simulation Center, Thomas Jefferson University, Philadelphia, Pennsylvania

Jessica L. Bienstock MD, MPH
Associate Professor, Residency Program Director, Director of the Division of Education, Department of Gynecology and Obstetrics, Johns Hopkins University School of Medicine, Baltimore, Maryland

Gary D. Blake MD
Maternal-Fetal Medicine, Sharp Mary Birch Hospital for Women; Maternal-Fetal Medicine, Scripps Mercy Medical Center, San Diego, California

Matthew P. Boente MD, FACOG
Physician, Gynecologic Oncology/Surgery, Minnesota Oncology, Edina, Minnesota

Stephanie B. Boswell MD
Resident, Internal Medicine, Mount Sinai Medical Center, New York, New York

Linda Bradley MD
Vice Chair, Obstetrics, Gynecology, and Women's Health Institute, Department of Obstetrics and Gynecology, Cleveland Clinic, Cleveland, Ohio

Norman A. Brest MD
Campus Chief, Obstetrics and Gynecology, Department of Obstetrics and Gynecology, Lankenau Hospital, Wynnewood, Pennsylvania

Ari D. Brooks MD
Associate Professor, Surgery, Drexel University College of Medicine; Chief, Surgical Oncology, Hahnemann University Hospital, Philadelphia, Pennsylvania

James F. Burke MD
Clinical Associate Professor of Medicine, Internal Medicine, Jefferson Medical College, Philadelphia, Pennsylvania; Designated Institutional Official, Graduate Medical Education, Lankenau Hospital; Director, Fellowship in Cardiovascular Disease, Lankenau Hospital, Wynnewood, Pennsylvania

Patricia I. Carney MD, FACOG
Deputy Director, Medical Affairs, Women's Health Care, Bayer HealthCare Pharmaceuticals, Wayne, New Jersey

Dmitri Chamchad MD
Visiting Assistant Professor, Anesthesiology, Drexel University, Hahnemann Hospital, Philadelphia, Pennsylvania; Assistant Professor, Anesthesiology, Lankenau Institute of Medical Research, Wynnewood, Pennsylvania; Anesthesia Research Director, Anesthesiology, Lankenau Hospital, Main Line Health System, Wynnewood, Pennsylvania; Obstetrics and Gynecology Research Associate, Obstetrics and Gynecology, Lankenau Hospital, Main Line Health System, Wynnewood, Pennsylvania

Robin M. Ciocca DO
Attending Surgeon, Department of Surgery, Lankenau Hospital, Wynnewood, Pennsylvania

Jonathan C. Cook MD
Department of Obstetrics and Gynecology, Thomas Jefferson University Hospital, Philadelphia, Pennsylvania

Michael F. Crutchlow MD
Adjunct Assistant Professor of Medicine, Division of Endocrinology/ Diabetes/Metabolism, University of Pennsylvania, Philadelphia; Associate Director, Clinical Pharmacology, Merck Research Laboratories, North Wales, Pennsylvania

Diana Curran MD
*Assistant Professor, Department of Obstetrics and Gynecology, University of Michigan Health System, Ann Arbor, Michigan
Obstetrics and Gynecology, SUNY Stony Brook School of Medicine, Stony Brook, New York*

Deborah M. Davenport MD, FACOG
Assistant Clinical Professor, Department of Obstetrics and Gynecology, SUNY Stony Brook School of Medicine, Stony Brook, New York

Ronit K. Devon MD
Attending Radiologist, Department of Radiology, Lankenau Hospital, Wynnewood, Pennsylvania

Philip J. DiGiacomo III MD
Resident, Department of Emergency Medicine, University of North Carolina Hospital, Chapel Hill, North Carolina

Alan E. Donnenfeld MD
Professor, Obstetrics and Gynecology, Thomas Jefferson University, Philadelphia, Pennsylvania; Partner, Main Line Perinatology, Obstetrics and Gynecology, Lankenau Hospital, Wynnewood, Pennsylvania; Medical Director, Genetics, Genzyme Genetics, Philadelphia, Pennsylvania

Mitchell I. Edelson MD
Attending Physician, Gynecologic Oncology Institute, Abington Memorial Hospital, Abington, Pennsylvania

Chad O. Edwards MS, RD
Clinical Nutrition Supervisor, Clinical Nutrition, Lodi Memorial Hospital, Lodi, California

Michelle M. Edwards DO
Associate Physician, Obstetrics and Gynecology/Women's Health, Kaiser Permanente Roseville Medical Center, Roseville, California

Ernest M. Enzien MD
Department of Medicine, Columbia Memorial Hospital, Hudson, New York; Department of Medicine, Northern Dutchess Hospital, Rhinebeck, New York

Michael S. Ferrell MD
Resident, Department of Radiology, Bryn Mawr Hospital, Bryn Mawr, Pennsylvania

Joseph S. Ferroni MD, FACOG
*Instructor, Obstetrics and Gynecology, Thomas Jefferson University, Philadelphia,
Pennsylvania; Department of Obstetrics and Gynecology, Paoli Memorial Hospital,
Paoli, Pennsylvania*

Sandra Fine MBA
*Vice President, Medical Education, Main Line Health System, Wynnewood,
Pennsylvania*

Mark O. Finnegan MD
*Attending Physician, Department of Obstetrics and Gynecology, Lankenau
Hospital, Wynnewood, Pennsylvania*

Benjamin Fogel MD
*Instructor of Pediatrics, University of Pennsylvania School of Medicine; Resident,
Pediatrics, Children's Hospital of Philadelphia, Philadelphia, Pennsylvania*

Donald G. Gallup MD
*Professor and Chair, Department of Obstetrics and Gynecology, Mercer University
School of Medicine; Obstetrics and Gynecology, Memorial University Medical
Center, Savannah, Georgia*

Andrew Gerson MD
*Clinical Associate Professor of Obstetrics and Gynecology, Thomas Jefferson
University School of Medicine, Philadelphia, Pennsylvania; Chief, Maternal-Fetal
Medicine, Main Line Health Hospitals, Wynnewood, Pennsylvania*

Brett C. Gilbert DO, FACOG
*Clinical Instructor, Infectious Diseases, Thomas Jefferson University,
Philadelphia, Pennsylvania; Medicine, Lankenau Hospital, Wynnewood,
Pennsylvania; Chair, Infectious Diseases, Medicine, Chestnut Hill Hospital,
Philadelphia, Pennsylvania*

Stephen E. Gordon MD, MBA
*Resident, Internal Medicine, Beth Israel Deaconess Medical Center, Boston,
Massachusetts*

Linnea S. Hauge PhD
*Assistant Professor and Educational Specialist, Department of Surgery and
Department of Medical Education, University of Michigan, Ann Arbor,
Michigan*

Randolph P. Heinzel MD
*Attending Physician, Department of Obstetrics and Gynecology, Lankenau
Hospital, Wynnewood, Pennsylvania*

David Holtz MD
*Clinical Assistant Professor, Obstetrics and Gynecology, Jefferson Medical College,
Philadelphia, Pennsylvania; Staff Physician, Obstetrics and Gynecology, Main Line
Gynecologic Oncology, Lankenau Hospital, Wynnewood, Pennsylvania;
Staff Physician, Obstetrics and Gynecology, Main Line Gynecologic Oncology,
Paoli Hospital, Paoli, Pennsylvania; Consulting Staff, Obstetrics and Gynecology,
Bryn Mawr Hospital, Bryn Mawr, Pennsylvania*

Mark J. Ingerman MD, FACP
*Chief, Infection Prevention and Control, Main Line Health System, Wynnewood,
Pennsylvania*

Keith Isaacson MD
Associate Professor, Obstetrics and Gynecology, Harvard Medical School, Boston, Massachusetts; Director of Minimally Invasive Surgery and Infertility, Obstetrics and Gynecology, Newton Wellesley Hospital, Newton, Massachusetts; Associate Gynecologist, Obstetrics and Gynecology, Brigham and Women's Hospital, Boston, Massachusetts; Associate, Gynecology, Obstetrics and Gynecology, Massachusetts General Hospital, Boston, Massachusetts

Gerald A. Isenberg MD
Associate Professor of Surgery, Jefferson Medical College; Director, Undergraduate Education, Surgery, Jefferson Medical College; Program Director, Colorectal Residency, Thomas Jefferson University Hospital, Philadelphia, Pennsylvania

Kirsten Jacobson MD
Physician, Healthquest, Poughkeepsie, New York

Daron A. Kahn MD
Resident, Internal Medicine, Thomas Jefferson University Hospital, Philadelphia, Pennsylvania

Joanne Kakaty-Monzo DO
Instructor of Education, Obstetrics and Gynecology, Philadelphia College of Osteopathic Medicine–Georgia Campus, Suwanee, Georgia; Attending Physician, Obstetrics and Gynecology, Jefferson University Hospital–Main Line Division, Lankenau Hospital, Wynnewood, Pennsylvania

Richard D. Kaplan MD
Chief, Ob/Gyn Service, Moses Cone Health System, Women's Hospital of Greensboro Moses Cone Health System, Greensboro, North Carolina

Joan A. Keegan DO
Resident, Obstetrics and Gynecology, Lankenau Hospital, Wynnewood, Pennsylvania

Carey L. Keiter DO
Family Medicine Resident, Family Medicine, Mercy Suburban Hospital, Norristown, Pennsylvania

Stephen P. Krell MD, FACOG
Staff Member, Obstetrics and Gynecology, Paoli Hospital, Main Line Health System, Paoli, Pennsylvania; President and Founder, Women's Health Care Group of Pennsylvania, Oaks, Pennsylvania

Leah Lande MD
Assistant Professor, Lankenau Institute for Medical Research; Pulmonary and Critical Care Medicine, Lankenau Hospital, Wynnewood, Pennsylvania

Kimberly M. Lenhardt MD, FACOG
Attending Obstetrician/Gynecologist, Obstetrics and Gynecology, Inova Fairfax Hospital, Falls Church, Virginia

Lawrence L. Livornese, Jr MD, FACP, FIDSA
Clinical Assistant Professor, Department of Medicine, Drexel University School of Medicine; Chair, Infection Control, Division of Infectious Diseases, Department of Medicine, Roxborough Hospital; Attending Physician, Division of Infectious Diseases, Department of Medicine, Chestnut Hill Hospital, Philadelphia, Pennsylvania

Barry D. Mann MD, FACS
Chief Academic Officer, Main Line Health System; Professor of Surgery, Jefferson Medical College; Executive Director, The Walter and Leonore Annenberg Conference Center for Medical Education; Program Director, Surgical Residency, Lankenau Hospital, Wynnewood, Pennsylvania; Adjunct Professor of Surgery, Drexel University College of Medicine, Philadelphia, Pennsylvania

Sara N. Mann
Writing Fellow, Brown University, Providence, Rhode Island

Gregory Margolin MD, MMS
Staff Physician, Department of Obstetrics and Gynecology, Our Lady of Lourdes Medical Center, Camden, New Jersey

Pinckney J. Maxwell IV MD
Assistant Professor of Surgery, Division of Colon and Rectal Surgery, Thomas Jefferson University, Philadelphia, Pennsylvania

Kristen M. McCullen MD
Physician, Department of Obstetrics and Gynecology, Virtua Health System, Voorhees, New Jersey

Garo Megerian MD
Maternal-Fetal Medicine, Main Line Health Hospitals, Pennsylvania

Shahab S. Minassian MD
Section Chief, Fertility and Reproductive Endocrinology, Department of Obstetrics and Gynecology, The Reading Hospital and Medical Center; IVF-Fertility Division, Women's Clinic, Ltd., West Reading, Pennsylvania

Gennady G. Miroshnichenko MD
Clinical Fellow, Department of Gynecologic Oncology, University of Toronto, Ontario, Canada

Benjamin E. Montgomery MD
Chair, Department of Obstetrics and Gynecology, The Bloomsburg Hospital, Bloomsburg, Pennsylvania

Jessica M. Mory DO
Physician, Obstetrics and Gynecology, Lankenau Hospital, Main Line Health, Wynnewood, Pennsylvania

Dionissios Neofytos MD, MPH
Assistant Professor, Medicine; Attending Physician, Medicine, The Johns Hopkins University School of Medicine, Baltimore, Maryland

Debra Nestel PhD
Professor of Medical Education, Gippsland Medical School, Monash University, Victoria, Australia

Suzanne S. Nogami MD
Resident, Obstetrics and Gynecology, Lankenau Hospital, Wynnewood, Pennsylvania

John J. Orris DO, MBA
Attending Reproductive Endocrinologist, Department of Obstetrics and Gynecology, Division of Reproductive Endocrinology and Infertility, Lankenau Hospital, Wynnewood; Paoli Hospital, Paoli; The Chester County Hospital, West Chester; Attending Reproductive Endocrinologist, Fellowship Director, Main Line Fertility and Reproductive Medicine, Bryn Mawr, Pennsylvania

Mehdi Parva MD
Resident, Obstetrics and Gynecology, Lankenau Hospital, Wynnewood, Pennsylvania

Gerald W. Peden MD, MA
Senior Medical Director, Claims Payment Policy, Independence Blue Cross, Philadelphia, Pennsylvania

Christian M. Perez MD
Attending Physician, Obstetrics and Gynecology, Virginia Beach General Hospital; Assistant Director, The New Hope Center for Reproductive Medicine, Virginia Beach, Virginia

William H. Pfeffer MD
Chief, Reproductive Endocrinology, Main Line Health System; Obstetrics and Gynecology, Lankenau Hospital, Wynnewood, Pennsylvania; Obstetrics and Gynecology, Bryn Mawr Hospital, Bryn Mawr, Pennsylvania; Active Staff, Paoli Hospital, Paoli; Active Staff, Riddle Memorial Hospital, Media, Pennsylvania; Courtesy Staff, Chester County Hospital, West Chester, Pennsylvania

Joel Port FACHE
Vice President of Planning and Business Development, Main Line Health System, Bryn Mawr, Pennsylvania

Paul S. Robbins DO
Division of Nephrology, Lankenau Hospital, Wynnewood, Pennsylvania

Nancy S. Roberts MD
Clinical Assistant Professor, Department of Obsetrics and Gynecology, Jefferson Medical College, Philadelphia; System Chairman, Obsetrics and Gynecology, Main Line Health System, Bryn Mawr, Pennsylvania

Norman G. Rosenblum MD, PhD
Professor and Director, Division of Gynecologic Oncology, Department of Obstetrics and Gynecology, Jefferson Medical College, Thomas Jefferson University Hospital, Philadelphia, Pennsylvania

Camilo A. Ruiz DO
Chief Resident, Department of Internal Medicine, Palmetto General Hospital, Hialeah, Florida

Sutthichai Sae-Tia MD, PhD
Physician, Department of Infectious Diseases, University of Pittsburgh Medical Center, Shadyside Hospital, Pittsburgh, Pennsylvania

Cynthia Carrole Sagullo MD, FACOG
Attending Physician, Obstetrics and Gynecology, The Valley Hospital, Ridgewood, New Jersey

Khaled H. Sakhel MD
Obstetrics and Gynecology, Synergy Medical Education Alliance, Michigan State University, Saginaw, Michigan

Peter A. Schwartz MD
Professor of Clinical Obstetrics and Gynecology, Obstetrics and Gynecology, Drexel University School of Medicine, Philadelphia; Attending Physician, Obstetrics and Gynecology, The Reading Hospital and Medical Center, West Reading, Pennsylvania

Anthony C. Sciscione DO
Professor, Obstetrics and Gynecology, Drexel University School of Medicine, Philadelphia, Pennsylvania; Director, Maternal-Fetal Medicine, Obstetrics and Gynecology; Residency Program Director, Obstetrics and Gynecology, Christiana Care Health Services, Newark, Delaware

David E. Seubert MD, JD
Director, Division of Maternal-Fetal Medicine; Vice Chief, Obstetrics, Department of Obstetrics and Gynecology, William Beaumont Hospital, Royal Oak, Michigan; Visiting Clinical Associate Professor, Department of Obstetrics and Gynecology, New York University School of Medicine, New York, New York

William R. Short MD, MPH
Assistant Professor of Medicine, Medicine/Infectious Diseases, Jefferson Medical College of Thomas Jefferson University; Infectious Diseases, Thomas Jefferson University Hospital, Philadelphia, Pennsylvania

Randi Silibovsky MD, FACP
Assistant Professor of Medicine, Division of Infectious Diseases, Thomas Jefferson University; Thomas Jefferson University Hospital, Philadelphia, Pennsylvania

Arlene Smalls MD
Outpatient Care Director, Department of Obstetrics and Gynecology, Lankenau Hospital, Wynnewood, Pennsylvania; Physician, Department of Obstetrics and Gynecology, Christiana Care, Newark, Delaware

Cynthia D. Smith MD
Clinical Assistant Professor, Department of Internal Medicine, Jefferson Medical College, Philadelphia, Pennsylvania; Program Director, Internal Medicine; Hospitalist, Department of Internal Medicine, Lankenau Hospital, Wynnewood, Pennsylvania

Kaighn Smith MD
Professor, Obstetrics and Gynecology, Thomas Jefferson University Medical School, Philadelphia, Pennsylvania; Emeritus Chair, Obstetrics and Gynecology, Lankenau Hospital, Wynnewood, Pennsylvania

Kathleen E. Squires MD
Professor of Medicine, Jefferson Medical College of Thomas Jefferson University; Director, Division of Infectious Diseases, Thomas Jefferson University Hospitals, Philadelphia, Pennsylvania

Caren M. Stalburg MD, MA
Clinical Assistant Professor, Obstetrics and Gynecology and Medical Education, University of Michigan Medical School, University of Michigan Health System, Ann Arbor, Michigan

Hindi E. Stohl MD
Resident, Department of Gynecology and Obstetrics, Johns Hopkins Medical Institutions, Johns Hopkins Hospital, Baltimore, Maryland

Vonetta T. Sylvestre MD
Resident, Department of Obstetrics and Gynecology, Lankenau Hospital, Wynnewood, Pennsylvania

Linda M. Szymanski MD, PhD
Fellow, Maternal-Fetal Medicine, Department of Gynecology and Obstetrics, Johns Hopkins University School of Medicine, Baltimore, Maryland

Paula M. Termuhlen MD, FACS
Program Director, General Surgery; Chief, Division of Surgical Oncology; Associate Professor of Surgery, Wright State University Boonshoft School of Medicine, Dayton, Ohio

Marc R. Toglia MD
Clinical Assistant Professor, Obstetrics and Gynecology, Thomas Jefferson School of Medicine, Philadelphia, Pennsylvania; Chief, Division of Urogynecology, Main Line Hospitals, Obstetrics and Gynecology, Main Line Hospital System, Wynnewood, Pennsylvania

Sue-Anne Toh MD
Fellow, Department of Medicine, University of Pennsylvania; Fellow, Endocrinology, Diabetes and Metabolism, University of Pennsylvania Health System; Fellow, Institute of Translational Medicine and Therapeutics, University of Pennsylvania, Philadelphia, Pennsylvania

Allan R. Tunkel MD, PhD
Chair, Department of Internal Medicine, Monmouth Medical Center, Saint Barnabas Health Care System, Long Branch, New Jersey

Beverly M. Vaughn MD
Clinical Assistant Professor, Obstetrics and Gynecology, Thomas Jefferson University, Philadelphia, Pennsylvania; Associate Program Director Obstetrics and Gynecology Residency, Obstetrics and Gynecology, Lankenau Hospital, Wynnewood, Pennsylvania

Michelle Vichnin MD
Director, Adolescent Medical Affairs, Merck Vaccines and Infectious Diseases, Merck & Co., Inc., West Point, Pennsylvania

Thomas A. Wadden PhD
Professor, Center for Weight and Eating Disorders, University of Pennsylvania, Philadelphia, Pennsylvania

Neelesh Welling MD
Research Assistant, Lankenau Hospital Cancer Center, Wynnewood, Pennsylvania

Mary Grady Walsh Esq.
Managing Attorney, Kevin H Wright and Associates, Lansdale, Pennsylvania

Frank J. White MD
Attending Physician, Department of Obstetrics and Gynecology, Riddle Memorial Hospital, Media, Pennsylvania

Mark B. Woodland MS, MD, FACOG
*Associate Dean, Program Director, and Clinical Professor, Obstetrics and
Gynecology and Graduate Medical Education, Drexel University College of
Medicine; Obstetrics and Gynecology, Hahnemann University Hospital;
Obstetrics and Gynecology, Pennsylvania Hospital, Philadelphia, Pennsylvania;
Obstetrics and Gynecology, Abington Memorial Hospital, Abington,
Pennsylvania*

Anthony Lee Yu
Medical Student, Jefferson Medical College, Philadelphia, Pennsylvania

Harry G. Zegel MD, FACR
*Clinical Associate Professor, Department of Radiology, Thomas Jefferson
University, Philadelphia, Pennsylvania; System Chair, Department of Radiology,
Main Line Health Hospitals, Wynnewood, Pennsylvania*

Contents

Section I
INTRODUCTION TO THE COMPETENCIES

Section Editor
Linnea S. Hauge PhD

Section Contents

Chapter 1
How to Study This Book

Michael Belden MD and Barry D. Mann MD

Obstetrics and Gynecology (Ob/Gyn) is one of the most broad and challenging of the medical specialties. This is due primarily to the varied aspects of care the obstetrician/gynecologist must be prepared to provide to a patient over the course of her lifetime. It is plausible that an obstetrician/gynecologist might begin caring for a patient as a young teen, continue to provide care for her throughout her reproductive life, and follow her through her postmenopausal years. The broad fund of knowledge required to provide this care may be intimidating for some, but can be a true joy to master. The goal of this book is to provide you with an introduction to Ob/Gyn, and to become your stepping stone toward the mastery of medical care for women. Becoming comfortable with the special aspects of provision of health care for women, including pregnancy-related care, is the overarching goal of your Ob/Gyn clerkship.

ORGANIZING STRUCTURE OF THE BOOK

In 1999, the Accreditation Council on Medical Education (the ACGME) instituted the six medical Competencies. The Council's goal was to standardize the elements of medical education in such a way that medical educators could move toward measurable goals, use a language that would be universal among educators, and ensure the competence of residency graduates in arenas broader than medical knowledge and technical competence. At the conclusion of each phase of your medical training, your teachers are now required to confirm that you are developing the requisite skills in the six Competencies: Patient Care, Medical Knowledge, Practice-Based Learning and Improvement, Interpersonal and Communication Skills, Professionalism, and Systems-Based Practice. You will find an introductory chapter describing the importance of each competency in this first section of this book. In the later, "case-based" chapters, you will find each competency addressed specifically, signaled by the following color coding:

Patient Care
Medical Knowledge
Practice-Based Learning and Improvement

Interpersonal and Communication Skills
Professionalism
Systems-Based Practice

Competency definitions according to the ACGME are provided in Appendix 1.

The contributors, chapter authors, and section editors have written and edited their work with an eye to making the field of Ob/Gyn easy to digest for the student. Think of the authors as speaking to you as if you were on teaching rounds. Each chapter begins with a case, followed by a differential diagnosis. Use the **Differential Diagnosis** section, as well as the **Clinical Entities,** to help you grasp the salient medical points. For information more detailed than that provided in the **Clinical Entities** boxes, use the textbook references that follow each clinical entity or click the helpful links at the end of each Clinical Entity box found on the book's website at www.StudentConsult.com.

The following obstetrics and gynecology textbooks have been chosen as part of the online resources available to you through Elsevier Publications for your continued study:

Obstetrics: Normal and Problem Pregnancies, 5th edition, by Steven G. Gabbe, et al.
Comprehensive Gynecology, 5th edition, by Vern L. Katz, et al.
Hacker and Moore's Essentials of Obstetrics and Gynecology, 5th edition, by Neville F. Hacker, et al.

CHAPTER ELEMENTS

In each chapter after a case and its differential diagnosis, a paragraph titled Speaking Intelligently will help you see the "big picture" and suggest a framework for sorting through the differential diagnosis in language that you might use with a colleague. Included under the Patient Care banner, Clinical Thinking, History, Physical Examination, Tests for Consideration, and Imaging Considerations comprise the most important aspects of the evaluation process.

The Clinical Entities boxes outline the entities considered in the differential diagnoses. The diagnoses listed for each case emphasize the most common medical conditions you may be faced with and are therefore typically fewer in number. Low-frequency diagnoses are described in the **Zebra Zone.**

Each case includes issues and solutions related specifically to the Practice-Based Learning and Improvement, Interpersonal and Communication Skills, Professionalism, and Systems-Based Practice competencies.

SUGGESTIONS FOR READING

Depending on how your clerkship rotation is structured, you could be assigned to the Obstetrics service, Gynecology service, or any of the subspecialties, including Gynecologic Oncology, Reproductive Endocrinology, or Maternal-Fetal Medicine. This text is subdivided into sections to facilitate your reading and preparation for these rotations. For example, if you are assigned to the Maternal-Fetal Medicine service and you are unclear about how to counsel patients regarding prenatal diagnosis testing, read that chapter first to get oriented. Then use your more comprehensive texts or websites to look up additional information as required.

TEACHING VISUALS

Sometimes, thinking about clinical problems in a more "visual" way can be the most instructive way to learn. There are five separate activities in this text, called "Teaching Visuals," that help facilitate this process. The five problems we address—fetal heart rate interpretation, managing postpartum hemorrhage, understanding the menstrual cycle, evaluating secondary amenorrhea, and ureteral anatomy—are vital to a complete understanding of obstetrics and gynecology. Complete these exercises to enhance your understanding of how to address these complex issues.

PROCEDURES

At the end of the book, there are two sections that describe the most important procedures commonly performed in obstetrics and gynecology. Major and minor Ob/Gyn procedures are described in easy-to-understand language. Read these as preparation for the operating room, as guides to understanding the requisite anatomy and technical skills of a procedure.

THE COMPETENCIES AND VERTICAL READS

The obstetrician/gynecologists who contributed to this book incorporated aspects of the Medical Knowledge, Patient Care, Practice-Based Learning and Improvement, Interpersonal and Communication Skills, Professionalism, and Systems-Based Practice competencies in the context of their cases. This book is organized to allow for a "vertical read," whereby readers may focus their study on each specific competency as it relates to Ob/Gyn. Vertical reads of the **Interpersonal and Communication Skills,** Professionalism, and **Systems-Based Practice** competencies are available online at www.StudentConsult.com.

Good luck on your rotation, and be sure to take advantage of every opportunity to learn as much as you can about this truly unique specialty.

Chapter 2
Medical Knowledge: An Essential Competency

James F. Burke MD *and Sandra Fine* MBA

He who studies medicine without books sails an uncharted sea, but he who studies medicine without patients does not go to sea at all.
—*William Osler, 1849–1919*

The Accreditation Council on Graduate Medical Education's six competencies—Patient Care, Medical Knowledge, Interpersonal and Communication Skills, Practice-Based Learning and Improvement, Professionalism, and Systems-Based Practice—are interdependent in the teaching and evaluation of physicians and physicians in training. Although each competency is essential and adds value in the total formation of a competent and compassionate physician, Medical Knowledge remains the cornerstone for the development of each of the other competencies. Although each competency has an impact on the quality of medicine practiced, Medical Knowledge still reigns supreme in its impact on safely administered patient care, the ultimate goal of every practicing clinician. Continuous acquisition of Medical Knowledge and development of one's own techniques in Practice-Based Learning and Improvement ensure that the competent and compassionate physician is a life-long learner who protects himself or herself from professional obsolescence.

The acquisition and assimilation of updated Medical Knowledge into the practice of current, evidence-based medicine is no simple task and is a never-ending journey. As the 21st century begins, it is estimated that greater than 50% of medical facts in published textbooks will be either incorrect or obsolete within 10 years. And there is every reason to assume that the rate of change of the knowledge base in medicine will continue to accelerate at a dizzying pace. Therein lies the challenge for educators and learners—how to stay current, grounded, and focused in managing the acquisition and application of new knowledge while basing one's practice on the many rich scientific truths upon which modern medicine is built. In essence, this is the concept of "keeping the baby" in "the bath water" while simultaneously refreshing the bath water as clinical medicine evolves.

One of the vital tools in the life-long mastery of Medical Knowledge is the ability to ask one's self and one's colleagues the "good question." Nurture your intellectual curiosity. The good question is more relevant to the continual mastery of Medical Knowledge than temporary knowledge of the right answer. As Medical Knowledge changes, good questions will always be pertinent. Right answers are ephemeral; right answers for today may become wrong answers for tomorrow. Life-long learners design their own paths for staying abreast of the changes in their chosen specialties. This requires developing an appetite for relevant, scientifically sound, continuing medical education, and also developing the skills to critically appraise the seemingly infinite body of research found in scholarly journals.

Recently recognized overt and subtle differences in disease states based on gender-specific symptoms (symptoms associated with myocardial infarction serve as an example[1,2]) present specific challenges to the field of obstetrics and gynecology. Moving at its exponential rate, Medical Knowledge will surely continue to challenge and contradict many long-standing medical "truths" based on gender-specific data yet to be explored. Because of educational issues such as this, learners who continue to acquire and assimilate ever-changing Medical Knowledge into their practices for the sake of their own intellectual curiosity and for the benefit of their patients will be best poised to inherit the future.

References

1. Robert B: Gender-specific aspects of cardiovascular disease. Available at http://www.womensheart.org/PDFs/2006-08-27_WomenHeartDisease_BR.pdf.
2. Zuzelo PR: Gender and acute myocardial infarction symptoms. MedSurg Nursing, June 2002. Available at http://findarticles.com/p/articles/mi_m0FSS/is_3_11/.

Chapter 3
Practice-Based Learning and Improvement

Linda M. Szymanski MD, PhD

DEFINING PRACTICE-BASED LEARNING AND IMPROVEMENT

Practice-Based Learning and Improvement (PBLI) is the challenge to set into place appropriate ongoing mechanisms so that you can improve your methods and outcomes throughout your years of practice. Physicians must monitor the quality of their own work, improve their practice processes, and keep up with developments in medicine.[1,2]

According to the Accreditation Council on Graduate Medical Education (ACGME) definition of PBLI,[1] residents and students must be able to investigate and evaluate their patient care practice, appraise and assimilate scientific evidence, and improve their patient care practices.

Residents and students are expected to

- Analyze practice experience and perform practice-based improvement activities using a systematic methodology.
- Locate, appraise, and assimilate evidence from scientific studies related to their patients' health problems.
- Obtain and use information about their own population of patients and the larger population from which their patients are drawn.
- Apply knowledge of study designs and statistical methods to the appraisal of clinical studies and other information on diagnostic and therapeutic effectiveness.
- Use information technology to manage information, access on-line medical information, and support their own education.
- Facilitate the learning of students and other health care professionals.[1]

For the purposes of this book, two important aspects of PBLI have been interspersed throughout the text: (1) the use of Evidence-Based Medicine, and (2) the need for ongoing self-assessment.

A major aspect of the PBLI competency is Evidence-Based Medicine. Accordingly, each contributor has chosen an important evidence-based article for inclusion in his or her chapter. The articles have been selected to demonstrate how a specific question relevant to Ob/Gyn practice has been posed and answered.

Because PBLI calls for the process of self-assessment, Competency-Based Self-Assessment Forms specific for obstetrics and gynecology cases have been developed; these are provided as Appendices 2 and 3 at the end of this section. These forms may be photocopied or downloaded from www.StudentConsult.com as Microsoft Word documents. It is hoped that these forms might serve as templates for student and resident self-assessment. At the discretion of Clerkship Directors and Program Directors, students may be encouraged to use these forms to create portfolios of their clinical encounters and educational experiences.

PRACTICE-BASED LEARNING AND IMPROVEMENT IN A CHANGING SYSTEM

Movements for change in the health care system have been prompted by the highly publicized report on medical errors, *To Err Is Human: Building a Safer Health System*, first released by The Institute of Medicine in 1999.[3] In this report, a comprehensive strategy was outlined to reduce preventable medical errors, including changes in medical education. Traditionally, accreditation of residency programs focused on *structure and process issues*, such as the availability of facilities and equipment, number of faculty, conferences held, and rotations offered. In parallel with the changing medical climate, the focus is shifting and more emphasis is now being placed on *outcomes*. In today's changing medical climate, health outcomes are being critically analyzed more than at any time in the past and more emphasis is being placed on evidence-based, cost-effective, patient-oriented care. Graduate medical education has become a particularly important arena for setting forth a model of PBLI.[4] Therefore, as a medical student and resident you are likely to participate in new approaches to individual and collective self-assessment implemented in your Ob/Gyn rotation. You might even take the initiative to introduce these approaches into your program. Some of these methods are not new to medicine and have been carried out informally. However, as we have become "outcome oriented," there is now greater impetus to assess the effectiveness of these measures. The ACGME has summarized a number of approaches that may be used in resident education to foster PBLI.[1] The following examples illustrate several of these approaches and ways in which they may be incorporated in your Ob-Gyn rotation.

Exit Rounds

In a group setting, with attending(s) present, a resident or student reviews a patient for whom he or she was responsible and describes what was learned from caring for that patient.

Practical Example: *Each morning on L&D, certain cases from the previous day are discussed. These may include all cesarean and operative deliveries, all preterm deliveries, and any other complications (e.g., postpartum hemorrhage, seizure). The resident involved presents the case to all other residents, medical students, and faculty (incoming and outgoing teams). Learning points are discussed and ways to improve outcome, if possible, are identified.*

See Chapter 16, Case 5.

Morbidity and Mortality Conferences

Morbidity and mortality (M&M) conferences typically involve patients who have experienced complications or death. The presenting resident describes the case and identifies what went wrong and what might have been done differently to improve the outcome. There is typically open discussion of the case. Although the specifics of M&M may differ from institution to institution and service to service, case reviews should be focused on an evidence-based review of the topic.

See Chapter 17, Case 6.

Practice-Based Small Group Learning Program

Residents and students meet to review current information about a specific clinical problem and to reflect on their experiences and challenges with the problem. Group discussion is stimulated by prepared material and led by a trained peer facilitator.

Practical Example: *Each week the residents meet with the Program Director or Department Chair for an hour to discuss programmatic issues. During the last 15 minutes, one of the residents briefly presents one of the American College of Obstetricians and Gynecologists (ACOG) Practice Bulletins.*

See Chapter 40, Case 25.

Evidence-Based Medicine Curriculum

Residents rotate as leaders of a group session to discuss the application of evidence-based medicine to one of their own patients. As preparation, residents develop a focused clinical question, conduct a literature search, critically appraise the evidence, and then apply it to the care of their own patients. Journal club is a practical example. Topics should be chosen to demonstrate important advances in care or new treatments.

See Chapter 45, Case 30.

Log and Learning Plan

Working with a mentor, residents keep a log of significant events or clinical surprises and develop a plan to address learning needs uncovered by these events.

See Chapter 18, Case 7.

Improvement Project

Residents work with a mentor to identify an aspect of their own practice that needs to be improved, implement the improvement, and determine its effectiveness during senior year.

See Chapter 54, Case 37.

Practice-Based Learning and Improvement pertains to improvements that can be made by both an individual physician and an educational community. The contributors and editors of this volume hope that its competency-based format will inspire the process of ongoing collective and individual self-assessment.

References

1. Accreditation Council for Graduate Medical Education (ACGME): The ACGME Outcome Project. Available at http://www.acgme.org/Outcome/.
2. Hayden SR, Dufel S, Shih R: Definitions and competencies for practice-based learning and improvement. Acad Emerg Med 2002;9:1242–1248.
3. Kohn L, Corrigan J, Donaldson M (eds): To Err Is Human: Building a Safer Health System. Washington, DC, Committee on Quality of Health Care in America, Institute of Medicine. National Academy Press, 2000.
4. Swing S: ACGME Launches Outcomes Assessment Project. JAMA 1998;279:1492.
5. Wu AW, Folkman S, McPhee SJ, Lo B: Do house officers learn from their mistakes? JAMA 1991;265:2089–2094.
6. Ziegelstein RC, Fiebach NH: "The mirror" and "the village": A new method for teaching practice-based learning and improvement and systems-based practice. Acad Med 2004;79:83–88.

Chapter 4
Interpersonal and Communication Skills

Debra Nestel PhD, *Katherine Berg* MD, *and Dale Berg* MD

The American College of Graduate Medical Education (ACGME) has defined the competency of **Interpersonal and Communication Skills** as:

Residents must be able to demonstrate interpersonal and communication skills that result in effective information exchange and teaming with patients, their patients' families, and professional associates.[1]

Communication is considered to be the core clinical skill. Everything in professional medical practice revolves around communication. The ability to communicate effectively is the skill by which patients will make judgments about you. Patients are competent to make such judgments, unlike other facets of medical work in which they usually do not have expertise. Patients want to be respected and have an opportunity to express their ideas, concerns, and expectations.

Although colleagues will make judgments on all facets of your medical work, communication will be a critical factor in forming their overall perception. Communicating sensitively, accurately, and in a timely fashion is essential for effective teamwork and safe clinical practice.

Developing effective interpersonal and communication skills is extremely important in your development and growth as a physician. Clinical practice is often highly demanding and takes place under conditions that are not conducive to easy communication. Consider the following:

- There are many stresses in clinical practice. When faced with a particularly frustrating, vexing, or challenging patient or circumstance, be mindful not to transfer that stress to others by being curt with patients and colleagues.
- Clinical practice is not time efficient. It is common to run behind schedule. Strive to be as punctual as possible with patients and colleagues. Acknowledging and apologizing for delays is respectful and may diffuse unhelpful emotions.
- Caring for patients regardless of their social standing, financial resources, or type of insurance is a defining feature of being a physician. These patients are often indigent, immigrant, and socially disadvantaged. To communicate well may require extra time and effort.
- Teaching students to become physicians is an extremely important component of medicine. The essence of effective teaching is an

ability to communicate. Use these interactions with students to further develop your communication and interpersonal skills.

■ Collegiality and kindness to colleagues and support staff is crucial to foster a culture that encourages the free transfer of information. An environment in which staff members feel empowered to speak up to one another is an environment likely to minimize medical errors.

Table 4-1 outlines a system, devised by the editors of this series, to identify various aspects of Interpersonal and Communication Skills that

Table 4-1 Interpersonal and Communication Skills	
Skill	**Case**
Listen actively with cultural, ethnic, gender, racial, age, and religious sensitivity	11, 24, 28, 32
Communicate effectively with patients	2–6, 8, 10, 12, 14, 20–22, 25, 29, 35, 36, 37
Empathy	8, 25
Considering the patient's perspective	4, 18, 29, 35
Choosing appropriate language	17, 37
Discussing unknowns	5, 16
Concern for health literacy, language, and cultural barriers	2, 12, 20
Delivering bad news	8, 22, 36
Avoiding communication traps	3, 21
Nonverbal communication	6, 7
Communicate effectively with families	9, 12, 33, 35
Communicate effectively with professional associates and staff members	7, 13
Begin patient encounters, educate and advise patients, and end encounters conveying sensitivity, compassion, and concern	1, 17, 23, 27
Discuss medical errors or professional mistakes honestly and openly in ways that promote patient learning	18
Convey key information accurately to the transition team assuming care	
Appreciate and discuss sensitive issues with patients, including:	16, 19, 23, 26, 27, 30, 31, 34, 38
Death and dying	31, 38
Health maintenance and disease prevention	19, 23, 26, 27
Substance abuse	30
Deliver accurate, clear, and concise oral presentations	

may be useful to the student, resident, and physician in dealing with the different cases presented in this book. The categories in the table have been derived from *Effective Patient-Physician Communication: Strengthening Relationships, Improving Patient Safety, Limiting Medical Liability* by Jane Ruddell,[2] and the American College of Surgeons' *Successfully Navigating the First Year of Surgical Residency: Essentials for Medical Students and PGY-1 Residents*.[3]

References

1. Accreditation Council for Graduate Medical Education (ACGME): General Competencies. Available at http://www.acgme.org/outcome/comp/compFull.asp.
2. Ruddell J: Effective Patient-Physician Communication: Strengthening Relationships, Improving Patient Safety, Limiting Medical Liability. Lebanon, Pa, Wescott Professional Publications, 2006.
3. American College of Surgeons: Successfully Navigating the First Year of Surgical Residency: Essentials for Medical Students and PGY-1 Residents. Chicago, American College of Surgeons, 2005.

Chapter 5
Professionalism from Hippocrates to the Residency Review Committee

Benjamin Fogel MD and Peter Schwartz MD

The defining aspects of "profession" include four characteristics:

- A calling requiring specialized knowledge, often with long and intensive preparation
- Instruction in specific skills and methods
- The demand to maintain the acquired knowledge
- The fundamental use of that knowledge and the derivative skills for the benefit of society

The responsibility (and privilege) to oversee and maintain the quality of the trust that society has placed in our profession, medicine, has been codified several times throughout the course of history:

- The Hippocratic Oath (460 BCE)
- The American Medical Association (AMA) Code of Ethics (1847)
- The Accreditation Council for Graduate Medical Education Professionalism Competency (2001)
- Medical Professionalism in the New Millennium: A Physician's Charter (2002)

It is worthwhile to look carefully at the concept of professionalism in medicine to see how it has evolved over time.

THE HIPPOCRATIC OATH

Almost 2550 years ago, sometime around 460 BCE, Hippocrates or his disciples formulated the Hippocratic Oath. The Oath elucidates professional responsibilities that have endured to this moment:

- Responsibility to the patient (beneficence)
- Responsibility to pass the profession on to the next generation
- Responsibility to do no harm
- Responsibility to maintain confidentiality
- Responsibility to maintain professional boundaries

THE AMERICAN MEDICAL ASSOCIATION CODE OF ETHICS

In 1803, Sir Thomas Percival published a "Code of Medical Ethics" in England, the most significant contribution to western medical ethics subsequent to Hippocrates.

The first American code of ethics was formulated by the AMA in 1847 and was based on Percival's Code. There were major revisions in 1903, 1912, 1947, and 1994; the latest rewrite of the Code of Ethics was adopted by the AMA in 2001 and includes the following nine principles[1]:

- Competent medical service
- Honesty
- Respect for the law
- Safeguarding of confidence
- Study, apply, and advance medical knowledge

- Freedom to choose whom to serve, and with whom to associate
- Responsibility to participate in improving community
- Paramount responsibility to the patient
- Access to medical care for all people

THE ACCREDITATION COUNCIL FOR GRADUATE MEDICAL EDUCATION PROFESSIONALISM COMPETENCY (2001)

Professionalism was defined by the Accreditation Council for Graduate Medical Education (ACGME) as follows: "Residents must demonstrate a commitment to carrying out professional responsibilities, adherence to ethical principles, and sensitivity to a diverse patient population." Furthermore, the ACGME recommends that:

- Residents are expected to demonstrate respect, compassion, and integrity; a responsiveness to the needs of patients and society that supercedes self interest; accountability to patients, society, and the profession; and a commitment to excellence and on-going professional development. Important aspects of this principle include the resident's need to put the patient first above his/her own self interest (patient primacy) and accountability to patients, society and the profession (not just oneself).
- Residents demonstrate a commitment to ethical principles pertaining to provision or withholding of clinical care, confidentiality of patient information, informed consent, and business practices.
- Residents demonstrate sensitivity and responsiveness to patient's culture, age, gender, and disabilities.

All three of these tenets address the issue of *conflict of interest*. Over the past two decades, the pharmaceutical industry and other parties intimately involved in the delivery of care have presented physicians with many opportunities that might have been considered reasonable marketing activities in the business world (e.g., dinners, gifts, trips, educational meetings). Physicians sometimes accepted these gifts. It is now recognized that gifts of any value have the tendency to provoke feelings of loyalty in the recipient. Solid ethical principle would suggest that physicians are expected to choose pharmaceuticals, instruments, and diagnostic tools and studies solely on the basis of their value for patients. Anything that might predispose the physician to select or appear to influence the decision for any other reason should be avoided.

MEDICAL PROFESSIONALISM IN THE NEW MILLENNIUM: A PHYSICIAN'S CHARTER (2002)

On February 9, 2002, as a response to many of the aforementioned concerns, a joint venture of the European Federation of Internal Medicine, The American College of Physicians, The American Society of Internal Medicine (ACP-ASM), and The American Board of Internal Medicine (ABIM) drafted "Medical Professionalism in the New Millennium: A Physician's Charter."[2] This document was published simultaneously in *The Lancet* and *Annals of Internal Medicine* and included *three fundamental principles* and a set of *ten professional responsibilities*. The editors of this textbook have used this schema of three principles and ten commitments to categorize the Professionalism teaching points for this book's case-based chapters.

Table 5-1 enables you to locate in the cases of this book concrete examples of the principles and commitments of the charter as they apply to the field of Ob/Gyn.

Table 5-1 Professionalism and Cases	
Professionalism Principles and Commitments	**Cases**
Principle of primacy of patient welfare	4, 7, 21, 22, 28, 33, 34
• Demonstrates dedication to serving the interest of the patient	
Principle of patient autonomy	2, 7, 8, 19, 26
• Demonstrates commitment to ethical principles pertaining to provision or withholding of care	
• Empowers patients to make informed decisions about their treatment	
Principle of social justice	8, 18, 25, 29
• Works actively to eliminate discrimination in health care	
Commitment to professional competence	6, 13, 16, 31, 37
• Demonstrates a commitment to excellence and life-long learning	

Table continues

Table 5-1 Professionalism and Cases—(cont'd)	
Professionalism Principles and Commitments	**Cases**
Commitment to honesty with patients • Demonstrates commitment to ethical principles pertaining to informed consent and business practices	7, 11, 36
Commitment to patient confidentiality • Demonstrates commitment to ethical principles pertaining to confidentiality of patient information	1, 17, 20–22
Commitment to maintaining appropriate relations with patients • Demonstrates sensitivity and responsiveness to patients' culture, age, gender, and disabilities	3, 10, 14, 30
Commitment to improving quality of care • Works collaboratively with other professionals to improve patient safety and optimize outcomes of care	35, 38
Commitment to improving access to care • Strives to reduce barriers to equitable health care	5, 27
Commitment to a just distribution of finite resources • Demonstrates commitment to cost-effective delivery of health care while meeting the needs of individual patients	12, 32
Commitment to scientific knowledge • Demonstrates commitment to promoting research and ensuring the appropriate use of new knowledge	13, 24
Commitment to maintaining trust by managing conflicts of interest • Demonstrates commitment to recognize, disclose, and deal with conflicts of interest	15
Commitment to professional responsibilities • Demonstrates commitment to maximizing patient care and respecting other health professionals • Demonstrates commitment to participating in self-regulation of the profession	9, 20, 23

THE FUTURE

For the past 15 years, the senior author of this chapter has asked resident candidates the following question: "If you agree that there might be a continuum between the following statements, where on that continuum are we currently, and are we in the appropriate place?"

- "Physicians are like priests whose service is the caring and comfort of their fellow person."
- "Physicians are businessmen who purvey health care."

Take a moment to consider how you might answer that question.

It is apparent that during the recent past, economic pressures on physicians have increased. This is a direct result of decreased reimbursements, increased costs including liability premiums, and pressure from managed care providers to reduce amount of services. All of these considerations have challenged the primacy of the ethical principle that care of the patient is paramount. This principle appears in *all* the codes of medical professionalism considered in this chapter.

The economics of health care reimbursement and managed care has made the physician a dual agent, responsible both to the patient and to the managed care provider. This has created an inevitable, inherent conflict of interest, particularly evident in the offering and provision of "appropriate services." This phenomenon also challenges the patient primacy medical ethic.

Pharmaceutical companies and other members of the "medical-industrial complex" have created real and potential conflicts of interest for physicians. This threatens the medical ethic of patient primacy as well.

Entrepreneurship and economic pressures challenge the professional obligations of competence and integrity. Some of our colleagues have acceded to providing expert witness testimony that their peers find untrue and improper. Some of our colleagues are experimenting with or providing services that appear outside their range of training, perhaps competence, or appropriate range of services (e.g., new technology, cosmesis, selling of products in the office). Among our colleagues there are many who believe that our interaction with industry is an appropriate evolution and we can be more effective by mastering the knowledge of business so we may better compete in the "marketplace." However, it should always be remembered that the *medical ethic* is a fiduciary one in which we are obligated to act in the patient's best interest even when it is contrary to our own. On the other hand, the *business ethic* is "caveat emptor," or let the buyer beware! It is difficult to rationalize the compatibility of these ethical frameworks.

Is there is a continuum between the priest and the businessman? Have we gone too far? Will we return to our historical foundations?

References

1. Principles of Medical Ethics, Adopted by the American Medical Association House of Delegates, June 2001.
2. ABIM Foundation, ACP Foundation, European Federation of Internal Medicine: Medical Professionalism in the New Millennium: A Physician Charter. Ann Intern Med 2002;136:243–246.

Chapter 6
The Systems-Based Practice Competency

Stephen A. Gordon MD and Gerald Peden MD

What is a system? The word "system" comes from both the Latin and Greek *systema*, meaning "an organized whole, a standing-together of parts or principles." *Webster's* defines a system as[1]:

A regularly interacting or interdependent group of items forming a unified whole.... an organization forming a network especially for distributing something or serving a common purpose.

Health care is frequently described as a system. Indeed, most of us have heard our patients describe a sense of frustration that they need help "navigating the system." As their physicians we are viewed (and, one hopes, view ourselves) as the captains of the ship, ready to help them navigate. As physician captains, we have a duty, to which we are bound by oath, to help them achieve the intended outcomes of their voyages. It is our ship: we charter the course, secure resources and supplies for the journey, direct the crew, and make sure that we reach our destination on time with as few delays and detours as possible. It is also our duty to make sure that the ship we are sailing is sound and up to accepted standards.

The implications of defining the delivery of health care as a *system* are numerous. Systems are formed to organize, standardize, and make efficient the delivery of a product. A system aims to standardize processes and procedures to achieve consistent and reproducible outcomes. Often the entire system focuses on a common goal. In our case, our patients' good health is the product.

Recognition that the processes for delivering care in various settings may be different is extremely pertinent to the field of Ob/Gyn. Different settings dictate different systems for direction and follow-through. Different standard procedures, for example, are required for admitting patients for inpatient acute care, outpatient diagnostic and therapeutic care, office-based care, preventive care, testing, screening, and so forth. In a hospital, physicians give direction by a written order that a nurse follows according to a defined system of care delivery; in the office setting, on the other hand, the physician may give direction verbally that is carried out without a written order. In still other settings, a computerized order entry system may be used to implement the physician's directives.

Patients will have expectations at each step along the way. They may have taken off from work to see a doctor in the office when they are ill, expecting to receive advice or treatment that will improve their immediate state of health. Sometimes expectations are met; sometimes they are not.

Indeed, there is evidence that our health care system does not function optimally and sometimes functions poorly. The Institute of Medicine's report *To Err Is Human* has brought medical errors to the forefront of our consciousness.[2]

And, as the numbers of uninsured continue to grow dramatically, the pressures on our system are increasing. Indigent patients tend to forego preventive care because they are unable to cope with the short-term expense. Eventually these patients require more costly acute care, which is inadequately reimbursed. This strains the system and its resources even further.

In the context of this volume, the competency editors for the Systems-Based Practice competency have attempted to deal with systems-based issues relevant to Ob/Gyn and the health care policy of today. Accordingly, we feel that it is appropriate as introduction to include comments about "the iron triangle of health care" and changes in national policy anticipated as a result of the change of administration at the time of the publication of this volume.

The fundamental constraints of health care policy are often referred to as the "iron triangle of health care." The argument is that the three goals of the health care system—high quality, broad access, and low cost—cannot all simultaneously be met: focusing on any one of them will necessarily require sacrificing one or both of the others. Accordingly, to expand coverage (access) requires either increasing total health care costs, or decreasing quality (in essence, spending less per person). Similarly, increasing the quality of care either requires raising total health care costs or providing fewer people with access to care. There is a compelling mathematical logic to this theory, and most policy experts agree that this rule holds true in many cases.

At present, the United States spends roughly $2 trillion a year on health care, or 16% to 17% of the gross domestic product, and fails to cover some 46 million uninsured people, or about 15% of the population. People who believe in the iron triangle argument believe that to cover the 46 million uninsured people in the United States will either require spending significantly more on health care or giving up the quality of care that most consider the hallmark of the U.S. health care system.

One of the most important exceptions to this rule, however, involves the considerable waste and inefficiency that seem to hamper our system. At the time of this writing we are entering a new political administration. A core tenet of the Obama administration's health care plan is that sufficient investment in *health information technology* will reduce unnecessary and wasteful spending by eliminating costs like extra hospital days due to medical errors or duplicative diagnostic tests ordered because the original results were not immediately available. Another core tenet of the administration's plan is that improving prevention and the management of chronic conditions will improve quality of care by eliminating the added costs of those who present for health care only after their conditions have progressed unnecessarily. Finally, the administration hopes that by increasing competition among insurers and pharmaceutical companies, we can reduce the costs of insurance coverage and drugs.

HOW CAN THIS BOOK HELP YOU LEARN ABOUT SYSTEMS-BASED PRACTICE?

For each case-based chapter, the authors were asked to contribute a paragraph on how a student or resident in Ob/Gyn might be made more aware of how to help the patient navigate the system more easily. The contributions have been categorized into three categories: (1) The System, (2) Improving the System, and (3) notes on Health Care Policy and Business (Table 6-1).

Table 6-1 Systems-Based Competency and Cases	
Systems-Based Concept	**Cases**
The System	
Provider operations and coordination	2, 8, 12, 14, 22, 36
Costs and cost drivers	3, 5, 15, 24, 27, 33, 35, 37
Reimbursement and insurance	13, 18, 20, 29, 33, 38
Improving System Function	
Systematization of practices	11, 30, 34
Utilization of information technology	10, 31
Process improvement	4, 26
Patient safety	1, 7, 26
Health Care Policy and Business	
Public health	6, 9, 14, 17, 23
Health care law	15, 16, 23
Business of medicine	2, 19, 21, 25, 28, 32, 35, 38

The system-based box in each chapter is a reminder: as the captains of the ship, we, as students, residents, and physicians, need to take the lead in understanding the system and working to improve it.

References

1. Merriam-Webster's Collegiate Dictionary, 11th ed. Springfield, Mass, Merriam-Webster Inc., 2003, p 1269.
2. Kohn L, Corrigan J, Donaldson M (eds): To Err Is Human: Building a Safer Health System. Washington, DC, Committee on Quality of Health Care in America, Institute of Medicine. National Academy Press, 2000.

Chapter 7
How to Succeed on the Ob/Gyn Clerkship

Philip J. DiGiacomo III MD

Although generally considered a difficult rotation, the Ob/Gyn clerkship can be one of the most rewarding times of your medical training.

The Ob/Gyn rotation can be intimidating because the world of Ob/Gyn seems to possesses its own "language," which often seems distinct from the standard terminology of medicine. This new language is full of abbreviations such as TAH/BSO (total abdominal hysterectomy/bilateral salpingo-oophorectomy), Pit (pitocin), and C/S (cesarean section). Your first few days on the rotation will most likely be spent deciphering these linguistic shortcuts. One way to streamline the learning process is to keep a readily accessible abbreviation guide on your person during the rotation and to be sure to actively review common Ob/Gyn terminology with the residents on your service in the first days of the rotation. (A brief set of the most common terms is provided in Table 7-1, at the end of this chapter.)

The sensitive and personal nature of both obstetric and gynecologic issues can make the rotation a challenge to your interpersonal skills and professionalism. You will be required to ask sensitive questions as part of your history taking, which will include inquiring about a patient's prior sexually transmitted diseases, number of lifetime sexual partners, and prior pregnancies and their outcomes. In addition, you will be required to learn how to perform pelvic and bimanual examinations. These examinations are highly personal and can sometimes be uncomfortable for patients. Nevertheless, these are important clinical skills to acquire. Do not shy away from an opportunity to interview a patient, to ask the necessary questions, and to perform the required examinations with appropriate supervision. It is important to develop confidence in yourself, for it is *your* confidence that is ultimately needed to put your patients at ease.

The Ob/Gyn rotation can be difficult because of the long and sometimes erratic hours you may be required to work. Maximize sleep when you can get it. If this means that you sleep most of the day after being up all night, then so be it. It usually takes a few days for your body to adjust to the new schedule, but have faith that it will indeed adjust! Although at times a nuisance, the odd hours of Ob/Gyn provide invaluable experience and learning opportunities. At night there are fewer health care personnel in the hospital, which means that students are often more directly involved in deliveries and emergency cesarean sections! Although the hours of the rotation can be difficult, it will give you an accurate glimpse of what life would be like if you choose Ob/Gyn as a career.

More than any other clerkship, the Ob/Gyn rotation exposes the student to the varied aspects of patient care: primary care and preventive care, as well as surgical aspects of care, including cesarean sections and gynecologic oncology. The uniqueness of the Ob/Gyn rotation is that it is the only arena in which you are actually able to participate in helping couples bring life into the world, one of the most important and memorable times in *their* lives. This is indeed a privilege. Delivering your first baby is an experience you will not soon forget.

To succeed on the Ob/Gyn clerkship you would be wise to demonstrate your *interest in learning* and your *enthusiasm for teamwork*.

The breadth of the specialty and your brief clerkship exposure to its many facets will demand that you read. So, read, read, read!

The contributors to this book hope that *Obstetrics and Gynecology: A Competency-Based Companion* will serve as a useful resource when you do so.

Gravity and Parity

One of the most commonly used notations in all of obstetrics and gynecology is Gravity and Parity, sometimes called "Gs & Ps". Gs and Ps refers to **G**ravity—the total number of times a patient has been pregnant, and **P**arity—how many living children a woman has delivered.

A G1P0 patient is pregnant with her first child, and has no living children. A G5P3 patient has been pregnant five times total, and has three living children. In some institutions Gs & Ps are further delineated in such a way that addresses specifics of parity. **G**ravity is listed in total, and **P**arity is broken down into **F**ull-term deliveries, **P**re-term deliveries, **A**bortions (including miscarriages and elective terminations of pregnancy), and **L**iving Children. For example, a G3 P2103 would have been pregnant three times, have two term deliveries, one pre-term delivery, no miscarriages or abortions, and three living children. A handy way to remember this notation is to use the first letter mnemonic: **F**lorida **P**ower **A**nd **L**ight.

Table 7-1 Commonly Used Abbreviations in Obstetrics and Gynecology

Like all fields of medicine, Obstetrics and Gynecology has its own unique language and nomenclature that can be frustrating to master at first. There is much regional variation, as well, which can add to the frustration. This is a relatively comprehensive list of the most commonly used abbreviations. Understand that not all of these may be used at your training site, and do not hesitate to ask for clarification if one of your instructors or associates uses an abbreviation or euphemism with which you are not acquainted.

AC	abdominal circumference
AFI	amniotic fluid index
AFP	alpha fetoprotein
AMA	advanced maternal age
AROM	artificial rupture of membranes
ASCUS	atypical squamous cells of undetermined significance
AUB	abnormal uterine bleeding
BCPs	birth control pills
BPD	biparietal diameter
BTL	bilateral tubal ligation
C/S	cesarean section
CST	contraction stress test
CTX	contractions
CX	cervix

Table continues

Table 7-1 Commonly Used Abbreviations in Obstetrics and Gynecology—(cont'd)

D&C	dilation and curettage
D&E	dilation and evacuation
DR	delivery room
DUB	dysfunctional uterine bleeding
EBL	estimated blood loss
ECC	endocervical curettage
EDC	estimated date of confinement
EGA	estimated gestational age
EMB	endometrial biopsy
FBS	fasting blood sugar
FH	fundal height
FHR	fetal heart rate
FHT	fetal heart tones
FL	femur length
FM	fetal movement
FSH	follicle-stimulating hormone
FTP	failure to progress
GBS	group B streptococcus
GC	gonococcus/gonorrhea
GHTN	gestational hypertension
HC	head circumference
hCG	human chorionic gonadotropin
HELLP	Hemolytic anemia, Elevated Liver enzymes, Low Platelet count
HPV	human papilloma virus
HSV	herpes simplex virus
IUD	intrauterine device
IUFD	intrauterine fetal demise
IUGR	intrauterine growth restriction
IUP	intrauterine pregnancy
IUPC	intrauterine pressure catheter
L&D	labor and delivery
LAVH	laparoscopically assisted vaginal hysterectomy
LH	luteinizing hormone
LMP	last menstrual period
LOF	leakage of fluid
L/S ratio	lecithin/sphingomyelin ratio
LTCS	low transverse cesarean section
NST	non-stress test
OA	occiput anterior
OCPs	oral contraceptive pills
OP	occiput posterior
PG	phosphatidyl glycerol
PID	pelvic inflammatory disease
PIH	pregnancy-induced hypertension
PMS	premenstrual syndrome

Table 7-1 Commonly Used Abbreviations in Obstetrics and Gynecology—(cont'd)

PML	premature labor
PNC	prenatal care
POC	products of conception
PPD	postpartum day
PPROM	preterm premature rupture of membranes
PROM	premature rupture of membranes
RDS	respiratory distress syndrome
SAB	spontaneous abortion
S<D	size less than dates
S>D	size greater than dates
SROM	spontaneous rupture of membranes
SSE	sterile speculum examination
STD	sexually transmitted disease
STI	sexually transmitted infection
SVD	spontaneous vaginal delivery
TAH/BSO	total abdominal hysterectomy/bilateral salpingo-oophorectomy
TL	tubal ligation
TOA	tubal ovarian abscess
TOL	trial of labor
T&S	type and screen
TVH	total vaginal hysterectomy
US	ultrasound
UTI	urinary tract infection
VB	vaginal bleeding
VBAC	vaginal birth after cesarean section
VTX	vertex

Chapter 8
Using the Competencies to Become an Effective Teacher

Hindi Stohl MD and Jessica L. Bienstock MD, MPH

Your Ob/Gyn rotation will, we hope, be an extremely rewarding experience. You will have the opportunity to see life being born, manage complex issues related to fertility and the menstrual cycle, and participate in operating room procedures. Perhaps more important, as a student, you can begin to think about how you will someday become an effective teacher. So, imagine yourself as an Ob/Gyn resident.

How we teach and learn medicine is constantly changing. One of the most recent changes has been the emphasis on Clinical Competencies. These competencies include Medical Knowledge, **Patient Care**, Practice-Based Learning and Improvement, Interpersonal and Communications Skills, Professionalism, and Systems-Based Practice. Needless to say, you will find yourself relying on and improving your Medical Knowledge and your Patient Care skills as you pursue your role as a teacher. Practice-Based Learning and Improvement and Interpersonal and Communication Skills are vital components of your role as a teacher.

When instructing residents to be team leaders, we use the following exercise as a guide to help them integrate competency awareness into the four roles that they will need to play on the Ob/Gyn service: **Communicator, Teacher, Coordinator,** and **Analyzer.**

If you are a resident, the following scenario and the guide to your four roles will be most pertinent. If you are a student, the guide will help you understand and empathize with the multifaceted tasks of the team leader. And should expectations not be made clear and when feedback is lacking, the following structure could help you negotiate your way by asking the appropriate questions.

OB/GYN RESIDENCY SCENARIO

Background

Imagine that you are currently the fourth-year chief resident on the labor and delivery (L&D) suite. With over 4000 deliveries per year, this is a very busy floor! You see a large volume of high-risk obstetric patients, and up to one fourth of your patients do not speak English as their primary language.

In addition to you, your team includes one Ob/Gyn attending, one nurse practitioner, an emergency medicine intern, a second-year and a third-year obstetrics resident, and three medical students. Together, you care for all of the patients on L&D as well as the antepartum and postpartum patients. You are also responsible for providing obstetric consultations to other services in the hospital and for performing male circumcisions for newborns in the nursery.

The Scenario

Three medical students will be rotating on your service beginning tomorrow:

- A first-year student, still in her preclinical years of training. She is eager to be inspired by a magical birth experience.
- A third-year student on his core clinical rotation, who is currently undecided about which field of medicine he wishes to pursue.
- A sub-intern from an outside institution hoping to be accepted to your residency program for the upcoming year.

Your Task

Your task is to guide each of these three students through their rotation and afford them an inspiring educational experience.

The Guide (your four roles)

The students currently rotating on your service have varying levels of medical training and are developing competence in the field of Obstetrics and Gynecology. Making this rotation a success for each of them will be a challenge. You will need to develop individualized objectives for each student, tailor your didactic approach based on the students' previous experiences, and be able to measure their performances according to level-appropriate standards.

First, you need to remember that to be an effective team leader you should try to incorporate into your leadership style the four qualities listed in the left column below. Attention to the related competencies listed in the right column can help you to be more effective.

Communicator	Interpersonal and Communication Skills
Teacher	Medical Knowledge
Coordinator	Systems-Based Practice
Analyzer	Practice-Based Learning and Improvement

The Specifics

Here are the skills you will need in each of these roles and some questions you should ask yourself to help guide you:

Communicator: Interpersonal and Communication Skills

- Clearly articulate the individual student's responsibilities.
- Explain your rationale for your decisions and actions.

- Take seriously and answer clearly the questions from your colleagues and your students.

Self-Directed Questions
- What are the most important elements of this patient's care that must be communicated to the entire team?
- Are all of my team members familiar with complex medical terminology or do I need to explain some of the common vocabulary to them?
- Are my team members communicating effectively with each other or do certain individuals tend always to be "the last to know?"
- Does everyone understand the reason(s) for specific patient care decisions?

Teacher: Medical Knowledge

- Provide an overview of the resources available to the members of your team.
- Set individualized goals and expectations for students.
- Dedicate time every week for teaching, using "down time" as an opportunity to review seminal topics.
- Remain attentive to your students' concerns.

Self-Directed Questions
- What are the important medical points for a student to have mastered upon completion of this rotation?
- Do the students know how to perform the tasks assigned to them? Do they know where to look if they do not?

Coordinator: Systems-Based Practice

- Maintain an accurate log of the patients on your service.
- Assign each student patients that he or she should follow.

Self-Directed Questions
- Are the students following patients who provide good learning opportunities?
- Do the students understand their roles in caring for their patients and know where they are supposed to be throughout the day?

- Does each student have the appropriate number of patients to follow?
- Are all of your team members familiar with each other and aware of each other's roles and responsibilities?
- What computer codes, passwords, or swipe access do the students need?

Analyzer: Practice-Based Learning and Improvement

- Accurately assess each student's knowledge and skills.
- Provide constructive feedback.
- Evaluate each student according to level-appropriate standards and expectations.

Self-Directed Questions

- Am I evaluating this student based on direct observation of his or her work or on hearsay?
- What is each of my students doing well and in what areas can they each improve?
- Am I providing helpful feedback or am I criticizing issues which cannot be changed?

Chapter 9
Oral Presentations in Obstetrics

Michael Belden MD

Developing skills to communicate effectively with colleagues regarding patients is crucial. This is certainly true when we communicate with each other regarding laboring patients.

You will find that the terminology and abbreviations we use can be confusing. It is best to master these shortcuts as soon as possible so that you can achieve a level of comfort using them (see Table 7-1 for a list of commonly used abbreviations). Until that point, there is no harm in using the formal medical terminology. For example, if a patient presents with preterm premature rupture of membranes (PPROM), it is acceptable to use the complete terminology until you are comfortable with the term PPROM. This is common sense, and will help you avoid errors in your presentations.

It is important to stay on point: we call this a "focused" presentation. When presenting a laboring patient to a senior resident or attending, concentrate on the obstetric issues at hand. Include only relevant medical problems or concerns that may be complicating the *pregnancy*. For example, the patient may have a strong family history of cardiovascular disease. For a healthy 25–year-old who presents in active labor, however, this is probably irrelevant. Again, this is common sense. Don't get bogged down with details that could best be omitted.

When presenting patients, think about your audience and tailor your presentation to your listener(s) and the circumstance. Your presentation of a patient will be different if done by telephone to an attending at 3:00 in the morning, at evening sign-out, or in a peer-review Morbidity and Mortality Conference. Consider the circumstances and use your clinical judgment to decide which details and relevant points need to be presented.

ADJUSTING THE LEVEL OF DETAIL

When giving a focused presentation of the patient, time is of the essence. Details should be relevant and germane to the case. Keep the presentation as short as possible and include points that are relevant to patient management decisions. Know all the aspects of the case, but distill down to the important points. Be prepared to elaborate on the case if needed. For example:

■ When presenting an uncomplicated patient, it is best to keep it short: "This is a 27-year-old G1P0 woman with an estimated date of confinement of February 2 who is 38 weeks' gestation. She presents with a chief complaint of contractions, which began 3 hours ago, are 5 minutes apart, and are extremely painful to her. Her last cervical exam was in the office 2 days ago, and she was 3 cm then. She is now 6 cm dilated. Her fetal heart tracing shows a baseline of 140 and is reactive. Her pregnancy has been uncomplicated. She would like to get an epidural."

■ When presenting a more complicated patient, more detail is required: "This is a 44-year-old G3P0Ab2 female with an estimated date of confinement of April 4 at 33 weeks' gestation who presents with a chief complaint of leakage of fluid. Her pregnancy is noteworthy for being conceived with in vitro fertilization of a donor egg. She has well-controlled gestational diabetes, but her last several blood pressures in the office have been elevated, about 140/90. Her fetus is being followed with twice-weekly nonstress tests because of intrauterine growth restriction. She describes a large "gush" of fluid about 2 hours ago, but is not having painful contractions. Her ruptured membranes have been confirmed with a sterile speculum exam. The fetal heart rate tracing shows a baseline of 150, with moderate variability. There are no contractions. Of note, she had an exploratory laparotomy 3 years ago for a pancreatic mass, which was benign, and had a partial small bowel obstruction after the surgery that resolved with conservative measures."

SYNTHESIZING THE INFORMATION AND DEVELOPING A PLAN

We take a complete history and perform a complete physical to get as much information as possible about the patient so that we can make intelligent decisions that will result in the best outcome for the patient. We present patients to each other orally to obtain additional opinions or to ensure the patient will be well taken care of when we are no longer primarily involved.

Synthesize the information from the history and physical so that you can develop a differential diagnosis. When you have a working differential diagnosis, think about the lab tests and radiologic studies you will need to confirm or rule out items in your differential. Develop a management plan. Be prepared to explain your thought process to everyone who is involved in the care of the patient.

In the sample case that follows you will find a woman who presents to the hospital in labor with a pregnancy of moderate complexity. High-priority findings appear in red type, and lower priority findings appear in blue type. After you read the history compare how a skilled presenter would present the same case in three different situations:

■ The 3 AM bedside presentation to the attending
■ Morning "sign-in" on the labor floor with the full obstetric team
■ A case presentation at a departmental conference

Typical Written History and Physical

NOTE THAT THE HISTORY AND PHYSICAL BELOW AND THE THREE DIFFERENT ORAL PRESENTATIONS THAT FOLLOW USE THE SAME DATA POINTS, PRESENTED IN DIFFERENT WAYS.

Chief complaint: Contractions.

History of present illness: The patient, A.G., is a 30-year-old G1P0 with a last menstrual period of December 26 and an estimated date of confinement of October 1 who is 39 weeks pregnant. Her due date was confirmed by a first-trimester ultrasound. She presents with contractions that began about 6 hours ago, and have been increasing in intensity. The contractions are now 3 minutes apart, and are extremely painful to her. She has had no leakage of amniotic fluid, and feels good fetal movement. She has had no vaginal bleeding.

The patient's pregnancy has been complicated recently by rising blood pressure. She had been seen twice the prior week in the office and her blood pressures had been 138/86 and 144/94 on those two occasions. She did not have proteinuria in the office. An ultrasound ordered 1 week ago because of her gestational hypertension revealed a fetus in the 36th percentile for growth with an amniotic fluid index of 12. The patient had a "normal" ultrasound at 20 weeks by her report, as well as a "normal" sequential screening test for Down syndrome and spina bifida. Her 1-hour glucose test and group B strep screen were both negative.

Past obstetric history: None

Past gynecologic history: A single abnormal Pap: atypical squamous cells of undetermined significance (ASCUS) at age 24, evaluated with colposcopy, which was negative for CIN

Past medical history: Hypothyroidism, migraine headaches

Past surgical history: Appendectomy at age 17

Medicines: Levothyroxine 0.088 mg PO q. day; ibuprofen as needed for migraines

Allergies: NKDA

Social history: She does not smoke, has an occasional glass of wine with her husband when she is not pregnant. She has been exercising for 45 minutes a day until her first elevated blood pressure 1 week ago.

Occupational history: She works in the marketing department for a skiing magazine.

Review of systems: Negative for cardiovascular, pulmonary, gastrointestinal, renal, urinary, or musculoskeletal problems

Physical exam: VS: T = 98.3, HR = 88, BP = 156/103, RR = 16, Wt. = 162 lbs

General appearance: A well-developed, well-nourished 30-year-old patient who is in distress when she has contractions

HEENT: Normal and intact
CV: Regular rhythm with a very soft systolic flow murmur
Lungs: Clear bilaterally
Abdomen: Gravid, uterine fundal height seemingly appropriate, nondistended, nontender, and soft, with palpable uterine contractions
Cervix: 7 cm dilated/95% effacement/+1 station
Fetal heart rate tracing: Baseline 140, moderate variability, reactive, with no decelerations
Toco: Regular contractions every 3 minutes
Extremities: +3 pitting ankle edema
Neuro: Very brisk patellar reflexes, no clonus
Labs: WBC = 12.2, Hb = 11.2, Hct = 33.0, Plts = 124, creatinine = 0.9, uric acid = 7.2, urinalysis with no WBCs or bacteria, with +3 proteinuria; AST = 26, ALT = 28, blood type O+, rubella immune
Bedside ultrasound: Vertex, AFI = 11, posterior placenta
Impression: A 30-year-old primiparous patient at full term, in labor, with likely preeclampsia
Plan:
1. Admit to labor floor and start an IV.
2. Administer epidural anesthesia at patient's request.
3. Begin IV magnesium drip for seizure prophylaxis.
4. Monitor fetus continuously.
5. Place a Foley catheter to measure urine output.
6. Check protein-to-creatinine ratio, or begin 24-hour urine collection for total protein.
7. Manage labor expectantly and intervene with amniotomy or oxytocin if required.

Oral Presentations Appropriate for Different Contexts

3 AM bedside presentation to attending	This is a 30-year-old G1P0 at full term who presents in labor, with no leakage of fluid. Her gestational dating is good, confirmed with an early ultrasound. She has been followed for increasing blood pressures for the last week, but with no proteinuria. Tonight her blood pressure is 156/103, and she has +3 proteinuria. I think she has preeclampsia, but her lab studies show no signs of HELLP syndrome. Her cervix is 7 cm dilated, very well effaced, with a favorable station. Her fetal heart rate tracing is reactive, and the baby is vertex both by my exam, and confirmed with ultrasound. I would like to let her get her epidural, and start a magnesium drip. She had an appy at age 17, in case we need to do a c-section.
Morning "sign-in" on the labor floor with the full obstetric team	In room no. 3 we have Ms. A.G., who is a 30-year-old G1P0 patient with an EDC of 10/1 and an EGA of 39 weeks who presented overnight with a chief complaint of contractions. She has had no leakage of fluid, and has had good fetal movement. She has been followed for the past week for increasing blood pressures, but has not had proteinuria in the office. Her pregnancy has been otherwise uncomplicated, with no GDM or other problems. Her GBS screen was negative. An ultrasound done last week revealed normal fetal growth, and a normal AFI. She has hypothyroidism, for which she takes levothyroxine, but is on no other meds. On exam her BP is 156/103, but she has no fever or tachycardia. She has +3 proteinuria on her urinalysis, but no signs of HELLP syndrome. Her fundal height is appropriate. Her cervical exam is now 9 cm, and she was 7 cm when she presented. Her fetal heart rate tracing has been reactive all along, with no decels. She has been contracting on her own every 3 minutes. My plan at this point is to continue to let her labor. We started magnesium at 2 g/hour at about 3:30 this morning. She has no signs of magnesium toxicity. I put in a Foley to measure her urine output. She has a pretty good shot at a vaginal delivery, but I am concerned about the possibility of a postpartum hemorrhage because of the magnesium.

Case presentation at a departmental conference

Ms. A.G. is an interesting patient who presented in labor 1 week ago. She is a 30-year-old G1P0 patient who arrived at the hospital at full term, in labor. Her pregnancy had been essentially uncomplicated but, interestingly, she had been followed for about a week before her presentation here for hypertension. We believed it was gestational hypertension because she did not have proteinuria. An ultrasound for fetal growth and AFI done at that time were entirely normal. When she presented to the hospital she was in labor, and did indeed have proteinuria. Thankfully, she did not develop HELLP syndrome, and her lab tests never deviated from normal. Ultimately she had a fast and normal labor, and delivered a healthy baby boy at 10:00 AM on the morning she presented. The baby weighed 7 lbs 1 oz, and had Apgar scores of 9 and 9. I am presenting Ms. A.G. because of the rapidity with which she developed preeclampsia. She had been followed closely as an outpatient, but only showed true preeclampsia after her arrival on the labor floor. We began a magnesium drip and she delivered uneventfully. We kept her on the magnesium for a full 24 hours after her delivery, and her pressures began to normalize by the time she was discharged to home, on postpartum day no. 3.

Editor's note: Each individual presentation emphasizes the most important points for the moment in time and the circumstances in which the patient is being presented. The first presentation focuses on the important task at hand: formulating a plan. The second presentation gives a summary of events up until that point, and further develops the plan of management. The third presentation brings to light an important point in the case, and develops a platform for further discussion and learning.

Appendix 1
ACGME General Competencies

ACGME GENERAL COMPETENCIES VERSION 1.3 (9.28.99)

The residency program must require its residents to develop the competencies in the six areas below to the level expected of a new practitioner. Toward this end, programs must define the specific knowledge, skills, and attitudes required and provide educational experiences as needed in order for their residents to demonstrate the competencies.

Patient Care

Residents must be able to provide patient care that is compassionate, appropriate, and effective for the treatment of health problems and the promotion of health. Residents are expected to:

- communicate effectively and demonstrate caring and respectful behaviors when interacting with patients and their families
- gather essential and accurate information about their patients
- make informed decisions about diagnostic and therapeutic interventions based on patient information and preferences, up-to-date scientific evidence, and clinical judgment
- develop and carry out patient management plans
- counsel and educate patients and their families
- use information technology to support patient care decisions and patient education
- perform competently all medical and invasive procedures considered essential for the area of practice
- provide health care services aimed at preventing health problems or maintaining health
- work with health care professionals, including those from other disciplines, to provide patient-focused care

Medical Knowledge

Residents must demonstrate knowledge about established and evolving biomedical, clinical, and cognate (e.g., epidemiological and social-behavioral) sciences and the application of this knowledge to patient care. Residents are expected to:

- demonstrate an investigatory and analytic thinking approach to clinical situations
- know and apply the basic and clinically supportive sciences which are appropriate to their discipline

Practice-Based Learning and Improvement

Residents must be able to investigate and evaluate their patient care practices, appraise and assimilate scientific evidence, and improve their patient care practices. Residents are expected to:

- analyze practice experience and perform practice-based improvement activities using a systematic methodology
- locate, appraise, and assimilate evidence from scientific studies related to their patients' health problems
- obtain and use information about their own population of patients and the larger population from which their patients are drawn
- apply knowledge of study designs and statistical methods to the appraisal of clinical studies and other information on diagnostic and therapeutic effectiveness
- use information technology to manage information, access on-line medical information, and support their own education
- facilitate the learning of students and other health care professionals

Interpersonal and Communication Skills

Residents must be able to demonstrate interpersonal and communication skills that result in effective information exchange and teaming with patients, their patients' families, and professional associates. Residents are expected to:

- create and sustain a therapeutic and ethically sound relationship with patients
- use effective listening skills and elicit and provide information using effective nonverbal, explanatory, questioning, and writing skills
- work effectively with others as a member or leader of a health care team or other professional group

Professionalism

Residents must demonstrate a commitment to carrying out professional responsibilities, adherence to ethical principles, and sensitivity to a diverse patient population. Residents are expected to:

- demonstrate respect, compassion, and integrity; a responsiveness to the needs of patients and society that supersedes self-interest; accountability to patients, society, and the profession; and a commitment to excellence and ongoing professional development
- demonstrate a commitment to ethical principles pertaining to provision or withholding of clinical care, confidentiality of patient information, informed consent, and business practices
- demonstrate sensitivity and responsiveness to patients' culture, age, gender, and disabilities

Systems-Based Practice

Residents must demonstrate an awareness of and responsiveness to the larger context and system of health care and the ability to effectively call on system resources to provide care that is of optimal value. Residents are expected to:

- understand how their patient care and other professional practices affect other health care professionals, the health care organization, and the larger society and how these elements of the system affect their own practice
- know how types of medical practice and delivery systems differ from one another, including methods of controlling health care costs and allocating resources
- practice cost-effective health care and resource allocation that does not compromise quality of care
- advocate for quality patient care and assist patients in dealing with system complexities
- know how to partner with health care managers and health care providers to assess, coordinate, and improve health care and know how these activities can affect system performance

From the Accreditation Council on Graduate Medical Education. Reprinted with permission.

Appendix 2
Competency Self-Assessment Form: Obstetrics

Competency Self-Assessment Form: Obstetrics

Patient Summary:

Dx:

Patient Care:

How and why did the patient present?
Was the patient in labor?
What was my plan of management?

Medical Knowledge

Did I know the basics well enough to participate in the patient's care? What knowledge points do I need to reinforce?

Practice-Based Learning and Improvement

Did I utilize evidence-based medicine? Did I increase my fund of knowledge regarding obstetrics?

Interpersonal and Communication Skills

Was I an effective member of the obstetrics team? Did I communicate well with my colleagues and ancillary staff? Did I communicate well with my patient and her family?

Professionalism

Did I function at the highest possible level? Was I professional in my interactions with the obstetrics team and the patient?

Systems-Based Practice

Did the medical system work at its best for the welfare of the patient? How can I facilitate improvements?

Appendix 3
Competency Self-Assessment Form: Gynecology

Competency Self-Assessment Form: Gynecology

Patient Summary:

Dx:

Patient Care:

Was I complete in my history and physical examination? Was my clinical reasoning appropriate and sound?

Medical Knowledge

Do I understand the basics of the patient's most likely disease processes?

Practice-Based Learning and Improvement

Did I utilize evidence-based medicine? Did I increase my fund of knowledge regarding gynecologic disease?

Interpersonal and Communication Skills

Did I work well with the team providing care? Was I respectful and compassionate in my interactions with the patient and her family?

Professionalism

Did I function at the highest possible level? What can I do to improve my medical professionalism?

Systems-Based Practice

Did the medical system work at its best for the welfare of the patient? How can I facilitate improvements?

Section II
CASES IN OBSTETRIC MANAGEMENT

Section Editor
Gary D. Blake MD

Chapter 10
Obstetric Tools: Prenatal Ultrasonography in Each Trimester

Andrew Gerson MD

Obstetric Ultrasonography and the Competencies

Patient Care	
Understand when obstetric ultrasonography can be beneficial to a patient.	
Medical Knowledge	
Learn how to use and interpret obstetric ultrasonography.	
Practice-Based Learning and Improvement	
Learn how to perform ultrasonography yourself (if possible), to acquire an invaluable skill for the timely evaluation of your patients.	
Interpersonal and Communication Skills	
Communicate to the patient why a test is needed, and what the results reveal.	
Professionalism	
Order the best test possible for the patient, at the best possible facility. Confer with a perinatologist or radiologist readily, whenever necessary.	
Systems-Based Practice	
Order tests in a cost-effective manner, keeping in mind it is often reasonable to order an expensive test first if it yields the most information and is best for the patient.	

Obstetric ultrasonography is *the* major tool for pregnancy assessment. Uses of ultrasonography in the first trimester include accurate pregnancy dating and assessment of viability, pregnancy location, and multiple gestation. Second-trimester ultrasonography is used primarily for confirmation of anatomic integrity. Third-trimester ultrasonography is useful for evaluation of growth and confirmation of fetal well-being. The following images illustrate these uses.

First-Trimester Ultrasonography

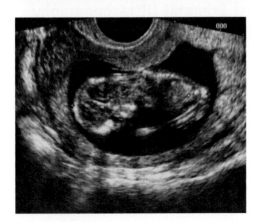

Figure 10-1
First-trimester ultrasonogram, at about 11 weeks.

Every ultrasonographic measurement describes a range of possible gestational ages. In the first trimester, the range is ±3 days. In the third trimester the range is ±3 weeks! Thus, an estimated date of confinement (EDC) can confidently be assigned after first-trimester ultrasonography, but not after third-trimester ultrasonography. First-trimester ultrasonography is also very useful for identification and evaluation of multiple gestations, fetal viability, and first-trimester bleeding.

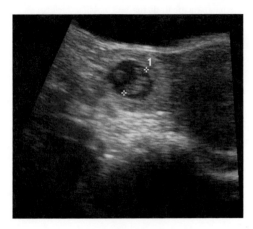

Figure 10-2
Ectopic pregnancy. Note the "doughnut sign," which identifies the pregnancy, and the adjacent empty uterine cavity.

First-trimester ultrasonography can be helpful in the evaluation of abdominal pain. Adnexal masses, ectopic pregnancies, uterine leiomyomata, and appendicitis are all part of the differential diagnosis of abdominal pain and an early pregnancy. Ultrasonography can often rule in or rule out the etiology of abdominal pain.

IMAGING CONSIDERATIONS

→**First-trimester ultrasonography:** Accurate pregnancy dating and assessment of viability, pregnancy location, and multiple gestation. $300

Second-Trimester Ultrasonography

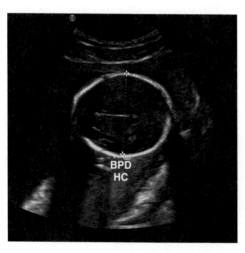

Figure 10-3
Second-trimester ultrasonogram showing accurate biparietal diameter (BPD) and head circumference (HC).

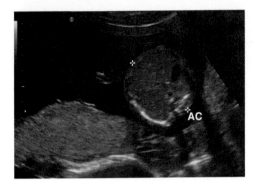

Figure 10-4
Second-trimester
ultrasonogram
showing accurate
abdominal
circumference (AC).

Ultrasonography is performed routinely in most medical communities at about 20 weeks of gestation. Benefits include accurate dating, placental location, and the diagnosis of multiple gestations and congenital abnormalities. Studies have suggested that competently performed ultrasonography will rule out 30% to 60% of congenital abnormalities. An additional benefit of routine ultrasonography is that it allows prospective parents to bond with their babies.

In a population at risk for having a fetus with an abnormal chromosome complement (e.g., patients of advanced maternal age or who have received abnormal screening test results), ultrasonography can be used as a means of reassurance. At least half of all chromosomally abnormal conceptions will show a clue or marker suggesting aneuploidy. These clues may include (but are not limited to) growth disturbances,

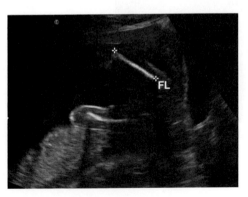

Figure 10-5
Second-trimester
ultrasonogram
showing accurate
femur length (FL).

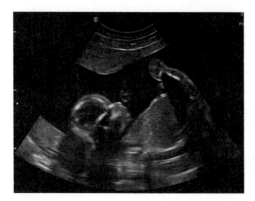

Figure 10-6 Normal second-trimester ultrasonogram with fetus in profile.

an obvious congenital abnormality, or a "soft" marker such as pyelectasis (fluid in the renal pelves), an echogenic cardiac focus (calcium deposit) in the heart, echogenic bowel, or short proximal limb bones. If these are present the chance of delivering an infant with an abnormal chromosome complement is increased. If these markers are absent, the chance is decreased. This should be communicated to the patient.

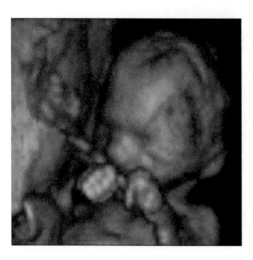

Figure 10-7 Three-dimensional ultrasonogram of a normal fetal face.

IMAGING CONSIDERATIONS

→**Second-trimester ultrasonography:** Accurate dating, placental location, and the diagnosis of multiple gestations and congenital abnormalities. $325

Third-Trimester Ultrasonography

Third-trimester ultrasonography is used primarily to assess amniotic fluid levels, placental location, and fetal position. The *amniotic fluid index* (AFI) is one of the components of the biophysical profile, which is an extremely useful tool to evaluate fetal well-being near full term (see Chapter 13, Antenatal Fetal Surveillance).

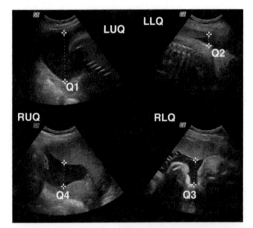

Figure 10-8
Assessment of amniotic fluid index in the third trimester.

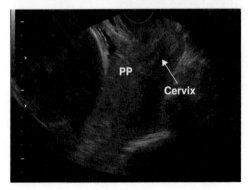

Figure 10-9
Placenta previa (PP) noted in the third trimester. Note that the placenta completely covers the cervix.

- In the third trimester, evaluation of fetal growth and size, placentation, and amniotic fluid are the most important uses of ultrasonography.
- Size is evaluated by measurements of the head, abdomen, and femur. An estimated weight can be calculated from these measurements. The single best predictor of fetal size is measurement of the abdominal circumference.
- Patients with hypertension are at risk of having small infants. In this group of patients the abdominal circumference will be significantly smaller than expected. Patients with diabetes are at risk of having fetuses with excessive growth. If growth is excessive, the abdominal circumference will be larger than anticipated.
- Estimation of fetal weight is also used to assess growth. It is plotted on a reference table versus gestational age to generate a percentile. Small fetuses are thought to be at or less than the 10th percentile. Large fetuses are considered to be at the 90th percentile or greater.
- Amniotic fluid is evaluated by the summation of the depths of pockets of free fluid in each of the four quadrants of the uterus. These measurements (in centimeters) are summed to generate an amniotic fluid index. An amniotic fluid index of 5 to 25 cm is considered normal. Greater than 25 cm defines *polyhydramnios* (an abnormally large volume of fluid), whereas less than 5 cm suggests *oligohydramnios* (low fluid).
- The general well-being of the fetus (which can be observed using the *biophysical profile*) is a direct evaluation of adequate placental function. Sustained fetal breathing (>30 seconds), gross body movements (>3 in a 30-minute period), tone (flexion and extension), and adequate amniotic fluid are observed using this test. If the four ultrasonographic parts of the profile—tone, gross movement, fetal breathing movements, and adequate fluid—are present, along with a "reactive" nonstress test, the fetus is considered to have a reassuring biophysical status.

IMAGING CONSIDERATIONS

→**Third-trimester ultrasonography:** Assess amniotic fluid levels, placental location, fetal position, and general fetal well-being. $225

Chapter 11
Routine Prenatal Care (Case 1)

Lucinda S. Antosh DO and Arlene Smalls MD

Case: A 27-year-old female G1P0 presents to clinic with a positive urine pregnancy test and an LMP that occurred 10 weeks before her presentation today.

Differential Diagnosis

Intrauterine pregnancy	Spontaneous abortion (miscarriage)	Ectopic pregnancy

Speaking Intelligently

The most important question you must ask with regard to a patient presenting with a positive pregnancy test is: "Is this a normal intrauterine pregnancy?" In the office setting, ultrasound provides the important information regarding pregnancy location and viability and assists in the confirmation of the EDC.

In an early intrauterine pregnancy, a gestational sac is the initial finding seen with a transvaginal ultrasound once the β-hCG level is greater than 1500 mIU/mL. A transvaginal ultrasound is a somewhat invasive procedure and the physician should always explain its use before proceeding. If the pregnancy cannot be visualized by ultrasound, obtain serial β-hCG levels to monitor the rate of β-hCG elevation. These levels should double every 48 hours. Plan to repeat the ultrasound evaluation in 1 to 2 weeks if the pregnancy cannot be visualized initially. The viability of a pregnancy is established once an embryo with a fetal heartbeat is observed within the uterine cavity.

Ultrasound is the most valuable tool to confirm pregnancy dating. First-trimester ultrasound measurements generally should agree with the clinical EDC determined by LMP, within 3 days. If the EDC established by the LMP and the ultrasound-established due date do not concur, the EDC established by the ultrasound should be chosen because it is more reliable, and menstrual history can be notoriously inaccurate. In the second trimester, the EDC by LMP and ultrasound should match within 10 to 14 days. Again, if there is no concurrence, the date established by the ultrasound is usually more accurate.

PATIENT CARE

Clinical Thinking
- Determination of an *intrauterine* pregnancy is essential.
- Accurate pregnancy dating is vital to providing good prenatal care throughout the pregnancy.
- The lab and screening studies that should be ordered depend on accurate pregnancy dating.
- Obtain a complete history to predict complications that might be encountered during this pregnancy.

History
- Date of the first day of LMP.
- Inquire about nausea and vomiting.
- Ask about abdominal pain and/or vaginal bleeding.
- History of previous pregnancy complications.
- **Past medical history** such as diabetes or thyroid disorders, which can affect the growth and development of the fetus.
- **Past surgical history** such as prior cesarean delivery, myomectomy, or other abdominal procedures that can affect the well-being of the pregnancy and mode of delivery.
- **Medications:** Inquire regarding exposures that may be potentially teratogenic.
- **Family history:** Inquire about genetic diseases known to be associated with ethnicity or personal family history that may predispose to certain diseases.

Physical Examination
- **Vital signs:** Blood pressure and pulse should be within normal range.
- **General appearance:** Assess patient's mood regarding pregnancy and her general health. Assess body habitus because obesity leads to increased incidence of pregnancy complications (e.g., chronic hypertension, gestational diabetes, preeclampsia, fetal macrosomia, higher rates of stillbirth, cesarean delivery, and postpartum complications).
- **Thyroid exam:** Assess for an enlarged thyroid gland or thyroid nodules.
- **Heart:** Listen for murmurs, gallops, and abnormal heart sounds. Functional systolic heart murmurs are common in pregnancy, but it is important not to miss true cardiac disease.
- **Lungs:** The lungs should be clear bilaterally. In asthmatic patients, listen carefully for wheezes.
- **Breast exam:** The breast exam should reveal normal breast tissue, with no masses or adenopathy noted.
- **Abdomen:** The abdomen should be soft without organomegaly. Assess the abdomen for tenderness.
- **Uterine fundal height** is measured from the pubic symphysis to the top of the uterus once the pregnancy is 20 weeks or greater. The

uterine fundal height should increase by 1 cm weekly thereafter, to match the gestational weeks.

- **Gynecologic exam:** A thorough pelvic exam, including a speculum and bimanual exam, is recommended for the initial visit. During the first trimester, uterine enlargement is measured and commented on by "weeks" of gestation. For example, a "6-week" uterus might feel about the same size as a baseball, and an "8-week" uterus might feel more like the size of a softball (this exam skill is difficult to master). Assess for the presence of any abnormal cervical or vaginal discharge via wet prep test. Obtain cultures for *Neisseria gonorrhoeae* and *Chlamydia trachomatis* and a Pap test.
- **Extremities:** Assess for pedal edema.

Tests for Consideration
- **Quantitative β-hCG:** Especially helpful if pregnancy is difficult to visualize on ultrasound or physical exam is inconsistent with dating. $35
- **Initial prenatal labs:**
  - CBC with platelet count to assess for anemia and thrombocytopenia $30
  - Blood type and Rh factor $85
  - Antibody screen $65
  - Hepatitis B screening for hepatitis B exposure $65
  - RPR for syphilis screening $42
  - Urinalysis, urine culture to assess for UTI $38
  - Rubella titer $21
  - Human immunodeficiency virus (HIV) $68
- **Other labs to consider:**
  - Hemoglobin electrophoresis, depending on patient's ethnicity $375
  - Cystic fibrosis screening $325
  - Toxoplasmosis titers $45
  - Early one hour glucose tolerance test (GTT) if patient is obese or has glucosuria on urine dip $80

IMAGING CONSIDERATIONS

→**First-trimester transvaginal ultrasound:** Provides accurate pregnancy dating, rules out ectopic pregnancy, and documents singleton or multiple gestation and ovarian pathology. Permits assessment of cervical length for increased risk of preterm labor. $225

→**Second-trimester transabdominal ultrasound:** Provides information regarding placental placement and fetal and uterine anatomy. $350

Clinical Entities	Medical Knowledge

Intrauterine Pregnancy

TP Amenorrhea is the cardinal sign of early pregnancy. Other early signs of pregnancy may be nausea with or without vomiting, breast tenderness, fatigue, and increased frequency of urination.

Dx Diagnosis is made by a combination of a positive β-hCG and transvaginal or abdominal ultrasound revealing an intrauterine pregnancy.

Tx It is wise for a woman to seek early prenatal care to help identify issues that may arise during her pregnancy. These concerns should be addressed at the first visit, and most clinicians will create a "problem list" and an overall plan for care at that time. As a matter of routine, prenatal care in the United States has been relatively standardized. Typically, patients are seen every 4 weeks in the first and second trimesters. At or about 28 weeks, the patient is seen every 2 weeks, and weekly beginning at 36 weeks and thereafter. A fetal anatomy ultrasound should be performed at about 20 weeks, and gestational diabetes screening should be done at or about 28 weeks. RhoGAM evaluations, as well as screening for maternal anemia, should be done at the 28-week visit as well. Group B strep screening is done at 36 weeks, and a treatment strategy can be developed if the culture is positive. Additional ultrasounds and targeted fetal surveillance are done as needed for specific patients who require these interventions. **See Gabbe 5, Hacker 7.**

Spontaneous Abortion (Miscarriage)

Pφ Spontaneous abortion, also known as *miscarriage*, typically occurs when the pregnancy is not viable. There are many variations, with relatively complex nomenclature. (See Chapter 20 on Early Pregnancy Loss and Miscarriage for a more comprehensive discussion.)

TP Spontaneous abortion is characterized by uterine bleeding or passage of products of conception, usually associated with a nonviable embryo. Keep in mind that in the circumstance of a "missed" abortion the patient will have a nonviable pregnancy with no vaginal bleeding or cramping.

Dx The diagnosis is made using history and physical exam, serial β-hCG levels (which are typically low or dropping), and ultrasound.

Tx The therapy can be expectant management, medical therapy with misoprostol, or a dilation and evacuation procedure (D&E). The D&E may be required to achieve the complete removal of all pregnancy-associated tissue. **See Katz 16, Hacker 7.**

Ectopic Pregnancy

Pφ An ectopic pregnancy is a gestation that implants outside the uterus. The most common location is within the fallopian tube. Less commonly, the fertilized ovum may implant on the ovary, in the abdomen, or in the cervix.

TP Typically a patient presents with first-trimester vaginal bleeding and/or abdominal pain. In many instances the abdominal pain can be severe, especially if the ectopic pregnancy has ruptured.

Dx The β-hCG is positive and the transvaginal ultrasound reveals no intrauterine pregnancy. Diagnosis is made by the combination of a positive β-hCG and a transvaginal ultrasound without evidence of an intrauterine pregnancy, combined with physical exam findings. Occasionally either a gestational sac or even an embryo can be visualized in the adnexal region by ultrasound.

Tx Treatment is either surgical or medical. Ectopic pregnancies are managed medically by giving methotrexate (see Practice-Based Learning and Improvement box, Chapter 36, Pelvic Pain). Specific indications for *surgical* therapy include (1) ruptured ectopic pregnancy, especially in a hemodynamically unstable patient; (2) inability/unwillingness to comply with or contraindications to medical therapy; (3) lack of timely access to a medical institution for management of tubal rupture, which can occur during medical therapy; and (4) failed medical therapy. In the absence of these criteria, medical therapy remains an option. **See Katz 17, Hacker 24.**

ZEBRA ZONE

a. **Molar Pregnancy:** A noninvasive, localized tumor of embryonic trophoblastic cells in the uterine cavity. Molar pregnancy should be suspected in a patient with uterine enlargement and a β-hCG level that is dramatically higher than expected. Ultrasound can help confirm the diagnosis. (See Chapter 55, Gestational Trophoblastic Disease.)

Practice-Based Learning and Improvement: Evidence-Based Medicine

Title
Diagnostic accuracy of the ultrasound above and below the β-hCG discriminatory zone

Authors
Barnhart KT, Simhan H, Kamelle SA

Institution
University of Pennsylvania

Reference
Obstetrics and Gynecology 1999;94:583–587

Comparison/control (quality of evidence)
Comparison of accurate diagnosis of intrauterine pregnancy versus ectopic pregnancy versus spontaneous abortion by transvaginal ultrasound in patients with a β-hCG level less than 1500 mIU or greater than 1500 mIU.

Outcome/effect
Transvaginal ultrasound used for diagnosis of intrauterine pregnancy versus ectopic pregnancy versus spontaneous abortion is less accurate when the β-hCG level is below 1500 mIU.

Historical significance
This study was one of the first to synthesize the values of β-hCG levels typically required to evaluate an intrauterine pregnancy with the associated findings provided by ultrasonography.

Interpersonal and Communication Skills

Be Careful about Assumptions; Build on a Patient's Knowledge
It is easy to make assumptions about what patients understand regarding health care delivery—especially in prenatal care. Even if the patient has been pregnant before, ask what she knows about the prenatal visits and care. Assessing the meaning of the pregnancy to the patient and her partner is critical in establishing rapport. Build on your patient's understanding as you explain what will happen over the course of time. Most patients appreciate insight into the purpose and process of subsequent visits. It is helpful to supplement this generic information with written notes such as a clinic-specific leaflet or booklet.

Professionalism

Principle: Commitment to Patient Confidentiality
As with all fields of medicine, in the practice of Ob/Gyn it is of primary importance to respect and maintain your patients' privacy. When a patient presents to you for her first prenatal visit and is accompanied by other individuals, including family or friends, it is prudent and appropriate to ask the patient privately if she feels comfortable discussing her history and undergoing a physical examination with these individuals present. The clinician must offer the patient the opportunity to have the others excuse themselves until the end of the examination. Often the patient may wish to have the ultrasound or Doppler auscultation of fetal heart tones component of the exam completed, then have members of the family return. Of course, every case is different and you must elicit and be sensitive to each patient's wishes.

Systems-Based Practice

Alternative Birthing: Home Birthing, Midwives, and Doulas
For most of human history, births have taken place in the home with the assistance of midwives. It was only during the 20th century that women started delivering in hospitals under the care of physicians. Since the 1970s in the United States, there has been a revival of midwifery coinciding with a nominal move towards so-called natural childbirth—giving birth without unnecessary medical intervention. Today, midwives are health care professionals who specialize in low-risk pregnancies as well as the provision of basic primary care to women. The American College of Nurse-Midwives (ACNM) and the American Midwifery Certification Board (AMCB) have created standards for training and certification that have given significant credibility to the profession, and have played an important role in the medical community's support for the use of midwives in the delivery of care. As a result, today, certified midwives are often found in hospitals and in practice with obstetricians, as well as in health care clinics, and many women choose to have a midwife involved in their delivery either in addition to or instead of an obstetrician. A doula, on the other hand, does not provide medical care. Their role is limited to providing physical and emotional support, as well as advice on making decisions during and after the childbirth process. In 1975, less than 1.0% of births in the United States were attended to by midwives, whereas by 2002 this proportion had risen to 8.1%.

Although the medical community has come to support the use of midwives in the delivery of care, the long-standing official stance of the American College of Obstetricians and Gynecologists (ACOG) has been against home births. The essence of their position on this issue is that although childbirth is a normal physiologic process that most women experience without problems, monitoring of both the woman and the fetus during labor and delivery in a hospital or accredited birthing center is essential because complications can arise with little or no warning even among women with low-risk pregnancies. ACOG acknowledges a woman's right to make informed decisions regarding her delivery and to have a choice in choosing her health care provider, but ACOG does not support programs that advocate for, or individuals who provide, home births.[1]

There have been a handful of studies on the safety of home births, and to date these studies have not demonstrated any increased risks of delivering at home. ACOG, however, believes that these studies are limited and lack scientific rigor. The organization contends that women delivering at home remain unable to access potentially life-saving medical and surgical interventions in the cases where the need arises.

Reference

1. American College of Obstetricians and Gynecologists: Home Births in the United States. ACOG Statement of Policy, ACOG Executive Board, Compendium of Selected Publications. Washington, DC, American College of Obstetricians and Gynecologists, 2007.

Chapter 12
Antenatal Screening and Prenatal Diagnosis for Fetal Genetic Disorders (Case 2)

Greg Margolin MD and Alan E. Donnenfeld MD

Case: A caucasian, 37-year-old G1P0 presents to her obstetrician/gynecologist for her first prenatal visit. She is at 10 weeks' gestation based on her last menstrual period. She is concerned about the risk of a chromosome abnormality in her fetus because she is of "advanced maternal age." She wants to know if her baby is going to have Down syndrome or any other genetic abnormalities. Both she and her husband are of Ashkenazi Jewish ancestry. They state they have no other significant family history of birth defects, genetic disorders, or multiple miscarriages.

Speaking Intelligently

All pregnancies are at some risk to have a congenital abnormality. The risk of birth defects in the general population is 2% to 3%. Certain factors such as maternal age, parental ethnicity, medication use, environmental exposures, family history of genetic disorders, or multiple miscarriages also affect the risk to have a child with a genetic abnormality. A thorough family history should therefore be obtained and information regarding medication and recreational drug exposures should be sought.

PATIENT CARE

Clinical Thinking

- Two general approaches are available to evaluate fetal health: screening tests and diagnostic tests.
- Screening tests determine if a patient is at an increased or a decreased risk to have a fetus with a particular abnormality.
- Diagnostic tests determine if a fetus is actually affected with a certain condition.
- Screening tests are typically risk free and include parental blood tests and prenatal ultrasonography.
- Diagnostic tests, such as amniocentesis and chorionic villus sampling (CVS), are typically invasive procedures and are associated with a small risk of pregnancy loss.
- Criteria for a useful prenatal genetic screening test are the following:
  - The test leads to the identification of a clinically significant disorder that is associated with morbidity or mortality.
  - The test is cost-effective and simple to perform.
  - The test is highly sensitive and highly specific.
  - The test is risk free or extremely low risk.
  - The test is associated with a low false-positive rate.
  - The test is reliable and reproducible.
  - Women with a positive screen (increased risk) can pursue a diagnostic test for definitive information.
  - An effective treatment or intervention can be instituted if a disorder is diagnosed. This can include consideration of pregnancy termination if, after genetic counseling, the patient elects this option.

History and Examination
- Obtaining a thorough family and genetic history is imperative.
- Often, a questionnaire is used that addresses key concerns such as maternal age, ethnicity of both parents, past obstetric history of the parents, and information on relatives with birth defects, multiple miscarriages, mental retardation, or genetic disorders.
- It is recommended that the father of the child be present when discussion of all pertinent information occurs. If complex issues or concerns arise, referral to a genetic counselor can be made.
- Invasive diagnostic testing via CVS or amniocentesis should be offered when appropriate. Screening for Down syndrome, trisomy 18, and neural tube defects should also be offered regardless of maternal age. CVS is a first-trimester procedure that involves taking a small sample of chorionic villi from the developing placenta for chromosome analysis. Amniocentesis is performed in the second trimester. Fetal epithelial cells floating in the amniotic fluid are retrieved and cultured, then analyzed for their chromosome complement.

Tests for Consideration
- **Screening:**
  - Maternal age — Free
  - Sequential screen — $175
  - Integrated screen — $165
  - Second-trimester screen — $86
  - Maternal serum alpha-fetoprotein — $48
  - Nuchal translucency ultrasonography — $225
- **Diagnostic:**
  - Amniocentesis — $432
  - CVS — $556
  - Ultrasonography — $225

Medical Knowledge

Screening Tests
Maternal Age: Historically, the first screening test devised to address the risk of a fetal chromosome abnormality was a simple question: How old will you be at delivery? If the response was 35 years of age or older, the patient would be considered screen positive because her risk of Down syndrome was greater than 1/270. She would therefore be offered a diagnostic test such as CVS or amniocentesis. However, screening based on maternal age detects only approximately 20% to 30% of all Down syndrome pregnancies. It is a poor screening test. A paradigm shift has emerged over the last few years that screening should no longer be based on maternal age alone, but should be

based on fetal risk. This risk is best determined by multiple parameters, such as maternal age, first-trimester sonographic evaluation of fetal nuchal translucency (see later), and both first- and second-trimester maternal serum testing.

Sequential and Integrated Screening: The American College of Obstetricians and Gynecologists has recommended that the ideal approach to screen for Down syndrome in patients who present in the first trimester involves evaluation of both first- and second-trimester parameters. This can be accomplished with either the sequential or integrated screening tests. Both incorporate maternal age, first-trimester sonographic evaluation of the fetal nuchal translucency (see later), first-trimester pregnancy-associated plasma protein A (PAPP-A), and second-trimester maternal serum alpha-fetoprotein (AFP), unconjugated estriol (uE3), human chorionic gonadotropin (hCG), and inhibin A. The difference between sequential and integrated screening is that with **sequential screening,** a preliminary risk is provided after analysis of the first-trimester parameters and a revised risk is provided (incorporating all seven variables) after all testing has been completed. With **integrated screening,** a first-trimester risk evaluation is not determined by the laboratory and therefore the patient does not receive a first-trimester risk analysis. Instead, information from the first trimester is held by the laboratory until all analytes are evaluated. Then, a single overall risk is provided in the second trimester. Both sequential (once completed) and integrated screening address risk to the fetus for Down syndrome, trisomy 18, and neural tube defects (NTDs). Critics of integrated screening assert that the laboratory is "withholding" first-trimester information. Proponents believe that the laboratory is simply "holding" the information until the single, most reliable overall risk can be determined, thus eliminating potentially conflicting first-trimester preliminary results followed by final second-trimester results that incorporate all variables. The first-trimester portion of the sequential screen detects 70% of all Down syndrome fetuses with a 1.2% FPR. The final risk assessment, which incorporates both the first- and second-trimester parameters, detects an additional 20% of Down syndrome pregnancies and increases the FPR by 2.5%. Overall, sequential screening detects 90% of Down syndrome pregnancies with a total FPR of 3.7%. The integrated screen detects 92% of Down syndrome pregnancies with a 5% FPR. When performing sequential screening, it is crucial that the second-trimester data be combined with the first-trimester information before determining Down syndrome risk. An approach that involves performing a first-trimester assessment followed by a separate second-trimester risk evaluation is known as **independent sequential screening.** This approach to aneuploidy screening is not recommended because the results of the two tests are not integrated; information from the first trimester is not included in the second-trimester analysis. Essentially, two successive and separate screening tests are performed instead of the recommended approach of following a screening test with a diagnostic test. Independent sequential screening leads to a very high Down syndrome detection rate (97%) but also yields a prohibitively high FPR of 19%.

Second-Trimester Screen: For patients who present after 14 weeks' gestation, second-trimester screening is the recommended Down syndrome, trisomy 18, and NTD screening option. Analysis of fetal risk is based on maternal age, AFP, uE3, hCG, and inhibin-A. Second-trimester screening using this quadruple-analyte screen enables detection of approximately 75% of Down syndrome pregnancies with an FPR of 5%.

Nuchal Translucency (NT): NT is defined as the subcutaneous fluid collection located at the back of the fetal neck identified on ultrasonography between 11 weeks and 13 weeks, 6 days of gestation. This fluid accumulation is thought to be excess lymphatic fluid or an early sign of congestive heart failure in a fetus with a congenital heart defect. The greater the NT size, the higher the risk of Down syndrome and trisomy 18. Measurements greater than 2.5 to 3.0 mm are considered elevated. Determining the risk of aneuploidy based on NT measurement alone is not recommended because the Down syndrome detection rate is inferior to that of both sequential and integrated screening. However, when the NT exceeds 2.5 to 3.0 mm, the risk of Down syndrome is unlikely to become screen negative once biochemical screening has subsequently been completed. Therefore, patients with NTs that exceed 2.5 to 3.0 mm should be offered invasive testing (CVS and amniocentesis) based on NT size alone. Using NT with first-trimester biochemical screening (called the *first-trimester combined test*) is a suboptimal screening approach compared with either sequential or integrated screening because the Down syndrome detection rate is approximately 83% and this test does not screen for NTDs.

Maternal Serum Alpha-Fetoprotein (MSAFP): This second-trimester maternal serum screening test is useful in determining the risk of fetal NTDs. An increase in circulating MSAFP is correlated with an elevated risk. The testing is optimally performed between 16 and 20 weeks' gestation. At a cutoff of 2 to 2.5 multiples of the median (MoM), the detection rate for anencephaly is approximately 95% and for open spina bifida, approximately 80%. The FPR is 2%. Some patients may decline screening for chromosome anomalies but wish to determine their risk for having a child with spina bifida. These patients may elect MSAFP screening as an isolated test. Because MSAFP is a component of the sequential, integrated, and second-trimester biochemical testing strategies, an assessment of NTD risk is provided for all patients electing any of these screening tests.

Ultrasonography: Ultrasonography is useful as a screening test for certain fetal anomalies, specifically chromosome abnormalities. In the first trimester, NT is the most useful parameter for trisomies 18 and 21 screening. In the second trimester, many sonographic findings are known to be associated with an increased risk of aneuploidy. These include excess nuchal skin fold thickness, short femur and humerus lengths, pyelectasis, an echogenic focus in the left ventricle of the heart, cardiac defects, echogenic bowel, ventriculomegaly of the brain, other two-vessel umbilical cord, hydramnios, choroid plexus cysts, a wide space between the first and second toes (sandal gap), and bowel atresia. In some situations, ultrasound can be a diagnostic test. An example is the sonographic detection of a neural tube or ventral wall defect.

Diagnostic Tests

Amniocentesis: Amniocentesis is an ultrasonographically guided procedure involving the transabdominal aspiration of a small amount of amniotic fluid. For the purpose of genetic diagnosis it is usually performed between 15 and 18 weeks' gestation. Amniocentesis before 15 weeks is not recommended because it is associated with an increased rate of postprocedure fetal loss and deformation (clubfoot). Amniotic fluid contains cells from fetal skin, respiratory tract, urinary tract, gastrointestinal tract, and placenta; this fluid is sent for cell culture and subsequent karyotyping. In experienced hands, mid-trimester amniocentesis is associated with an approximate 1/300 risk of pregnancy loss.

Chorionic Villus Sampling: This prenatal diagnosis procedure is performed between 10 and 13 weeks' gestation. Two approaches can be used. The transabdominal approach is similar to amniocentesis. Using sonographic guidance, a thin needle is passed into the developing placenta and chorionic villi are aspirated into a 20-mL syringe containing culture medium. The transcervical approach involves the introduction of a small catheter into the vagina and through the cervix. Ultrasonography is used to help guide the catheter into the placenta and a small amount of placental tissue is aspirated for culturing and subsequent karyotyping. CVS carries an approximate 1% risk of fetal loss. CVS should not be performed before 10 weeks' gestation because it may be associated with an increased risk of fetal limb reduction defects at this early gestational age.

Clinical Entities   **Medical Knowledge**

Down Syndrome

Pφ Down syndrome is caused by an extra copy of chromosome 21. Ninety-six percent of cases involve trisomy 21 (three separate chromosome 21s) as a result of nondisjunction during oogenesis (most commonly) or spermatogenesis (rarely). Two percent of cases arise from chromosome translocations and 2% involve mosaicism (a mixture of normal and Down syndrome cells).

TP Affected individuals have mental retardation (average IQ 40), poor coordination, short stature, distinct physical characteristics including upslanting palpebral fissures, a protruding tongue, epicanthal folds, simian creases in the hands, hypotonia, excess skin at the posterior nape of the neck, and prominent cheeks, a 40% risk of congenital heart defects, an increased risk of duodenal atresia, Hirschsprung's disease, leukemia, and premature development of Alzheimer's disease. Average life expectancy is 50 to 70 years.

Dx Although screening tests can identify patients at increased risk of carrying a fetus with Down syndrome, a reliable diagnosis requires chromosome analysis. Prenatally, this can be achieved through CVS or amniocentesis. Postnatally, peripheral blood chromosome analysis is available.

Tx No treatment to correct the mental retardation associated with Down syndrome is available. If the prenatal diagnosis is made before 24 weeks, the couple has the option to terminate the pregnancy. After birth, therapy is based on the congenital anomalies that are present. For example, some infants may require cardiac surgery to correct congenital heart defects. See **Gabbe 6, Hacker 7.**

Trisomy 18

Pφ Trisomy 18 is caused by an extra copy of chromosome 18.

TP Affected individuals have severe and profound mental retardation. Congenital anomalies include heart defects, choroid plexus cysts, a two-vessel umbilical cord, fetal growth restriction, diaphragmatic hernia, ventral wall defects, NTDs, and skeletal anomalies such as radial aplasia. Fifty percent of affected infants die by 1 week of age and 90% die within 5 months of birth. Approximately 5% survive their first year. Long-term survival is unusual.

Dx Although screening tests can identify patients at increased risk of carrying a fetus with trisomy 18 (80% to 90% detection rate), a reliable diagnosis requires chromosome analysis. Prenatally, this can be achieved through CVS or amniocentesis. Postnatally, peripheral blood chromosome analysis is available.

Tx No treatment to correct the mental retardation associated with trisomy 18 is available. Correction of congenital anomalies such as brain, cardiac, skeletal, and other defects, although possible, is not recommended given the dismal prognosis for survival. If the prenatal diagnosis of trisomy 18 is made before 24 weeks, the couple has an option to terminate an affected pregnancy. After birth, therapy is based on providing comfort and supportive care. Support groups to provide assistance to parents caring for a child with trisomy 18 are available. See **Gabbe 6, Hacker 7.**

Neural Tube Defects

Pφ NTDs are caused by failure of closure of the neural tube between the third and fourth weeks after conception. This birth defect occurs in 1 to 2 per 1000 pregnancies. A defect at the cranial end leads to anencephaly. Failure of closure at the inferior end of the spinal canal results in spina bifida. Eighty percent are open defects in which neural tissue is exposed; 20% are classified as closed (skin-covered) defects.

TP MSAFP screening leads to the detection of 80% of open NTDs. The diagnosis of an NTD can be made with either ultrasonography or amniocentesis. Risk factors for this multifactorial disorder include low socioeconomic status, Irish ancestry, poor nutritional intake, and vitamin deficiency.

Dx Prenatal ultrasonography is highly sensitive and specific in the detection of NTDs. For anencephaly, absence of the calvarium and a prominent supraorbital ridge are evident. For spina bifida, ultrasonography typically reveals a smaller-than-expected head diameter as well as ventriculomegaly of the brain, an abnormal shape to the skull (lemon sign), and an anterior curvature of the cerebellum (banana sign). These signs are all due to brain stem herniation (Arnold-Chiari malformation). The spinal defect can be visualized on transverse and sagittal imaging of the fetal spine.

Tx Treatment is primarily focused on the prevention of NTDs by adequate supplementation with folic acid. All women who consider embarking on a pregnancy should take 1 mg of folic acid daily at least 3 months before planning conception. Those with a family history of NTDs should be supplemented with 4 mg of folic acid per day. Folic acid supplementation is expected to reduce the frequency of NTDs by 75%. If, however, a fetus is diagnosed with an NTD, the option of pregnancy termination is available. Anencephaly is uniformly fatal. There is significant morbidity associated with spina bifida but the prognosis depends on the size of the defect and its location (the most inferior defects have the best prognosis). Problems may include lower extremity paralysis, bowel and bladder dysfunction, mental retardation, and cerebral palsy. Experimental fetal surgery to correct the defect during pregnancy is offered in a few select programs. It is unclear if fetal surgery improves prognosis because prospective, randomized studies on the efficacy of fetal surgery to correct spina bifida have not yet been completed. See **Gabbe 9, Hacker 7.**

Genetic Diseases in the Ashkenazi Jewish Population

Pφ Several autosomal recessive genetic diseases are more common in the Ashkenazi Jewish population than other ethnic groups. Some of these disorders are severe and untreatable and are associated with death during childhood (e.g., Tay-Sachs disease, Canavan's disease, Niemann-Pick disease type A). Others result in significant morbidity but are not always fatal during childhood (e.g., cystic fibrosis, Bloom's syndrome, familial dysautonomia, Fanconi anemia type C, Gaucher's disease, mucolipidosis IV) and some are treatable with dietary restriction (e.g., glycogen storage disease type 1a, maple syrup urine disease).

TP Any expectant couple in which one partner has any Jewish ancestry should be offered carrier screening for these disorders. A fetus can be affected only if both parents are carriers of a mutation for the same disorder. Unfortunately, carrier detection is not 100% accurate because not all carriers have an identifiable mutation.

Dx The diagnosis of an affected fetus or infant is based on DNA analysis or enzyme assay from a CVS or amniocentesis. Invasive prenatal diagnosis should be offered only if both parents are known carriers or if one parent is a carrier and the other is not available for testing.

Tx There are no fetal treatments available for any of these disorders. After birth, some disorders are treatable or controllable with pharmacologic therapy (e.g., Gaucher's disease, familial dysautonomia) or with dietary restriction (e.g., glycogen storage disease type 1a, maple syrup urine disease). Some disorders are untreatable and lethal (e.g., Tay-Sachs disease, Canavan's disease). The option of pregnancy termination should be discussed after the prenatal diagnosis of one of these disorders. Preimplantation genetic diagnosis with transfer of unaffected embryos is an option for couples at risk for one of these disorders. See **Gabbe 6 and 7, Hacker 7.**

ZEBRA ZONE

a. **Congenital Finnish nephrosis:** The prenatal screening process occasionally identifies pregnancies with particular analyte levels that indicate an increased risk of certain rare genetic disorders. One example is a lethal renal disorder, which is associated with an extremely high level of Maternal Serum-AFP.

b. **Smith-Lemli-Opitz syndrome:** A multiple congenital anomaly syndrome associated with a cholesterol synthesis enzyme defect. This disorder presents with undetectable estriol levels.

c. **Inaccurate gestational dating:** Some analyte patterns may initially be interpreted as revealing an increased risk of aneuploidy or NTD. However, after ultrasonography, incorrect gestational age or multiple gestation may be identified and indicate a negative screening test once the test is reinterpreted using proper information.

Practice-Based Learning and Improvement: Evidence-Based Medicine

Title
First-trimester or second-trimester screening, or both, for Down syndrome. First- and Second-Trimester Evaluation of Risk (FASTER) Research Consortium

Authors
Malone F, Canick JA, Ball RH, et al.

Institution
FASTER Research Consortium

Reference
New England Journal of Medicine 2005;353:2001–2011

Problem
To determine the optimal Down syndrome screening strategy.

Intervention
Prenatal screening for Down syndrome, trisomy 18, and neural tube defects.

Comparison/control (quality of evidence)
Prospective, multicenter, interventional analysis.

Outcome/effect
Detection and false-positive rates for all permutations of prenatal screening for aneuploidy, including first-trimester combined screening, second-trimester screening, and integrated screening, were determined.

Historical significance/comments
This study, involving over 33,000 patients, concluded that the optimal approach to prenatal screening for Down syndrome, trisomy 18, and neural tube defects uses a strategy that includes both first- and second-trimester parameters (integrated or sequential screening).

Interpersonal and Communication Skills

The Importance of Understanding a Test before Having It
Communicating the results of screening tests is different from discussing the results of diagnostic tests. This is a subtlety that requires clear explanation to patients. Commonly, expectant parents assume that a positive screening test indicates that their fetus has a congenital anomaly. This is incorrect. A positive screening test simply means the parents are at an increased risk of having a child with a particular disorder and that further diagnostic testing, such as CVS or amniocentesis, is indicated. For example, when first introducing the

concept of a screening test for Down syndrome to patients, it is crucial to explain clearly the concept of screening. Should a Down syndrome screen reveal an increased risk (e.g., a 1/100 risk), *parents should be counseled that there is still a 99% probability that their fetus does **not** have Down syndrome*. They should also be informed that to determine the chromosomal status of the pregnancy, a diagnostic test such as CVS or amniocentesis is necessary. Only after genetic counseling to discuss the risks and potential benefits of invasive testing can parents make an informed decision as to whether they wish to pursue such testing.

The key interpersonal skills to successfully communicating in this setting are patience, clarity, and willingness to repeat the important concepts. You should demonstrate to your patient that you understand that these can be difficult, complicated conversations.

Professionalism

Principle: Patient Autonomy

As medical professionals, it is our obligation to provide information to patients that will allow them to make informed decisions and to be supportive of the decisions they have made. We must, for example, discuss the option of prenatal screening for genetic disorders such as Down syndrome, trisomy 18, and NTDs with all patients. Many patients, based on religious and personal perspectives, will decline such screening tests; they do not want to know if they are at increased risk to deliver a fetus with a genetic disorder because they would never consider pregnancy termination. Knowing that they are at increased risk would only heighten their anxiety. Such a decision should be supported. Prenatal screening for genetic disorders is optional and it is a patient's prerogative to either accept or decline such testing.

When a fetus is diagnosed with a congenital anomaly such as spina bifida, genetic counseling regarding the prognosis and management of infants with this condition should be addressed. Only after the parents are fully educated regarding the significance of this abnormality should the option of pregnancy termination be raised. Given the unpredictable prognosis and the advances in medical care, many parents will elect to continue their pregnancy. Some patients who would never consider pregnancy termination may choose to pursue prenatal screening for fetal disorders for the following reasons: (1) prenatal diagnosis most often confirms the fetus to be *un*affected with a particular disorder, providing relief and reassurance; (2) if the fetus is found to be affected, parents have time to adjust to having a child with special needs; and (3) subsequent medical involvement may be altered based on the prenatal diagnosis. For instance, parents may elect to avoid a cesarean section for *fetal* indications if an infant has a known lethal condition such as anencephaly.

The clinician must be prepared for some parents changing their minds and electing to terminate an affected pregnancy once they understand the implications of a disorder and are confronted with the reality that their fetus is affected. The autonomy of the patient-couple must be supported at each step of this process.

Systems-Based Practice

Using Genetic Counseling Services

For women considering invasive prenatal diagnosis or for those with a significant family history of a genetic disorder, referral to a **genetic counselor** is indicated. Board-certified genetic counselors are Master's-level genetic professionals. They are specially trained to obtain a thorough, three-generation pedigree, interpret the family history to determine risks to the fetus, and provide an analysis of these risks. Genetic counselors communicate the benefits and limitations of screening and prenatal diagnosis and are a superb resource for physicians to help address patient concerns regarding the genetic health of their fetus. When discussing screening tests, genetic counselors address detection rates (percentage of all pregnancies with a particular disorder that are detected with the screening test) and the false-positive rate (FPR) of tests. The FPR is defined as the percentage of patients who undergo screening and are informed they are at an increased risk even though they are carrying an unaffected fetus. During a genetic counseling consultation, patients are provided with a risk assessment of chromosome abnormalities and informed about available screening and diagnostic tests that are appropriate to consider. It is recommended that all expectant couples be offered the option of both screening and diagnostic testing for fetal chromosome abnormalities.

Chapter 13
Antenatal Fetal Surveillance (Case 3)

Vonetta Sylvestre MD and Garo Megerian MD

Case: A 35-year-old G3P1011 with a singleton intrauterine pregnancy at 30 5/7 weeks presents to the High-Risk Obstetrics Clinic for a prenatal visit. Her pregnancy is complicated by chronic hypertension, for which she takes alpha methyldopa. Prior ultrasonography has revealed intrauterine growth restriction (IUGR) with an estimated fetal weight less than the 10th percentile. Measurement of her uterine fundal height reveals that she measures smaller than estimated gestational age. Today, her blood pressure is 120/78. Fetal heart tones are in the 140s as measured by Doppler. During her exam, she asks whether she will need any special tests as her pregnancy progresses. What conditions require fetal surveillance and what tests are available to the clinician to evaluate fetal well-being?

Common Indications for Antenatal Testing: A Condensed Differential Diagnosis

Hypertension: chronic or gestational		Intrauterine growth restriction (IUGR)		Post-term pregnancy
Type 1 diabetes mellitus	Oligohydramnios		Preeclampsia	Decreased fetal movement

Speaking Intelligently

Every pregnant patient needs to be evaluated in the context of her underlying medical problems or conditions. We often call this the "problem list." If any of these problems are known to increase the risk for intrauterine fetal morbidity or mortality, the patient is a candidate to undergo **antenatal fetal surveillance.** The purpose of this testing is to identify a fetus that displays problematic physiologic changes so that intervention can be initiated before the onset of fetal compromise. Once identified, the fetus can be delivered promptly, before the occurrence of intrauterine hypoxia or cellular injury. There are multiple published algorithms and protocols that address when to start surveillance tests and how frequently to perform them. Unfortunately, fetal death may sometimes occur in women with no identifiable underlying risk factors. It is important to note that there are many maternal and fetal conditions that do not lend themselves specifically to a rigorous surveillance protocol.

PATIENT CARE

Clinical Thinking
- The initial evaluation of a patient who may require antenatal surveillance involves identifying those risk factors that increase the chance of intrauterine fetal compromise.
- Fetal testing is implemented for patients who are deemed to be at risk and permits intervention before the occurrence of fetal injury.

History
- The initial approach to a patient who presents for antenatal testing is to determine which factors put her at increased risk for fetal compromise.
- Review the family history of the patient.
- Review the obstetric history to determine the progression of the pregnancy and how the coexisting medical conditions have been managed to date.
- Screen the patient for complications that may have resulted from long-standing medical problems, such as diabetes or hypertension.

Physical Examination
- **Vital signs:** Pay special attention to blood pressure measurements. Pregnancy usually reduces maternal blood pressure. Therefore, elevated pressures are especially worrisome.
- **Uterine fundal height:** Fundal height is measured in centimeters and generally corresponds to gestational age between 20 and 34 weeks. Measure the distance between the symphysis pubis and the uppermost part of the uterine fundus. Fundal height measurements can be influenced by maternal body habitus and bladder filling.
- **Urine dipstick:** (Technically a "lab" test, but done as part of the physical examination at a routine obstetrics visit in the office setting.) Assesses the presence of proteinuria (an indicator of possible evolving preeclampsia).

Tests for Consideration
- **Nonstress test (NST):** Assesses uteroplacental function by the presence of accelerations of fetal heart rate associated with fetal movement. A nonstress test is considered **reactive** if, within a 20-minute period, there are 2 accelerations of at least 15 beats per minute (BPM) above the established baseline lasting at least 15 seconds in a fetus greater than 32 weeks' gestation, or 10 BPM above baseline lasting at least 10 seconds in a fetus less than 32 weeks' gestation. $50
- **Contraction stress test (CST):** Assesses utero-placental function by measuring the fetal response to induced or spontaneous contractions. A positive CST occurs when late decelerations occur with more than half of the contractions in a ten-minute time window. $250
- **Biophysical profile (BPP):** Assesses fetal well-being using five biophysical components, four findings determined by ultrasonography in combination with a fetal heart rate nonstress test. Normal measurements are scored as 2 points and abnormal measurements are scored as zero points. $250
  - Scoring criteria:
    Reactive NST = 2 points.
    Fetal breathing: One episode of rhythmic breathing lasting 30 seconds or greater in 30 minutes = 2 points.
    Fetal movement: Three or more discrete body movements in 30 minutes = 2 points.
    Fetal tone: One or more flexion and extension motions of a fetal extremity or opening and closing of a hand in 30 minutes = 2 points.
    Amniotic fluid index (AFI): A single vertical pocket measuring at least 2 cm, or a sum total of 5 cm measured in each of the four quadrants (right lower quadrant, right upper quadrant, left lower quadrant, and left upper quadrant) = 2 points.
  - Intervention based on scoring:
    A score of 8 or 10 on BPP is accepted as reassuring and monitoring is repeated only if there is a clinician indication.
    A score of 6 warrants repeat testing in 24 hours if the fetus is preterm or delivery if the fetus is term.
    A score of 4 or less warrants delivery.
- **Modified biophysical profile:** A modified BPP consists of an NST and AFI. $225
- **Umbilical artery Doppler velocimetry:** Assesses umbilical artery blood flow by measuring vascular impedance. Umbilical artery Doppler flow velocimetry

is a particularly useful tool in cases of intrauterine growth restriction. The systolic-to-diastolic ratio is abnormal when it is greater than the 95th percentile for gestational age or if diastolic flow is either absent or reversed. $375

Antenatal Testing Algorithm

- **Nonstress test (NST)** is readily available and is generally considered a first-line test.
- **Biophysical profile (BPP)** can be done as a follow-up if the NST is not reactive.
- **Contraction stress tests (CSTs)** have to some degree been replaced with the BPP, but there are certain instances when the CST can be of great value. The CST is still considered one of the gold standard tests of fetal well-being.
- **Umbilical Doppler velocimetry** is useful in cases of IUGR.

Clinical Entities	Medical Knowledge

Hypertension: Chronic or Gestational

Pφ Essential, or chronic, hypertension occurs when the patient's blood pressure elevation antedates the pregnancy. Its pathogenesis is thought to be due to alterations in the renin-angiotensin system. Rare secondary causes include renal artery stenosis or hyperaldosteronism. On occasion, a normotensive patient can develop hypertension without proteinuria during the pregnancy. This is called *gestational hypertension*. (See Chapter 21 for a more comprehensive discussion of hypertension in pregnancy.)

TP Patients are usually asymptomatic and are diagnosed by blood pressure determination.

Dx Diagnosis is based on three sequential blood pressure readings greater than 140/90. In pregnant patients, any hypertension occurring before 20 weeks' gestational age is considered chronic hypertension.

Tx Chronic hypertension is managed with judicial use of medication and antenatal surveillance. Patients are followed closely to diagnose the development of superimposed preeclampsia. Antenatal surveillance is essential to monitor fetal well-being. **See Gabbe 33, Hacker 14.**

Type 1 Diabetes Mellitus

Pφ Type 1 diabetes mellitus (DM) is due to insulin deficiency secondary to destruction of pancreatic beta cells. (See Chapter 22 for a more comprehensive discussion of diabetes in pregnancy.)

TP Diabetic ketoacidosis commonly occurs and is often the initial presentation of patients with type 1 DM.

Dx Virtually all patients with type 1 DM already carry this diagnosis when they present for prenatal care. Pediatricians generally use a fasting glucose level of greater than 126 as the threshold for diagnosis. The child is then usually referred to a pediatric endocrinologist for further care.

Tx Tight glycemic control with insulin and diet modification is the cornerstone of treatment. Periodic glycohemoglobin testing measures the average blood sugar over the previous 4 to 6 weeks. As the physiologic changes of pregnancy progressively antagonize insulin effectiveness, increased insulin requirements can be anticipated throughout the gestation. **See Gabbe 37, Hacker 16.**

Preeclampsia

Pφ Preeclampsia is a disorder of the arterial vascular endothelium that results in increased vascular constriction. It is characterized by the onset of hypertension and proteinuria during the second half of the gestation. (See Chapter 21 for a more comprehensive discussion of hypertensive disorders in pregnancy.)

TP Patients may present with complaints of headache, blurry vision, or epigastric pain. However, often a patient is asymptomatic on presentation and the clinician makes the diagnosis on screening during a routine prenatal visit.

Dx Diagnosis is made by assessment of vital signs and a 24-hour urine collection for proteinuria. Mild preeclampsia occurs when blood pressure is greater than 140/90 with greater than 300 mg of proteinuria/24 hours. Severe preeclampsia is characterized by blood pressure greater than 160/110 or greater than 5 g of proteinuria/24 hours. HELLP syndrome is a particularly malignant form of severe preeclampsia characterized by **H**emolysis, **E**levated **L**iver Enzymes, and **L**ow **P**latelets.

Tx Treatment of mild preeclampsia depends on gestational age. If a patient is near term, delivery is indicated. Before term, stable patients can be placed on bed rest and followed with repeat laboratory studies and antenatal testing. Delivery is indicated in cases of severe preeclampsia or HELLP syndrome. **See Gabbe 33, Hacker 14.**

Post-term Pregnancy

Pφ Post-term pregnancy refers to pregnancies that extend beyond 42 weeks of gestation. Risk factors include primiparity, male sex, anencephaly, history of prior post-term pregnancy, and genetic predisposition.

TP As the placenta ages beyond 42 weeks, gradual deterioration of fetal perfusion occurs, leading to an increased risk of intrauterine hypoxia and stillbirth. Antenatal surveillance assesses current fetoplacental integrity.

Dx Accurate assessment of gestational age is an important aspect of prenatal care.

Tx Because of the risks associated with post-term pregnancies, a patient should not be allowed to go beyond 42 weeks' gestation. The choice of method of induction is primarily determined by the patient's Bishop score (assess cervical ripeness for induction). If there are signs of fetal compromise or uteroplacental insufficiency, such as nonreassuring antenatal testing results or oligohydramnios, immediate delivery is indicated. **See Gabbe 11, Hacker 12.**

Oligohydramnios

Pφ Oligohydramnios (decreased amniotic fluid) is most often a result of decreased fetal urine production secondary to decreased uteroplacental perfusion. There are several other conditions that can lead to oligohydramnios, including premature preterm rupture of membranes (PPROM), renal hypoplasia (Potter's syndrome), and urinary tract outlet obstruction.

TP A common presentation occurs when the patient presents for a routine prenatal visit and is noted to have a fundal height that measures significantly less than her gestational age.

Dx Oligohydramnios is diagnosed by assessment of the AFI. An AFI of less than 5 is considered diagnostic of oligohydramnios.

Tx If the patient is near term, delivery is indicated. Before term, the patient is followed with ultrasonography to assess AFI, and NSTs. If oligohydramnios occurs in association with IUGR, this is a particularly ominous situation requiring intervention. **See Gabbe 31.**

Intrauterine Growth Restriction

Pφ Lagging fetal growth (<10th percentile for gestational age) can result from a variety of different maternal, placental, or fetal abnormalities. The most common causes of IUGR include placental insufficiency, poor maternal nutrition, cigarette smoking, and congenital fetal viral infection.

TP A uterine fundal height measurement 2 or more cm **less than** gestational weeks by dates is an indication for a sonographic examination of fetal weight.

Dx Confirmation of IUGR is determined by measurement of fetal head circumference, abdominal circumference, and femur length. Estimated fetal weight (EFW) found to be less than the 10th percentile for gestational age on ultrasonography requires careful additional follow-up, or intervention.

Tx Full-term pregnancies should be delivered, either with induction of labor or cesarean section. Fetuses remote from delivery should be followed with aggressive surveillance and delivered when a reasonable gestational age is reached, or if surveillance becomes nonreassuring. **See Gabbe 29, Hacker 12.**

Decreased Fetal Movement

Pφ A diminution of fetal movement as perceived by the mother, usually as a result of placental insufficiency or cord compression.

TP The mother perceives the fetus moving less frequently than previously, or less than what she would consider normal. Ten fetal movements in a 2-hour time period is a common baseline determination of normal fetal activity.

Dx Decreased fetal movement can be indicative of fetal compromise. However, a common cause of decreased movement is fetal sleep. Antepartum surveillance will help distinguish true fetal jeopardy from physiologic fetal sleep patterns.

Tx There are many false alarms with this subjective complaint. A reassuring NST or BPP is usually sufficient to rule out fetal compromise.

ZEBRA ZONE

Uncommon indications for antenatal testing include the following:

a. **Antiphospholipid syndrome:** an autoantibody-associated syndrome which predisposes the pregnant patient to hypercoagulability and fetal loss as a consequence of placental insufficiency.

b. **Poorly controlled hyperthyroidism:** uncontrolled hyperthyroidism during pregnancy is associated with gestational hypertension, congestive heart failure, preterm delivery, and placental abruption.

c. **Hemoglobinopathies:** abnormalities of maternal hemoglobin synthesis, particularly sickle cell disease, increase the likelihood of stillbirth.

d. **Systemic lupus erythematosus:** predisposes a patient to increased risk of preeclampsia, intrauterine growth restriction, preterm birth, congenital fetal heart block, pregnancy loss, and stillbirth.

e. **Isoimmunization:** Rh isoimmunization can result in significant fetal anemia; merits close evaluation, including, at times, consideration of intrauterine blood transfusion.

f. **Prior fetal demise:** Up to 50% of intrauterine fetal deaths will be unexplained. Patients who have had a prior stillbirth, whether unexplained or not, should be followed carefully during the third trimester.

g. **Multiple gestations:** Twin and higher order multiple pregnancies are much more likely to result in preterm delivery and non-concordant fetal growth.

Practice-Based Learning and Improvement: Evidence-Based Medicine

Title

Fetal pulse oximetry and cesarean delivery

Authors

Bloom SL, Spong CY, Thom E, Varner MW, Rouse DJ, Weininger S, Ramin SM, Caritis SN, Peaceman A, Sorokin Y, Sciscione A, Carpenter M, Mercer B, Thorp J, Malone F, Harper M, Iams J, Anderson G; National Institute of Child Health and Human Development Maternal-Fetal Medicine Units Network

Institution

University of Texas Southwestern Medical Center

Reference
New England Journal of Medicine 2006;355:2195–2202

Problem
Does knowledge of fetal pulse oximetry affect the rate of cesarean section?

Intervention
Placement of fetal pulse oximeter during labor with results either known to the attendant versus withheld during the course of labor. In theory, the measurement of fetal oxygen status in labor would give a more accurate assessment of fetal well-being than heart rate monitoring alone.

Comparison/control (quality of evidence)
Multicenter, randomized clinical trial (level I).

Outcome/effect
No significant difference was noted in the rates of cesarean section between the groups that did or did receive fetal pulse oximetry monitoring. Fetal pulse oximetry monitoring did not lower the cesarean section rate in the monitored group.

Historical significance/comments
This study was the first large-scale trial examining whether fetal pulse oximetry would improve outcomes or lower cesarean section rates. This was the first time that a method of antenatal testing was subjected to rigorous study before its implementation.

Interpersonal and Communication Skills

Setting Expectations: Explaining the Importance of Tests
It is important to explain the reasons for tests during pregnancy. A thorough explanation reduces patient anxiety, establishes appropriate expectations, and focuses the responsibility for the patient's participation in her own care. Consider, for example, the following two versions of explaining the NST, perhaps the most common test for fetal well-being:

- "I would like you to have an NST weekly because your baby is measuring a bit smaller than we expect, and I am worried that the baby may be at risk for a stillbirth."
- "I think we should start with some more vigilant prenatal surveillance testing. When I measure the size of your abdomen it seems that the baby is measuring a bit smaller than I would expect, and sometimes this can be a problem. Usually, when babies measure on the 'smaller side,' this simply means that it is a small baby ... nothing more. On the other hand, sometimes when a fetus is smaller than expected it can be a sign that the placenta

is beginning to lose its ability to function well and to provide oxygen and nutrients to the baby. A nonstress test is an easy and safe way to ensure that the baby's heart rate is not showing signs of stress ... it will almost always be normal, but if it is not, then we can know right then and there that something needs to be done."

Both explanations make the same point: it is important to follow this patient's fetus closely in the hopes of diminishing the possibility of stillbirth. The second explanation, however, seems preferable. It lets the patient know that while there may be a potential cause for concern, you are aware of it and you are being proactive.

Professionalism

Principle: Commitment to Maintaining Appropriate Relations with Patients

The practice of medicine is truly unique in many ways. One of the most interesting aspects of medicine, and Obstetrics and Gynecology in particular, is the level of access you are permitted into your patients' personal lives. As you care for patients over time, you will become familiar with their medical concerns, and you will also come to know them as individuals. Your patients may comment on, or ask for your opinion regarding topics ranging from child-rearing to marital infidelity. The scope of each patient's personal concerns is indeed vast. It is extremely important that you always maintain the most appropriate professional decorum possible. It can be tempting, sometimes, when patients "open up" to such a degree, to respond in kind. This is not always the best course of action. Instead, keep in mind the principle of maintaining appropriate relations with patients. The doctor–patient relationship is indeed very privileged, and you must be careful always to keep the patient's best interest at heart. Always act with the highest standard of professionalism and pride in your work.

Systems-Based Practice

Ordering Tests Appropriately

It is customary for a patient to undergo laboratory tests after her first prenatal visit and at selected points later in the pregnancy. Prenatal screening for fetal disorders associated with significant fetal problems is desired by the majority of expectant parents. The introduction of a comprehensive screening program that includes ultrasonography and biochemical analyses provides vital information to expectant parents regarding the health of their unborn child and may significantly affect the final outcome for the patient and child. It is important to know which tests are recommended and when. As a general principle, it is best to be aware of and to follow the recommendations of the American College of Obstetricians and Gynecologists with regard to prenatal evaluation and testing (see The American Academy of Pediatrics and American College of Obstetricians and Gynecologists, *Guidelines for Perinatal Care*, 6th edition [2007]).

Limit antenatal testing to patients for whom it is truly indicated. It can be tempting—indeed, you may even feel pressured—to order sonograms, NSTs, or even BPPs in an attempt to reassure the patient or yourself that "everything is fine with the baby." Be sure to understand that for the vast majority of the low-risk pregnant population, there is little evidence that hypervigilant antenatal testing improves outcome.

Chapter 14
Teaching Visual: Fetal Heart Rate Interpretation

Stephanie Boswell MD, Emily Abramson MD, Daron Kahn MD, and Michael Belden MD

Objectives

- Recognize a normal reactive fetal heart tracing (FHT).
- Identify the various patterns and causes of decelerations on FHTs.
- Help your patient understand how FHTs reflect fetal well-being and how their interpretation aids in determination of possible interventions.

Medical Knowledge

Fetal heart rate monitoring is a tool to help evaluate fetal oxygen status and general well-being during labor. Through Doppler signaling, the fetal heart rate is graphed on a beat-to-beat basis alongside maternal contraction monitoring for complete analysis. Although the fetal heart rate has many characteristics that are used to assess well-being, the three major parameters to consider for analysis are baseline heart rate, variability, and periodic changes.

Baseline Heart Rate

Baseline fetal heart rate is the first factor to consider. It refers to the overall mean fetal heart rate rounded to increments of five beats per minute for a minimum of 2 minutes during a 10-minute segment. A normal baseline fetal heart rate ranges from 110 to 160 beats per minute. Baseline rates above 160 beats per minute are referred to as *fetal tachycardia*, and rates below 110 beats per minute are called *fetal bradycardia*.

Baseline Variability

Baseline variability is the beat-to-beat fluctuation in the fetal heart rate of two cycles per minute or greater. Visually, this is the amplitude of peak-to-trough in beats per minute, and defined in terms of length of beats:

- **Absent variability** indicates that the amplitude range is undetectable.
- **Minimal variability** indicates an amplitude range that is detectable, but five beats per minute or fewer.
- **Moderate, or normal variability** shows an amplitude range 6 to 25 beats per minute.
- **Marked variability** is characterized by an amplitude range greater than 25 beats per minute.

The presence of variability denotes a mature nervous system, with the sympathetic nervous system increasing the heart rate and the parasympathetic nervous system decreasing the heart rate.

Periodic Changes: Accelerations and Decelerations

Periodic changes are transient changes of the fetal heart rate of brief duration that eventually return to baseline. They are classified as either **accelerations** or **decelerations.**

- **Accelerations** are sustained increases of heart rate above the baseline and are physiologic responses to fetal movement. The onset to the peak of an acceleration should be less than 30 seconds from the previous baseline. The duration of an acceleration is defined as the time from the initial change in fetal heart rate from the baseline to the return of the fetal heart rate to the baseline. At 32 weeks' gestation and beyond, an acceleration should be 15 beats per minute or more above baseline, with a duration of 15 seconds or more but less than 2 minutes. Before 32 weeks' gestation, an acceleration should be 10 beats per minute or more above baseline, with a duration of 10 seconds or more but less than 2 minutes. If an acceleration lasts 10 minutes or longer, it is a baseline change.

- ■ **Decelerations** are sustained decreases of the heart rate below the baseline. They are further subdivided into early, variable, and late, depending on their timing, their relationship to contractions, and their shape. Decelerations are discussed in further detail in the following.

Reactive/Reassuring Pattern:
This pattern has a baseline heart rate between 110 and 160 beats per minute, shows good variability, and has 2 accelerations of at least 15 beats above the baseline heart rate that last for at least 15 seconds each in a 20-minute period.

Clinical Correlation:
This pattern is reassuring as it demonstrates a normally reactive fetus.

Fetal Heart Tracing

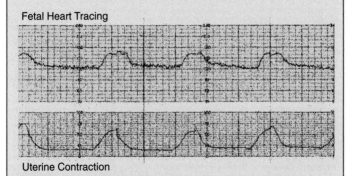

Uterine Contraction

Figure 14-1

Note that fetal reactions are accelerations with return to baseline.

Early Decelerations:
These are decelerations that begin with the contraction, reach their nadir at the peak of the contraction, and return to baseline as the contraction concludes. They are shallow and symmetric with a gradual drop and return to baseline.

Clinical Correlation:
Early decelerations are a result of fetal head compression, which causes a vagal reflex that slows the heart rate. They are not considered pathologic. An example is shown in Figure 14-2.

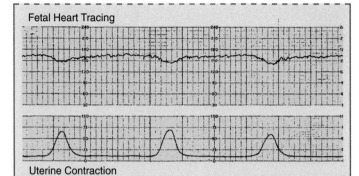

Fetal Heart Tracing

Uterine Contraction

Figure 14-2 Early decelerations.

Variable Decelerations:

Variable decelerations can occur at any time throughout the course of fetal monitoring and do not necessarily show any relationship to maternal contractions, although they are sometimes precipitated by contractions. The onset of a variable deceleration is usually more precipitous than in other types of decelerations, with an onset to nadir of less than 30 seconds. The duration of these decelerations is variable, and brief accelerations may often be seen immediately before and after these decelerations. Looking at a tracing quantitatively, the decrease in fetal heart rate is 15 beats per minute or more, with a duration of 15 seconds or more but less than 2 minutes.

A prolonged deceleration is characterized by a decrease of the fetal heart rate below the baseline of 15 beats or more, lasting 2 minutes or more, but with a return to baseline in less than 10 minutes from onset. An example of variable decelerations is shown in Figure 14-3.

Clinical Correlation:

Variable decelerations are thought to be a result of umbilical cord compression, which results in decreased blood flow to the fetus. If these decelerations are prolonged, show a large drop from the baseline heart rate, or are repetitive, this may be a sign of fetal distress.

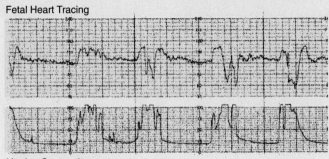

Fetal Heart Tracing

Uterine Contraction

Figure 14-3 Variable decelerations.

Late Decelerations:

These decelerations begin at the peak of a contraction and gradually recover back to baseline after the contraction has completed. The drop is symmetric and gradual with an onset to nadir of 30 seconds or more. Eventually there is a return to baseline.

Clinical Correlation:

Late decelerations suggest the possibility of uteroplacental insufficiency. An example is shown in Figure 14-4.

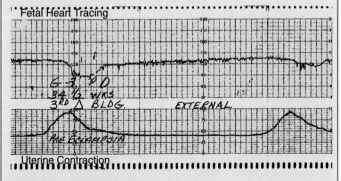

Figure 14-4 Late decelerations.

Systems-Based Practice

Using Standardized Descriptions of Fetal Heart Rate Tracings: The Three-Tiered Fetal Heart Rate Interpretation System

Over the course of the past decade there has been further consideration of fetal heart rate (FHR) tracing patterns and their impact on fetal and maternal outcomes. Unfortunately, controversy still exists, particularly in regard to efficacy, nomenclature, and interpretation of patterns. In 2009 the *Eunice Kennedy Shriver* National Institute of Child Health and Human Development, along with the American College of Obstetricians and Gynecologists and the

Society for Maternal-Fetal Medicine established a more uniform nomenclature and codification system that is rapidly gaining widespread acceptance:

Category I FHR tracings are normal. Category I tracings include all normal tracings, along with normal tracings that show early decelerations. Category I tracings are highly predictive of normal fetal acid-base status, and may be followed routinely.

Category II FHR tracings are indeterminate. Category II tracings include all FHR tracings that are not Category I or Category III, but are not predictive of abnormal fetal acid-base status. Nevertheless, these tracings require active surveillance, and clinical circumstances must also be considered. Intrauterine resuscitative measures may be considered. Non-repetitive variable decelerations, or intermittent periods of minimal variability would fall into this category.

Category III FHR tracings are abnormal. Category III tracings are strongly suggestive of abnormal fetal acid-base status, and require evaluation. Resuscitative measures should be provided, including intravenous fluids, maternal position changes, discontinuation of augmentation or induction of labor, and possibly the administration of tocolytic therapy if uterine tachysystole is occurring. If the Category III tracing does not resolve, prompt delivery should be a consideration. Persistent late or variable decelerations, or absent variability are examples of Category III FHR tracings.

See: Compendium of Selected Publications, ACOG Practice Bulletin 106, Intrapartum Fetal Heart Rate Monitoring: Nomenclature, Interpretation, and General Management Principles, The American College of Obstetrics and Gynecology, July 2009, 324-34 for a more complete discussion of this new categorization system.

Interpersonal and Communication Skills

Discussing the Fetal Heart Tracing with the Mother
Expectant mothers are generally aware that the fetal heart tracing monitors the health and safety of their babies, but they are usually unaware of the significance of the different patterns seen on the FHT. Because continuous fetal heart rate monitoring is the primary tool we use to assess general fetal well-being, communication of our interpretation of the heart rate pattern to a laboring woman is crucial. When a tracing is reassuring, this knowledge will be a source of comfort; however, when you see a nonreassuring pattern, you should begin a discussion with the mother about its causes and the possible implications of this information.

Medical Knowledge

Nonreassuring Patterns
Nonreassuring patterns include fetal bradycardia, fetal tachycardia, loss of short-term variability, late decelerations, and persistent late variable decelerations. These abnormalities cannot be immediately interpreted as indicating fetal distress. The more frequent the abnormality, the greater the quantity of different abnormalities, and

the lack of response to interventions such as maternal positioning, maternal oxygen administration, and intravenous fluids all point to the possibility of the development of fetal acidemia.

Even though a nonreassuring tracing may be a sign of fetal distress, including hypoxia, acidemia, or infection, the likelihood of false-positive findings with regard to fetal well-being is high. Regardless of the high likelihood of false-positive fetal monitoring, nonreassuring fetal tracings require intervention. These interventions include:

- *Watchful waiting:* A single late or variable deceleration can be monitored to see if it becomes repetitive or persistent.
- *Minimal/moderate interventions:* Such interventions can often correct nonreassuring patterns, although increased vigilance is subsequently warranted. These include:
  - Reposition the mother.
  - Give supplemental oxygen to the mother.
  - Give intravenous fluids to the mother.
  - Stop medications that increase contractions.
  - Give the mother medications to weaken contractions/relax the uterus.
  - Stimulate the fetal scalp.
- *Major intervention:* Emergency cesarean section.

Interpersonal and Communication Skills

Discussing an Emergency Cesarean Section with Parents

When fetal heart tracings show persistent, nonreassuring patterns regardless of previous interventions, an emergency cesarean section may become necessary. This possibility must be communicated as early as possible and the risks and benefits of the procedure explained. These conversations may be difficult with a laboring patient, and, though honesty must prevail, care must be taken not be overwhelm patients with the information that the baby may be in danger. Be prepared to answer any questions that come up in the moment or later. Keeping open communications with the patient is vital to achieve the best outcome for both the mother and baby.

Exercises

The interpretation of fetal heart rate monitoring tracings can be a challenge for even experienced obstetricians. A useful way to become comfortable with the concept of fetal heart rate tracing interpretation is to draw the different patterns in order to better understand the temporal relations between contractions and the various types of decelerations. On the following pages you will find three separate, but blank, fetal monitoring grids, each suggestive of a deceleration. For each case, the first deceleration has been suggested by dots. Complete the dotted line and draw additional decelerations. After each example, remind yourself of the clinical correlation in the space provided.

Late Deceleration

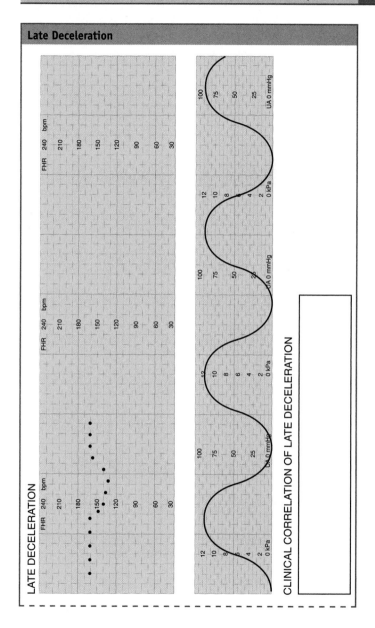

LATE DECELERATION

CLINICAL CORRELATION OF LATE DECELERATION

Early Decelerations

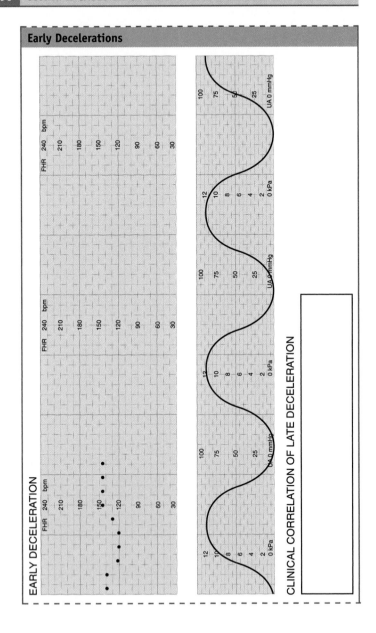

EARLY DECELERATION

CLINICAL CORRELATION OF LATE DECELERATION

Variable Deceleration

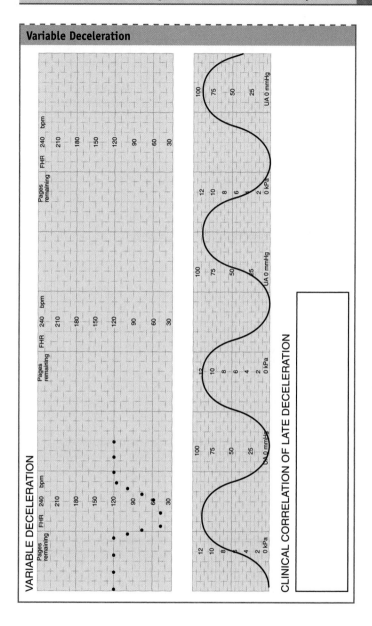

VARIABLE DECELERATION

CLINICAL CORRELATION OF LATE DECELERATION

Reference

1. American College of Obstetricians and Gynecologists: Intrapartum fetal heart rate monitoring nomenclature, interpretation, and general management principles. ACOG Practice Bulletin #106, Clinical Management Guidelines of Obstetrician-Gynecologists. Washington, DC, American College of Obstetricians and Gynecologists, 2009.

Chapter 15
Obstetric Anesthesia (Case 4)

Dmitri Chamchad MD

Case: A 36-year-old G1P0 at 39 weeks' gestation presents to the hospital in labor. Her contractions are regular and strong, her membranes are ruptured, and her cervix is 3 cm dilated. She is very uncomfortable. She would like something for pain, but is unsure of the options available and what she might ultimately prefer. She asks to speak briefly with the obstetric anesthesiologist to consider her choices.

Options for Obstetric Anesthesia and Analgesia

Narcotics for analgesia	Spinal anesthesia
Epidural anesthesia	General anesthesia

Speaking Intelligently

The challenges presented by a parturient requiring anesthesia or analgesia make the role of the obstetric anesthesiologist both challenging and rewarding. Physicians and others providing anesthetic services to the labor and delivery suite must be familiar with the unique physiology of the parturient and the effects of numerous drugs and techniques on the parturient and fetus.

PATIENT CARE

Clinical Thinking

- We can divide anesthesia for parturients into three subgroups:
  - Anesthesia for labor and vaginal delivery such as epidural anesthesia, spinal analgesia, and combined spinal/epidural anesthesia.
  - Anesthesia for cesarean sections such as epidural, spinal anesthesia, combined spinal/epidural anesthesia, and general anesthesia.
  - Anesthesia for nonobstetric surgery during pregnancy.
- We must also consider anesthesia needs for less common procedures and interventions, such as trauma, laparoscopic surgery, and external cephalic version.
- Although rare and performed only in selected centers, considerations for fetal surgery may sometimes be necessary.
- Realistically, we must concentrate on anesthesia for labor and vaginal delivery and anesthesia for cesarean section.
- Maternal physiologic changes during pregnancy influence virtually all organ systems, and a thorough knowledge of these changes becomes the foundation of thoughtful and competent anesthesia care.

Medical Knowledge

Physiologic Alterations of Pregnancy the Anesthesiologist Must Consider

System	Change	Anesthetic Considerations
Respiratory	Upper airway edema	Difficult intubation
	Upper airway friability	Bleeding with nasal tubes
	↑Ventilation and respiratory rate	Rapid induction/emergence
	↓Functional residual capacity	Rapid desaturation
	↑Myocardial oxygen consumption ($M\dot{V}_{O_2}$)	
Cardiovascular	↑Cardiac output	Slows induction for inhaled agents
	↑Intravascular volume	Hematologic reserve for hemorrhage
	↓Resistance	Low mean blood pressure
	Aortocaval compression (>20 wk)	Left lateral tilt

System	Change	Anesthetic Considerations
Neurologic	↑Sensitivity of peripheral nerves to local anesthetic ↑Sensitivity of central nervous system to general anesthetics	↓Dose required for epidural/spinal
Hematologic	↓Hemoglobin ↑Coagulation factors ↓Serum proteins	↓Oxygen carrying capacity ↑Risk of deep vein thrombosis ↑Edema ↑Sensitivity to drug toxicity
Musculoskeletal	↑Joint and ligament laxity	↑Risk of dural puncture
Gastrointestinal	↓Gastroesophageal junction integrity Slowed gastric emptying during active labor	↑Reflux and possible aspiration under general anesthesia

History
- All patients entering the obstetric suite may potentially require anesthesia, whether planned or emergent. The anesthesiologist should be aware of the presence and relevant history of all patients in the labor and delivery suite.
- Pertinent historic items include age, parity, duration of the pregnancy, and any complicating factors.
- Patients definitely requiring anesthetic care (for labor or cesarean section) should undergo a preanesthetic evaluation as early as possible.

Physical Examination
- Vital signs must be evaluated first. Are the patient's pulse and blood pressure within normal limits? Is her respiratory rate normal?
- Does she have an adequate airway? Will she be difficult to intubate if the need arises?
- What is her body habitus and body mass index (BMI)? On many occasions drugs may need to be titrated to meet increased or decreased needs.

- Is her spine normal? Does the patient have scoliosis or indwelling hardware?
- What is the cervical examination status? Providing regional anesthesia before the patient is in active labor can prolong labor duration.
- Is the fetal heart rate tracing appropriate and reassuring?

Tests for Consideration
- **CBC:** A very important baseline test to consider. Virtually every patient should have a CBC ordered. $35
- **PT/PTT/INR:** Is the patient at risk for a coagulopathy or bleeding during a procedure? $25
- **Fibrinogen/D-dimer:** These tests become relevant if there is a risk or clinical likelihood of disseminated intravascular coagulation (DIC). Do we need to give additional blood products? $60
- **Type and screen:** Keep on hand in case transfusion is required. $125
- **ECG:** Required if the patient has known cardiac issues. $25
- **CXR:** May be helpful if pulmonary status is a problem. $75

Management Considerations
- Virtually all women in true labor should be managed with intravenous fluids to prevent dehydration. An 18-gauge intravenous catheter should be placed should transfusion become necessary.
- Blood should be sent for typing and screening.
- Regardless of the time of last oral intake, all pregnant patients are considered to have a full stomach and to be at risk for pulmonary aspiration.
- Because the duration of labor may be prolonged, guidelines often allow small amounts of clear liquid for uncomplicated labor. The minimum fasting period for elective cesarean section should be 6 to 8 hours.
- All patients should ideally have tocodynamometry (uterine contraction monitoring) and fetal heart rate monitoring.
- The supine position should be avoided unless a left uterine displacement device (>15-degree wedge) is placed under the right hip.

Clinical Anesthetic Choices	Medical Knowledge

I = Indication
T = Technique
B = Benefits
SE = Side effects and risks

Narcotics for Analgesia

I   Labor pain.

T   Narcotic pain medication, usually administered with a potentiating sedative (such as promethazine), given intravenously or intramuscularly.

B   Quick-acting agents, with no need for an anesthesiologist to administer. This technique has compared favorably with other forms of obstetric anesthesia/analgesia in past.

SE   Occasional oversedation is the most worrisome risk, as well as small risk of fetal oversedation because narcotics typically cross the placenta readily. **See Gabbe 16, Hacker 8.**

Epidural Anesthesia

I   Labor pain, or as a technique for cesarean section anesthesia/ analgesia.

T   The epidural potential space is infiltrated with a mixture of anesthetic agent, typically ropivacaine, lidocaine, or bupivacaine, and sometimes a narcotic agent as well. After an initial bolus injection, an indwelling catheter on a pump is the usual method of administration.

B   Excellent and ongoing pain relief with good patient satisfaction. Literature suggests there is no increased risk of cesarean section and no medication effects on the fetus.

SE   May nominally increase rate of instrumental delivery, thus potentially increasing the risk of maternal trauma. Transient hypotension is common and usually self-limited. The risks of a "high spinal" or spinal headache (much less common than with spinal anesthesia; see later) are slight. Infection is extremely rare. **See Gabbe 16, Hacker 8.**

Spinal Anesthesia

I   Typically chosen as a technique for cesarean sections, or sometimes for surgery during pregnancy. Used on occasion for instrumental deliveries.

T   Local anesthetic agents, sometimes with narcotics added, are injected into the subarachnoid space.

B   Very fast acting, with excellent analgesia.

SE   Ongoing risk of spinal headache. A "high spinal" can impede ventilation which may result in the need for intubation. Infection is extremely rare. **See Gabbe 16, Hacker 8.**

General Anesthesia	
I	Used typically in true emergencies, when the patient does not have satisfactory regional anesthesia and requires immediate cesarean delivery. Also used for other surgical procedures in pregnancy.
T	Endotracheal intubation, with a combination of inhaled anesthetics and intravenous muscle relaxants and powerful sedatives.
B	Excellent anesthesia and analgesia.
SE	May increase risk of bleeding or hemorrhage due to uterine relaxation. Maternal hypotension is uncommon and usually promptly reversible. If prolonged, however, this may increase the risk of fetal compromise. Maternal aspiration is a small risk, but with proper antiaspiration prophylaxis this is rare. **See Gabbe 16, Hacker 8.**

ZEBRA ZONE

Unexpected Anesthesia Complications

a. **Failed intubation:** Rare, but raises the risk of aspiration.

b. **Maternal convulsions:** A rare side effect of unintended intravascular injection of regional anesthesia.

Practice-Based Learning and Improvement: Evidence-Based Medicine

Title

Effect of epidural vs parenteral opioid analgesia on the progress of labor: A meta-analysis

Authors

Halpern SH, Leighton BL, Ohlsson A, Barrett JF, Rice A

Institution

Department of Anaesthesia, University of Toronto and Women's College Hospital, Toronto, Ontario, Canada

Reference

Journal of the American Medical Association 1998;280:2105–2110

Problem

Does epidural anesthesia increase the risk of cesarean section?

Intervention

Epidural anesthesia versus parenteral opioid anesthesia.

Comparison/control (quality of evidence)
Meta-analysis of several studies.

Outcome/effect
No increased risk of cesarean delivery associated with administration of epidural anesthesia, although epidural anesthesia did increase the risk of instrumental deliveries and did lengthen the duration of labor.

Historical significance/comments
This historic meta-analysis confirmed the long-held belief that epidural anesthesia did not increase the risk of cesarean section, and was generally very safe.

Interpersonal and Communication Skills

Communication while Performing a Procedure

Most communication teaching has traditionally focused on interactions between physicians and patients during history taking. There has been much less focus on communicating with patients while performing procedures. As more procedures and complex operations are performed on conscious patients, acquiring these skills becomes increasingly important.

There are obvious reasons why it is important to communicate. You can gain the patient's cooperation, assess their progress, and continue to build your relationship. Although this may seem obvious, when you are concentrating on a procedure, it can be easy to overlook the patient. This is especially the case if you are inexperienced or if things don't go as expected.

The administration of epidural anesthesia during labor is a commonly performed procedure that lends itself to an interactive relationship between the physician and the patient. During placement of the epidural catheter you will see that the anesthesiologist will intermittently look at the patient's face for nonverbal cues. Anesthesiologists will observe the patient's posture for excessive tension, and try to put the patient at ease. Usually, it is important for patients to relax so that they can maintain their positioning. If there are periods when the physician may want to work in silence, she or he will typically let the patient know rather than just going quiet. Some physicians find it helpful to talk through the steps of the procedure, but remember that not all patients will want such a commentary.

Many anesthesiologists will give clear instructions to the patient so they know what they have to do:

- "It is very important that you stay as still as possible during the time it takes to complete the procedure."

- "If you think you will have to move, then say so and I can stop what I am doing."
- "This drape is what we call *sterile* so it means that the area around the site of needle entry is clean. It is very important that you do not touch it."
- "The procedure should be only minimally uncomfortable to you. If you experience any severe pain or discomfort it is important to tell me."

On completion of the procedure, remember to thank patients for their cooperation and briefly go over what you have just done and what happens next.

Professionalism

Principle: Primacy of Patient Welfare

The ethical principle of beneficence comes into consideration every time you care for a laboring patient who is in pain. As a care provider you would like to make the patient as comfortable as possible. You must also weigh the risks of early oversedation, such as prolonging labor, against the patient's need for pain relief. It would be unacceptable, for example, to administer epidural anesthesia to a woman who presents with a few painful contractions, but is not yet showing signs of cervical change or impending active labor. Although an epidural could potentially make her very comfortable, it would not be in her best interest because true labor, with painful contractions and cervical dilation, could be days or even weeks away. As always, the clinician must do what is best for the patient based on clinical judgment and assessment of the situation at hand.

Systems-Based Practice

Fetal Heart Rate Monitoring

Fetal heart rate (FHR) monitoring was first introduced in 1958 as a way to monitor fetal well-being during labor and delivery, and has become virtually ubiquitous in labor and delivery units in developed nations. The rise of evidence-based medicine and its demands that clinical practice be based on actual evidence has brought a new set of challenges to FHR monitoring. To date, there is little to no evidence that FHR monitoring actually improves either fetal or maternal well-being. Although most clinicians agree that there is some correlation between FHR tracings and fetal well-being, the widespread use of FHR monitors has failed to reduce the rates of cerebral palsy or neurologic injury among newborns. Significantly, FHR monitoring has become popular at the same time as cesarean section rates have dramatically risen, and many believe that the widespread use of FHR monitoring, combined with an overly litigious environment in medicine, has led to unnecessarily high cesarean section rates. As most clinicians will agree, it is quite common to perform a caesarean section for a nonreassuring FHR tracing, only to find a newborn who is healthy and in no distress. This is because the positive predictive value of a test is directly proportional to the prevalence, and because the prevalence of asphyxia in labor is low, despite the high sensitivity of FHR monitoring, its positive predictive value is still quite low. Although there is still considerable controversy over this practice, many clinicians agree that pending more conclusive randomized, controlled studies, and given the current legal climate, it is inadvisable to abandon the use of FHR monitors.

Chapter 16
Normal Labor (Case 5)

Vonetta Sylvestre MD

Case: A 22-year-old G2 P1001 presents to Labor and Delivery at 39 and 5/7 weeks' gestation complaining of painful contractions. She noted that the contractions started to increase in frequency and became painful 6 hours before coming to the hospital. She has had no leakage of fluid and no vaginal bleeding and she has noted good fetal movement. Her obstetric history is significant for one prior uncomplicated full-term vaginal delivery of a 6-pound, 2-ounce infant. She is contracting every 4 minutes. Her cervical examination: 4 cm dilated, 50% effaced, and −1 station. The fetal vertex is palpated on cervical examination. Fetal heart monitoring is reassuring and reactive.

The patient requests an epidural for pain relief. Two hours later, the cervical examination is 6 cm dilated, 100 % effaced, and −1 station, and artificial rupture of membranes is accomplished. The amniotic fluid is clear. Four hours later, the cervical examination reveals 8 cm of dilation. After an additional hour, the patient is found to have a fully dilated cervix, and begins pushing. After 45 minutes of pushing, the infant delivers easily.

Differential Diagnosis

Normal labor

Speaking Intelligently

My first question is always, "Is this a normal labor?" The patient initially presented at 4 cm of dilation and progressed to 6 cm, which is the appropriate rate of dilation for a multiparous patient over a 2-hour interval. In the face of a routine first pregnancy and uneventful first delivery, it is reasonable to expect that the patient will have a similar course during the conduct of her current labor. As long as the fetal heart tracing continues to show reassuring fetal status, the most prudent course of events is to let the process continue with no additional intervention. Of course, oxytocin remains an available option for labor augmentation if required.

PATIENT CARE

Clinical Thinking

- When a patient presents in labor it is important to have an expectation of the normal course of events. If the patient achieves the anticipated milestones, then frequently no obstetric intervention is warranted. However, if the patient deviates from the expected course, then an appropriate management schema is necessary. Developing a coherent plan and using appropriate interventions as needed have been established to be the most safe and effective way to achieve optimal obstetric outcomes. This general strategy is often called the *active management of labor*.
- Effective management of labor requires knowledge of the basic mechanisms of labor and the progression of normal labor. In addition, it is important to evaluate the patient for any factors that might affect her labor progress.

- If not already done, review the obstetric history of the patient to determine if her prior labor(s) progressed normally. Inquire if any obstetric instrumentation, such as a vacuum extractor or obstetric forceps, was used during the prior delivery or if any obstetric complications occurred at that time.
- An evaluation of the maternal pelvis, as well as an estimation of the fetal size, can be extremely helpful as you begin to formulate a plan for the management of a patient's labor. Recent sonograms can provide an estimation of the fetal weight. In addition, the clinician can assess fetal weight based on the bedside physical examination.

History
- Review of prenatal records: Determine if the patient has had any obstetric, fetal, or maternal complications that may affect her delivery or may require special management during delivery or in the postpartum period.
- Keep in mind that prenatal records are basically standardized across the United States. These documents are typically easy to read in an emergency.
- The patient described in the preceding case has had an uncomplicated prenatal course. Her prior delivery was straightforward. The delivery of her current pregnancy can, in general, be anticipated to be straightforward as well.

Physical Examination
- **Assessment of fetal presentation and position:** It is important to assess the presenting part of the fetus because a nonvertex presentation frequently will require a cesarean delivery.
- **Presentation** refers to the fetal part that is palpated in the birth canal. This can be assessed either by vaginal examination or by Leopold's maneuvers on abdominal examination (Leopold's maneuvers are a time-honored physical examination skill that allows the clinician to make an assessment regarding the presentation of the fetus). If necessary, the clinician can also assess fetal presentation by ultrasonography (most modern obstetric units have a mobile ultrasound machine available for bedside use).
- **Position** refers to the relationship of the presenting part to the birth canal. When the fetus is vertex, the head is usually flexed and the fetal occiput is the presenting part.
- **Vaginal Examination:** The decision to perform an immediate digital vaginal/cervical examination on a patient who presents in labor should be influenced by the patient's presenting symptoms and chief complaint.

If the patient is simply having labor contractions, or appears to be in active labor, a timely examination is indicated to assess the progress of the labor and to evaluate for the possible initiation of regional anesthesia, if the patient so desires. ***On the other hand, if the laboring patient notes either leakage of fluid or vaginal bleeding, you must first evaluate the patient for signs of ruptured membranes and/or vaginal bleeding.***

- **Evaluate for rupture of membranes:** It is important to evaluate for rupture of membranes, because prolonged rupture can increase the risk of infection. If rupture of membranes has occurred, the clinician may choose to limit cervical exams, since an increased number of cervical exams can increase the risk of infection in these patients. Rupture of membranes is assessed by means of a sterile speculum exam. Signs of rupture on speculum exam include pooling of amniotic fluid in the vaginal vault, pH of 7.0 as indicated by use of nitrazine paper, and "ferning" of amniotic fluid.
- **Evaluate for vaginal bleeding:** Patients in labor often present with "bloody show". If the vaginal bleeding is deemed abnormally excessive (particularly in a patient who is not known to have a preexisting placenta previa), a bedside ultrasound should be performed to rule out previa before a digital cervical examination is performed.
- **Cervical examination:** A cervical examination is accomplished by the insertion of two gloved fingers into the vagina. The dilation, effacement, station, and position of the cervix can be assessed.
  - **Cervical dilation** is determined by measuring the distance from the margin of the cervical opening on one side to the margin on the opposite side. Cervical dilation ranges from 0 cm (closed) to 10 cm (complete dilation).
  - **Cervical effacement** (thinning) refers to the length of the cervical os compared with an uneffaced cervix. A normal cervical length is 3 to 4 cm. Measurement of cervical effacement ranges from 0% to 100%. A cervix completely thinned would be described as 100% effaced.
  - **Station** refers to the level of the presenting fetal part in relation to the ischial spines of the maternal pelvis. The station can range from −5 to −1 (above the ischial spines) to 0 station (at the ischial spines), to +1 to +5 (below the ischial spines). When the presenting part is at +5, it is visible at the introitus. (Some clinicians use a −3 to +3 system of measuring station.)
  - **Position of the cervix** refers to the location of the cervix in relation to the maternal vaginal apex. The cervix can be described as posterior, mid-position, or anterior.

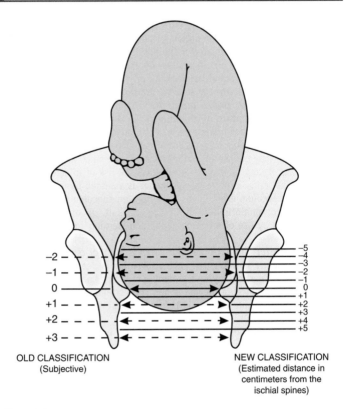

OLD CLASSIFICATION
(Subjective)

NEW CLASSIFICATION
(Estimated distance in
centimeters from the
ischial spines)

Figure 16-1
The relationship of the leading edge of the presenting part of the fetus to the
plane of the maternal ischial spines determines the station. Station +1/+3 (old
classification) or +2/+5 (new classification) is illustrated.

IMAGING CONSIDERATIONS

→**Obstetric ultrasonography:** Performed in the delivery
room, obstetric ultrasonography can reveal useful
information about the position and presentation of
the fetus. Many modern delivery rooms have a
"dedicated" ultrasound machine available for this
purpose $225

Clinical Entities **Medical Knowledge**

Normal Labor: Cardinal Movements	
Cardinal movements of labor	A normal labor is characterized by the **cardinal movements of labor.** These classic movements are a construct that can be used to describe a process that typically happens seamlessly and spontaneously. Think of these movements happening over the course of a normal labor with each movement flowing elegantly into the next. These movements ultimately allow the presenting part to progress through the maternal pelvis.
Engagement	The biparietal diameter (measured ear to ear) is the widest transverse diameter of the fetal head. Engagement refers to the descent of the biparietal diameter as it passes through the pelvic inlet. Engagement may occur weeks before delivery (typical in primigravidas) or during labor (typical of multigravidas).
Descent	Descent is the movement of the presenting part down through the pelvis.
Flexion	The fetal head may meet resistance as it descends, usually resulting in flexion of the head. The chin is brought closer to the fetal thorax.
Internal rotation	The head turns in such a manner that the fetal occiput moves toward the symphysis pubis, resulting in an occiput anterior position. The occiput may rarely rotate towards the sacrum such that the occiput is posterior.
Extension	The flexed fetal head comes in contact with the pelvic floor and the force of the uterine contractions combined with the resistance of the pelvic floor result in extension of the fetal head.
External rotation or restitution	The head is delivered and the pelvic forces that resulted in internal rotation now work to turn the fetal body toward its original anatomic position.
Expulsion	The anterior shoulder appears under the symphysis pubis and shortly thereafter the posterior shoulder delivers. The remainder of the fetus follows.

Normal Labor: Stages of Labor

First stage of labor	The first stage of labor begins with the onset of regular contractions in association with cervical change. It concludes when cervical dilation is complete. The first stage is divided into the latent phase and the active phase. • The latent phase starts when the mother perceives regular contractions. The latent phase usually ends at 3 to 5 cm of cervical dilation. The length of the latent phase can be extremely variable from patient to patient. • The active phase starts thereafter. The rate of cervical dilation is considerably faster during the active phase. In a primipara, the minimal rate of dilation is 1.2 cm per hour in the active phase. In a multipara, dilation should proceed at 1.5 cm per hour.
Second stage of labor	The second stage of labor starts when cervical dilation is complete and ends with delivery of the fetus. The second stage of labor is typically thought of as the "pushing" phase.
Third stage of labor	The third stage of labor starts after delivery of the fetus and ends with delivery of the placenta. Although usually brief, the third stage can last as long as 30 minutes.
Fourth stage of labor	The fourth stage of labor begins immediately after the delivery of the placenta, and is usually considered to end 2 hours later. **See Gabbe 12, Hacker 8.**

ZEBRA ZONE

a. **Prolonged latent phase (sometimes also called "false labor"):** This can often be confused with true labor. It is important to understand that during the latent phase, in the face of a reassuring fetal heart rate tracing, it is sometimes best to assume an expectant approach.

b. **Braxton-Hicks contractions:** These sporadic contractions, although sometimes quite painful for the patient, do not cause cervical dilation.

Practice-Based Learning and Improvement: Evidence-Based Medicine

Title
A clinical trial of active management of labor

Authors
Frigoletto FD Jr, Lieberman E, Lang JM, et al.

Institution
Brigham and Women's Hospital, Boston, Massachusetts

Reference
New England Journal of Medicine 1995;333:745–750

Problem
Would active management of labor reduce rates of cesarean section?

Intervention
Active management of labor using frequent cervical examinations, amniotomy, and oxytocin augmentation.

Comparison/control (quality of evidence)
Randomized clinical trial; level I evidence.

Outcome/effect
Active management of labor was associated with shorter labor times and lower rates of infections but had no effect on the rates of cesarean section.

Historical significance/comments
This was one of the seminal studies confirming that active management of labor reduces poor maternal and fetal outcomes. Active management of labor is now widely accepted to be the standard of care.

Exit Rounds

Consider using the Labor and Delivery Room as a place to incorporate the Practice-Based Learning and Improvement exercise described as follows: in a group setting, with attending(s) present, a resident reviews a patient for whom he or she was responsible and describes what was learned from caring for that patient.

   Practical Example: Each morning on L&D, certain cases from the previous day are discussed. These may include all cesarean and operative deliveries, preterm deliveries, and any other complications (postpartum hemorrhage, seizure, etc.). The resident involved presents the case to all other residents, medical students, and faculty (incoming and outgoing teams). Learning points are discussed and ways to improve outcome, if possible, are discussed.

Interpersonal and Communication Skills

Introducing the Setting, the Procedures, and the Team
It is important to establish a relationship with your patient who presents in labor. Introduce yourself when she first arrives on the labor floor so that she is aware that you will be observing and managing her labor and delivery. Once the patient has been evaluated, review the chart and make sure that you are aware of and understand the plan for her delivery. Explain to her the management plan of her labor. Patients find a knowledgeable and coordinated medical team reassuring. Words of encouragement during labor are also helpful. Use language with positive connotations. Try not to appear judgmental or rushed. For example, if a patient's labor seems protracted, reassure the patient that this is a common occurrence and that oxytocin can be used to augment the process. Be mindful not to make the patient feel that a slow or protracted labor is somehow her fault. Take the time necessary to explain the importance of intravenous fluid management, fetal monitoring, contraction monitoring, and the need for frequent vital signs. Explain that there are other important members of the team who may be involved in her care. Introduce nurses, residents, students, neonatologists, and anesthesiologists as appropriate.

Professionalism

Principle: Commitment to Improving Access to Care
An estimated 300,000 children of illegal immigrants are born in the United States every year, many of them qualifying for emergency Medicaid and incurring real costs on taxpayer-funded health care.*
Immigration reform, which is essentially a political issue, plays a major role in access to health care of people living in the United States. In this population it is essential to begin education about early pediatric issues even during the birth admission. Fear of deportation can deter parents from bringing children for subsequent well-baby care, often preventing children from receiving appropriate vaccinations. It is our responsibility as medical professionals to be politically involved and make our voices heard in government on this and related issues.

*For more information see: Illegal immigrant births—At your expense. CBS Evening News. Available at http://www.cbsnews.com/stories/2008/04/07/eveningnews/main4000401.shtml.

Systems-Based Practice

Cesarean Section Rates and Clinical Outcomes
In general, vaginal deliveries are still widely considered to be the safest mode of delivery for both mother and fetus. Vaginal delivery is

associated with faster recovery times, lower risk of hemorrhage, lower rates of infection, and shorter hospital stays compared with cesarean section. The combination of these factors results in significantly decreased cost and in lower mortality and morbidity for the mother. Although these factors appear to hold true for healthy mothers and fetuses, it is widely believed that distressed fetuses require cesarean sections to expedite delivery.

Over the last few decades, increasing concern over litigation (usually relating to cases of cerebral palsy) as well as increased rates of maternal obesity and fetal macrosomia have led to rising cesarean section rates across the world. Whether fetal and maternal outcomes are improving as a result of this trend is unclear. Most interestingly, there seems to be a growing body of evidence suggesting that the occurrence of cerebral palsy has remained very stable in the past several decades, even in the face of rising cesarean rates. As a professional practice, obstetrician/gynecologists have readily embraced continuous electronic fetal monitoring, with a low threshold for cesarean section, in the hope that this strategy would diminish the number of children born with cerebral palsy. Unfortunately, this has not been borne out by the current evidence. In fact, it now seems that cerebral palsy is most likely multifactorial in nature, and may arise most commonly as a consequence of prematurity and undiagnosed maternal infection. Absent further studies, it seems that cesarean sections alone are not successful in preventing fetal neurologic injury.

Chapter 17
Abnormalities of Labor and Their Management (Case 6)

Michael Belden MD

Case: A 26-year-old G1P0 at 38 weeks' gestation presents to the hospital in labor. She is noted to have had a normal prenatal course, with no identified problems. She presents in active labor, at 4 cm cervical dilation. She receives epidural anesthesia, and her membranes are artificially ruptured. Her labor progresses slowly, and after a 2-hour period at 9 cm of dilation she receives oxytocin augmentation. She then progresses to full dilation and begins pushing. After 3 hours in the second stage of labor, her fetus was found to be at the +3/5 station.

The estimated fetal weight was 6 lbs, and the patient's pelvis seems adequate clinically.

Differential Diagnosis

Arrest and protraction disorders	Fetal malpresentation	Inadequate or infrequent uterine contractions	Cephalopelvic disproportion

Speaking Intelligently

This case presents one of the most common problems we face in obstetrics: how to manage a patient whose labor and delivery initially appears to be proceeding smoothly, but ultimately becomes difficult. The obstetric term for "difficult labor" is **dystocia.** Abnormalities of labor, especially protraction and descent disorders, can usually be attributed to one of three problems, which are often referred to as the "Three P's": abnormalities of the **passenger, passage, and power** of the labor. Reaching the correct diagnosis enables us to choose the safest possible intervention to insure a safe outcome for both the fetus and mother.

PATIENT CARE

Clinical Thinking

The three P's noted in Speaking Intelligently help us think about the common problems in a simple and methodical way:

- **Passenger:** Fetal malpresentations present a problem caused by the (baby) **passenger.**
- **Passage:** Cephalopelvic disproportion represents a mismatch between the size of the fetus and the maternal pelvis; the problem is the **passage.**
- **Power:** Inadequate or infrequent uterine contractions represent a problem of uterine **power.**

Thinking of these complicated problems in simple terms enables us to quickly and accurately formulate best solutions to these problems.

History

- The most important component of the history is evaluating the progress of labor over time.
- Has the patient been making normal progress? For a nulliparous patient, one would generally expect the cervix to be dilating at not less than 1.2 cm/hour. Has our patient met these criteria?
- Has the patient had a recent sonogram predicting the estimated fetal weight?

- Was the patient ever told her pelvis felt inadequate for a vaginal delivery on physical examination?

Physical Examination
- The physical examination in such cases depends on bedside skills that are difficult to acquire, and to a great degree come only with experience.
- What is the estimated fetal weight obtained by physical examination? For the experienced examiner, this estimate can be quite accurate.
- What is the position of the fetus? Occiput posterior or occiput transverse fetal positions are the most commonly identified causes of malpresentation.
- Do the patient's contractions seem clinically powerful? Would an intrauterine pressure catheter measuring Montevideo units (see below) be helpful?

Tests for Consideration
- **Measurement of Montevideo units:** A reproducible measure of the power of uterine contractions. An intrauterine pressure catheter must be in place. $250

IMAGING CONSIDERATIONS

→**Obstetric ultrasonography:** Third-trimester ultrasonography, focusing on the estimated fetal weight, can sometimes be helpful. $225

Clinical Entities   Medical Knowledge

Arrest and Protraction Disorders of Labor

Pφ A **protraction disorder** occurs when the rate of cervical dilation is less than expected in the active phase of labor (see Chapter 16 for a discussion of normal progress in labor).

An **arrest disorder** can be divided into two types: arrest of descent and arrest of dilation.
- **Arrest of descent** refers to a complete cessation of descent of the presenting part. In the second stage of labor, arrest of descent is diagnosed in a multiparous patient after 2 hours with an epidural and 1 hour without an epidural. A primiparous patient is considered to have arrest of descent if there is no downward movement of the fetal vertex during the second stage for up to 3 hours if she has an epidural or 2 hours if she does not have an epidural.

- **Arrest of dilation** occurs when there is complete cessation of dilation over a 2-hour period in the presence of adequate contractions.

TP Typically, the patient's sequential cervical examinations will show no change in dilation, effacement, or station.

Dx Abnormal progress during labor can be caused by multiple factors (see the additional clinical entities boxes in this chapter for further discussion).
- **Inadequate contractions:** If a patient has inadequate contractions, either in frequency or intensity, then labor will not progress. The adequacy of contractions can be assessed with the use of an intrauterine pressure catheter and the calculation of Montevideo units. Montevideo units are calculated by adding up the peak contraction pressures in millimeters of mercury (mm Hg), in a series of contractions over a 10-minute period as charted on the toco tracing. The baseline pressure is then subtracted. A Montevideo unit total of over 200 for a 10-minute window of time is considered adequate.
- **Epidural anesthesia:** Epidural anesthesia can on occasion affect labor by increasing the length of the first and second stages of labor. Some studies note that epidural anesthesia may prolong labor by 40 to 90 minutes. Epidural anesthesia may also reduce maternal expulsive forces, lengthening the second stage.
- **Cephalopelvic disproportion:** A successful labor depends on the ability of the fetus to pass through the maternal pelvis. If the fetus is too large or the maternal pelvis is contracted, then cephalopelvic disproportion occurs. Clinical pelvimetry is a useful tool to assess the maternal pelvis, but has not been shown to predict a successful vaginal delivery when used alone.

Tx If the cause of the protraction disorder is inadequate contractions, this can usually be overcome by amniotomy (if the membranes are not already ruptured) and/or augmentation with oxytocin to strengthen uterine contractile force. In the presence of an arrest of dilation or descent, cephalopelvic disproportion needs to be considered before oxytocin augmentation is begun. Ultimately, an operative delivery (forceps, vacuum, or cesarean section) may be necessary for disorders of arrest of descent. Cesarean section is the only appropriate intervention for disorders of arrest of dilation. **See Gabbe 13, Hacker 11.**

Fetal Malpresentation

Pφ Malpresentations are believed to be caused by the bony architecture of the pelvis, most commonly of the platypelloid or android type. Cephalopelvic disproportion (see later) may also be the cause. The two most common malpresentations are the occiput posterior position and the deep transverse arrest.

TP The fetal vertex does not flex properly, thus presenting a much larger diameter to the pelvis. This disrupts the "cardinal movements of labor" (see Chapter 16, Normal Labor).

Dx Diagnosis can be made (preferentially) by physical examination of the fetal sutures, or as a diagnosis of exclusion, if the fetal architecture is obscured by moulding or edema and fetal sutures cannot be palpated.

Tx Management is dictated by the position of the fetus in the pelvis. If the fetus is at +2/5 to +3/5 station and close to delivery, manual or instrumental rotations can be helpful. Choosing the appropriate forceps is a matter of great debate. Kielland forceps were designed to help manage malpresentations, specifically deep transverse arrests and occiput posterior presentations—both of which may benefit from rotational maneuvers. More standard forceps, such as Tucker-McLean or Simpson forceps, can also be used (see Operative Delivery Procedure 2: Forceps-Assisted Vaginal Delivery). **See Gabbe 14, 17; Hacker 11.**

Inadequate Uterine Contractions

Pφ Inadequate contractions are common. The true pathophysiologic process behind them is not well understood. For whatever reason, the power of uterine contractions is inadequate to move the fetus safely and expeditiously through the birth canal. On occasion, conduction (epidural) anesthesia or oversedation has been implicated as the cause of inadequate contractions, but this is controversial.

TP Inadequate contractions are characterized by a protraction of the active phase of labor (cervical dilation less than 1.2 cm/hour in nulliparous patients, or 1.5 cm/hour in multiparous patients), or of the second stage (the "pushing" stage, after the patient reaches full cervical dilation).

Dx Diagnosis is made by careful and vigilant observation of the patient and her labor progress.

Tx Treatment typically begins with ambulation or amniotomy. Usually oxytocin augmentation will strengthen contractions sufficiently to result in cervical change. **See Gabbe 13, Hacker 11.**

Cephalopelvic Disproportion

Pφ **Fetal macrosomia**—a fetus too large for the mother to deliver safely vaginally—is becoming a more common problem owing to increasing obesity in the general population. Of course, the causes of cephalopelvic disproportion are multifactorial, involving parental genetics, increasing gestational age, and maternal diet and physiology. Gestational diabetes is one of the more common causes of fetal macrosomia.

TP Typically, macrosomia is somewhat difficult to predict, and estimations of fetal weight can be notoriously inaccurate, even with ultrasonography.

Dx The diagnosis of cephalopelvic disproportion can be made by clinical or sonographic evaluation of the estimated fetal weight and a clinical evaluation of the adequacy of the maternal pelvis. Keep in mind, however, that there can be a large margin of error when using ultrasonographic fetal weights as the primary criterion for this diagnosis. In fact, as obstetrics is currently practiced, the only way to truly make the diagnosis of cephalopelvic disproportion is to allow a trial of labor.

Tx Treatment usually requires delivery by cesarean section (see Operative Delivery Procedure 4: Cesarean Section). **See Gabbe 17, 19; Hacker 11.**

ZEBRA ZONE

a. **Breech, brow,** and **face presentations** are rare. Often they resolve with watchful waiting, or the fetus delivers vaginally in spite of the malpresentation. At times, arrested labor necessitates cesarean section.

Practice-Based Learning and Improvement: Evidence-Based Medicine

Title
Effect of mode of delivery in nulliparous women on neonatal intracranial injury

Authors
Towner D, Castro MA, Eby-Wilkens E, Gilbert WM

Institution
Department of Obstetrics and Gynecology, University of California Davis

Reference
New England Journal of Medicine 1999;341:1709–1714

Problem
Which mode of delivery is most likely to cause intracranial injury in the fetus?

Intervention
This study compares **spontaneous delivery** versus **vacuum-assisted delivery** versus forceps delivery versus **cesarean section**.

Comparison/control (quality of evidence)
A well-done study that looks at the likelihood of maternal and fetal injury when using the common obstetric interventions for dystocia.

Outcome/effect
This study demonstrated that forceps, vacuum-assisted, and cesarean deliveries all have about the same risk for intracranial injury.

Historical significance/comments
This seminal article suggests that the common risk factor for intracranial injury is not an instrumental delivery, but more likely to be an abnormal labor.

Practice-Based Learning and Improvement

Morbidity and Mortality Conference
Morbidity and Mortality (M&M) conference is the setting for presenting the cases in which patients have experienced complications or death. Typically, in a teaching hospital a senior resident presents the case and identifies what went wrong and what might have been done differently to improve the outcome. There should be open discussion of the case.

For a case in which abnormalities of labor are considered, a typical M & M might address the particular reasons a cesarean section was performed for a patient in labor. The presenting resident should describe the course of the patient's labor and should facilitate the discussion of alternative management plans. Discussion of complications to the patient or child should be based on evidence-based practice with the hope of improving care for future patients.

M & M conferences are typically "peer-review" protected, which means that the discussion should not leave the room, and that the dialogue of the meeting cannot be used in court in a prosecutory fashion.

Interpersonal and Communication Skills

Reassurance during Times of Frustration in Labor
It can be very disconcerting to a patient when she begins to show signs that her labor is not progressing normally. Commonly, through her frustration, she will jump to the conclusion that cesarean section is perhaps the only solution. At these times it is important to offer reassurance both verbally and nonverbally.

Consider your tone of voice and your body language. Verbally, explain in clear language what you think the problem might be. In this situation it is always best to be as focused as possible. You may need to explain the medical rationale for your diagnosis. For example, "I believe your labor is not progressing well because of likely cephalopelvic disproportion—the baby's head is simply too large for your pelvis" sounds much better than "Your baby is huge! You have no chance of a vaginal delivery!" Try to be nonjudgmental, and understand that a large number of patients will initially be frustrated when faced with the high likelihood of cesarean section as a result of labor dystocia. Discuss the options and allow the patient to participate in the decision-making process. If it is likely that the patient and fetus will do well regardless of the mode of the delivery, be sure to tell her this. Your tone of voice and other paralinguistic characteristics are important in conveying reassurance. Adjust your volume and pace of speech to show your concern, confidence, and commitment.

Nonverbally, also be aware of your posture and body movements. It may be appropriate to use touch to convey your reassurance too. Although there are sensitivities about touching patients, you are likely to be a good judge of when a simple gesture will reassure.

Professionalism

Principle: Commitment to Professional Competence

Remember that in virtually all obstetric cases, you are caring for two (or more in the case of multiple gestation) patients. Selecting interventions and mode of delivery must be weighed carefully against evidence describing the safest and "best" practices. Both physician and patient should understand that cesarean section is not without risk and is not to be considered the solution to all dystocia problems. On the other hand, a vaginal delivery should not be viewed as the ideal end point in and of itself, with no regard for the possibility of fetal or maternal trauma. In obstetrics/gynecology, as in other fields of medicine, the clinician must be able to select the appropriate method of intervention based on the best available evidence. This knowledge and its practical application must be mastered to help make emergent decisions with the patient and patient-couple.

Systems-Based Practice

Global Health Perspective: Obstetric Fistulas in Developing Countries

Obstetric fistula is a common childbirth injury among women living in poverty in the developing world. The injury results from prolonged obstructed labor, and can be largely prevented by the appropriate use of cesarean sections. Overall rates vary, but are highest in resource-poor nations in Africa and Asia, with rates as high as 350 per 100,000 reported in Eritrea. Obstetric fistulas can be vesicovaginal or rectovaginal, with the former leading to urinary incontinence and increased rates of urinary tract infections and the latter leading to fecal incontinence and increased rates of vaginal infections. As a result of their severe incontinence, women suffering from this injury are often socially debilitated. It is not uncommon for women suffering from severe obstetric fistulas to live secluded lives at home, unwilling to go out in public for fear of humiliation, and to be shunned by family and friends and abandoned by their husbands. Because the injury almost always results from a prolonged and obstructed labor, sufferers are too often left without a living child from the delivery. Obstetric fistulas are largely treatable with surgery, which is relatively simple and successful in 90% of cases, at relatively minimal cost. Lack of access to health care facilities and lack of health care providers trained in repairing fistulas are the major obstacles preventing more widespread treatment.

Chapter 18
Postpartum Hemorrhage (Case 7)

Renee M. Bassaly DO *and Norman A. Brest* MD

Case: A 39-year-old G4P3003 patient at 40 3/7 weeks' gestation presents to the labor and delivery floor in labor. Because of a prolonged course, the patient's labor is augmented with oxytocin. Ultimately, the mother undergoes a forceps-assisted vaginal delivery of an 8-lb, 9-oz infant. The placenta delivers shortly after the infant. After delivery of the placenta, the mother is noted to have a greater than expected amount of brisk vaginal bleeding.

Differential Diagnosis

Uterine atony	Obstetrical trauma (uterine, cervical or vaginal)	Retained placenta
Abnormal placental implantation	Coagulation disorder	

Speaking Intelligently

The evaluation of postpartum hemorrhage begins with a thorough pelvic examination looking for evidence of lacerations. Be sure to include visualization of the vaginal apex and cervix. Carefully inspect the placenta, looking for missing cotyledons that may have been retained in the uterine cavity. Palpation and massage of the uterine fundus will indicate if uterine atony is present. With atony, the uterus will feel soft and boggy to the examiner. Bleeding from other remote locations such as intravenous sites, the bladder, or skin petechiae may suggest disseminated intravascular coagulation (DIC).

After the initial evaluation our first action is to instruct the nursing staff to administer uterotonic agents to help the uterus contract and slow uterine bleeding. The initial drug of choice is intravenous oxytocin, but rectal misoprostol or intramuscular methylergonovine are also beneficial. In cases of hemorrhage, during the immediate postdelivery period the nursing staff should be checking the patient's vital signs frequently and ensuring that intravenous access is available and adequate. A second wide-bore intravenous line should be started. Emptying the bladder will often assist in facilitating uterine contractility. If retained placental tissue is suspected, manual removal, with or without curettage, is performed. Bedside ultrasonography may be used to assist with this procedure, so that it can be done with direct real-time visualization.

PATIENT CARE

Clinical Thinking

- Identify the source, and control the bleeding!
- Examine the vagina and cervix for any lacerations requiring repair.
- Perform vigorous uterine massage and administer uterotonics such as oxytocin, methylergonovine, carboprost tromethamine, or misoprostol.
- What if these measures do not work and the bleeding continues? If the patient has been given all of the various uterotonic medications in proper order and there are no obvious lacerations, you will need to call for anesthesia assistance and move the patient to the operating room.
- Order baseline lab studies, including a CBC and coagulation panel. Type and cross the patient for packed red blood cells (at least 2 units). Make sure that fresh-frozen plasma and/or cryoprecipitate are available. Intravenous access with a large-bore catheter must be available for proper fluid resuscitation.

History

- Uterine atony is the most common cause of postpartum bleeding. Accordingly, look for the risk factors of uterine atony: a full bladder, multiple gestation, fetal macrosomia, polyhydramnios, prolonged labor, oxytocin augmentation, chorioamnionitis, and multiparity.

- Has the patient been using anticoagulants, such as heparin, enoxaparin (Lovenox), warfarin, or aspirin?
- Regarding this delivery, was the length of the first or second stages of labor prolonged? What did the baby weigh? Was oxytocin used? If so, how much and for how long?
- Past medical history should include questions about personal and family history of bleeding or coagulation disorders, and history of heavy menses.
- Inquire about medical problems, especially hypertension and asthma. Past surgical history is also important.
- A detailed past obstetric history includes previous postpartum hemorrhage, parity, history of cesarean section, and any previous problems with pregnancy or delivery.

Physical Examination
- **Vital signs:** Tachycardia is the earliest sign of hemorrhagic shock. Hypotension follows as shock becomes more severe. Fever may be a sign of chorioamnionitis.
- The examination should focus on locating the source of bleeding. Palpation of the uterus can help identify atony; an enlarging uterus suggests intrauterine bleeding.
- Good exposure and ample lighting are needed for observation of vaginal, cervical, or periurethral lacerations, or retained placenta.
- Palpate the vagina and vulva for hematomas.
- Examine the patient overall, and intravenous sites in particular for signs of oozing suggestive of DIC.

Tests for Consideration
- **CBC:** To determine hemoglobin and hematocrit levels and to look for thrombocytopenia, white blood cell count to look for infection. $35
- **Prothrombin time (PT)/partial thromboplastin time (PTT)/international normalized ratio (INR):** To assess for possible DIC. $60
- **Fibrinogen/D-dimer:** To assess for possible DIC. $60
- **Type and screen:** To prepare for possible transfusion. $125

IMAGING CONSIDERATIONS

→**Ultrasonography:** Look for evidence of retained placenta. $225

→**CT scan:** Look for uterine rupture, intra-abdominal or retroperitoneal hematoma, and hemoperitoneum. $800

→**Angiography:** Can often identify the bleeding vessel and interventional techniques can be used to occlude it. $1500

Clinical Entities	**Medical Knowledge**

Uterine Atony

Pφ Uterine atony is the most common cause of postpartum hemorrhage. When placental separation occurs, myometrial contractions constrict vascular sinuses, which prevents hemorrhage. Uterine atony occurs when the uterus fails to contract, allowing continued flow of blood through the spiral arterioles after delivery.

TP Hemorrhage occurs after delivery of the placenta and is associated with a large and boggy uterus.

Dx Diagnosis is made by clinical examination with estimated blood loss of greater than 500 mL for a vaginal delivery and greater than 1000 mL for a cesarean section.

Tx Treatment is first attempted with uterine massage and emptying of the bladder. If bleeding continues, uterotonic agents are used. **Oxytocin (Pitocin)** is usually given intravenously as a first-line agent. If oxytocin fails to produce adequate uterine tone, second-line therapies should be initiated. Methylergonovine (Methergine), carboprost tromethamine (Hemabate), and misoprostol (Cytotec) are all effective therapy. The choice of second-line therapy depends upon the particular side effects and contraindications of each drug. If medical therapy is unsuccessful, surgical management will be required. The two major principles that underlie the surgical options are (1) uterine compression and (2) interruption of the uterine blood supply. (1) Compressive surgical options include uterine packing using a gauze pack or a specialized uterine (Bakri) balloon, or a B-Lynch compression stitch. (2) Surgical uterine artery or hypogastric artery ligations are effective. Angiographic occlusion (instead of surgical ligation) of pelvic vessels can be effective if the patient is stable enough to be transferred safely to the angiographic suite. Hysterectomy will be definitive for bleeding, but is considered as a last resort. **See Gabbe 18, Hacker 10.**

Agent	**Side Effects**	**Contraindications**
Oxytocin (Pitocin)	Nausea, emesis	None
Methylergonovine (Methergine)	Hypertension, hypotension, nausea, emesis	Hypertension, Pre-eclampsia
Carboprost Tromethamine (Hemabate)	Nausea, emesis, diarrhea, flushing, chills	Active cardiac, pulmonary, renal, hepatic disease
Misoprostol (Cytotec)	Tachycardia, fever	None

Trauma

Pφ Maternal pelvic trauma can occur with a spontaneous vaginal delivery or, more often, in the case of a forceps- or vacuum-assisted vaginal delivery. The risk of trauma is increased by fetal macrosomia.

TP Trauma presents after delivery with blood loss arising from the site of the laceration.

Dx Diagnosis is made by direct visualization. Careful inspection of the perineum, vagina, and cervix is required. A hematoma in the perineal area or the vaginal mucosa may be appreciated by palpation.

Tx Treatment is a site-specific repair of the laceration. Hematomas can be observed for increasing size. Often they are treated by packing the vagina with gauze. **See Gabbe 18, Hacker 10.**

Retained Placenta

Pφ The average time from delivery to expulsion of the placenta is 8 to 9 minutes. A placenta is considered retained if it fails to deliver within 30 minutes after the birth. More commonly, the term *retained placenta* refers to a fragment of the placenta that remains in the uterus (rather than the whole placenta), preventing adequate contraction of the postpartum uterus.

TP Presentation is characterized by failure to deliver the entire placenta. A portion of placental tissue may be seen at the cervix, or noted to be missing on inspection of the placenta after it has been delivered. Similar to uterine atony, a large amount of bleeding is seen coming from the uterine cavity and a boggy uterus is palpated.

Dx Diagnosis is made by clinical presentation and by manual palpation of placental tissue in the uterus. Ultrasonography can be used to aid in this diagnosis.

Tx When the entire placenta remains inside the uterus, administration of uterotonics aids in uterine contraction leading to expulsion of the placenta. Rectal misoprostol is commonly used for this indication. If this is unsuccessful, manual extraction of the placenta can be accomplished if adequate anesthesia is present. If small portions of placenta or membranes remain in the uterus, curettage of the cavity or exploration with ring forceps can aid in removal of tissue. If large portions of placenta are retained, suction curettage can be performed for evacuation of tissue. These techniques are usually performed under ultrasonographic guidance, and the patient must have adequate anesthesia. **See Gabbe 18, Hacker 10.**

Abnormal Placental Implantation

Pφ Placental implantation is abnormal when the placenta has embedded in the myometrium (the muscular wall of the uterus) without a cleavage plane for separation. A *placenta accreta* superficially invades the myometrium. A *placenta increta* penetrates deeply into the myometrium. If placental tissue grows through the full thickness of the myometrium it is called a *placenta percreta*. Risk factors for abnormal placental implantation include prior instrumentation (i.e., D&E), multiple pregnancies, prior manual extraction of a placenta, increased maternal age, and prior cesarean delivery.

TP Abnormal implantation can sometimes be identified at the time of delivery when the placenta cannot be completely removed even using the previously described maneuvers. There is usually a large amount of bleeding. Bleeding is from the placental implantation site.

Dx Abnormal placental implantation, such as placenta accreta, can often be seen on ultrasonography as well as MRI before the delivery. Direct visualization of invasion of the placenta into the bladder, bowel, or other abdominal structures at time of surgery is pathognomonic for placenta percreta. Bleeding can never be controlled and hysterectomy is usually necessary. The final diagnosis is confirmed by the pathologist.

Tx Treatment of choice when abnormal placentation is identified before delivery is cesarean section with hysterectomy. Conservative management by leaving placental fragments in situ and giving weekly methotrexate has been successful in a limited number of cases. **See Gabbe 18, Hacker 10.**

Coagulation Disorders

Pφ Coagulation disorders directly affect the patient's ability to form clots and slow bleeding. These include thrombocytopenia, von Willebrand disease, and hemophilia.

TP Presentation is uncontrollable hemorrhage after delivery from the uterus or other puncture sites. Frequently, uterine tone seems adequate in spite of continued bleeding.

Dx Diagnosis is made with lab studies. Diagnosis of von Willebrand disease includes slight to moderate reduction of activated PTT, a factor VIII level 15% to 30% of normal, a prolonged bleeding time. This diagnosis is sometimes made before delivery by eliciting a history of heavy menses. Diagnosis of a coagulopathy is suspected in patients with a history of menorrhagia, hemarthroses, bleeding gums, and the like. Genetic testing can be performed on these patients.

Tx Treatment, such as replacement of platelets and administration of desmopressin acetate (DDAVP), cryoprecipitate, or fresh-frozen plasma is based on the specific deficiency. **See Gabbe 18, Hacker 10.**

ZEBRA ZONE

a. **Uterine rupture:** A patient with a history of a previous cesarean section is at increased risk for uterine rupture when attempting a vaginal delivery. This phenomenon is very rare, but not impossible, in an unscarred uterus.

b. **Uterine inversion:** Although rare, uterine inversion can occur with excessive traction on the still attached umbilical cord when attempting to deliver the placenta.

c. **Amniotic fluid embolism:** This rare and often fatal event occurs when amniotic fluid or fetal debris travels through venous return into the pulmonary vasculature. The patient immediately complains of chest pain and shortness of breath, followed by cardiovascular collapse and DIC.

Practice-Based Learning and Improvement: Evidence-Based Medicine

Title
Is rectal misoprostol really effective in the treatment of third stage of labor? A randomized controlled trial

Authors
Caliskan E, Meydanli MM, Dilbaz B, et al.

Institution
Social Security Council: Maternity and Women's Health Teaching Hospital, Ankara, Turkey

Reference
American Journal of Obstetrics and Gynecology 2002;187:1038–1045

Problem
Postpartum hemorrhage.

Intervention
(1) Oxytocin 10 IU plus rectal misoprostol; (2) rectal misoprostol; (3) oxytocin 10 IU; and (4) oxytocin 10 IU plus methylergonovine (Methergine) 0.2 mg.

Comparison/control (quality of evidence)
Level I, randomized, controlled trial.

Outcome/effect
The incidence of postpartum hemorrhage was 9.8% in the rectal misoprostol therapy group versus 3.5% in the oxytocin and Methergine therapy group ($P = .001$). There were no significant differences among the four groups with regard to a drop in hemoglobin concentrations. Significantly more women needed additional oxytocin in the group that received only rectal misoprostol therapy, compared with the group that received oxytocin and Methergine therapy (8.3% vs. 2.2%; $P < .001$). The primary outcome measures were similar in rectal misoprostol therapy and oxytocin-only therapy.

Historical significance/comments
Because of its ease of administration, low cost, and lack of need for refrigeration, misoprostol was expected to be a very good option for the treatment of postpartum hemorrhage, especially in developing countries. However, rectal misoprostol was found to be significantly less effective than oxytocin plus Methergine for the prevention of postpartum hemorrhage.

Practice-Based Learning and Improvement: Log and Learning Plan

This is an excellent example of team-based practice-based learning and improvement.

Log and learning plan: Working with a mentor, residents keep a log of significant events or clinical surprises and develop a plan to address learning needs uncovered by these events.

The postpartum floor provides an opportunity to review the course of a patient's labor and to involve her at the bedside, if necessary. Hemorrhage, arrest of dilation, need for cesarean section, or need for instrumental delivery can all be reviewed in this setting.

Interpersonal and Communication Skills

Mental Rehearsal for Maintaining One's "Cool"

Postpartum hemorrhage is a potentially life-threatening event. Because of the severity of the situation it is of utmost importance to communicate calmly and clearly with the patient and the staff. After long hours of pushing and finally celebrating the birth of the child, the patient must now be made to realize that if her postpartum bleeding cannot be controlled with first-line medical therapies, operative measures may be rapidly required. Explaining the situation to the patient and her family in the most honest but calm and reassuring manner, while continuing to treat the patient, can be a difficult challenge. It important that you demonstrate leadership by setting the emotional tone. Remaining calm and composed is essential and helps others in the room not to "lose their cool." This scenario is fortunately infrequent, but is clearly one of the most stressful in obstetrics. Mental rehearsal of what you would do and how you would respond is a very effective strategy to prepare for any number of stressful medical situations. That is, think through systematically the possible outcomes and actions you would take, including when you would call for further help. Just as for medical "codes," mental rehearsal of postpartum hemorrhage (and similar emergent scenarios) can be extremely beneficial. If you have an opportunity to participate in simulation-based team training then it is important to practice in a controlled environment in which there is no consequence for patients. Rarely do we have an opportunity to see how we perform as a member of a team. Many simulation-based training programs provide opportunities for you to see yourself as others do. This is a powerful learning experience.

Professionalism

Principles: Patient Autonomy, Commitment to Honesty, and Primacy of Patient Welfare

Postpartum hemorrhage can be a life-threatening emergency and the obstetrician needs to act quickly. Whenever possible, however, the patient must be informed about the risks and benefits of the interventions required to stop the bleeding. She and her significant other need to understand the acute issues and the possible etiologies of the bleeding, and the potential ramifications of the therapies contemplated. Although it is of great importance to explain all of this, in a life-threatening emergency the medical needs of the patient may override the need for fully informed consent. Once the emergency has been appropriately managed it is very important that the nature of the emergency, any procedures that took place, and the long-term sequelae of these procedures be explained to the patient. Based on each individual situation, the obstetrician must decide on the proper order of informing patient and family, allowing for patient decision making and appropriate therapy.

Systems-Based Practice

Medical Errors versus Adverse Events

One in 25 vaginal deliveries (4%) will result in a postpartum hemorrhage, and 25% of all maternal deaths related to childbirth are due to postpartum hemorrhage. Although the consequences can be tragic and fatal, does fatal postpartum hemorrhage represent a medical error?

In 1999, the Institute of Medicine issued its landmark report entitled *To Err Is Human: Building a Safer Health System*, which, among other things, received considerable press attention for highlighting the fact (gleaned from two individual studies) that as many as 44,000 to 98,000 people die each year in hospitals due to medical errors.

It is important in medicine to differentiate between **adverse outcomes** and **medical errors**. The Institute of Medicine defines a medical error as "the failure to complete a planned action as intended or the use of a wrong plan to achieve an aim." An adverse event, however, is defined as "an injury caused by medical management rather than by the underlying disease or condition of the patient." Not all adverse events are preventable: these are the inherent risks associated with treatment, and these are not considered medical errors. Consider a patient, for example, who dies from an unknown allergic reaction to an antibiotic. The patient is fatally injured by the treatment, and not the underlying disease, and thus this constitutes an adverse event. If, however, the patient's drug allergy was already known, this represents a preventable adverse event and therefore a medical error. Accordingly, a subset (some studies suggest the majority) of adverse events are preventable and thus considered medical errors. Conversely, only a small subset of medical errors actually results in adverse events.

By these definitions, postpartum hemorrhage after vaginal delivery is not an adverse event because it is not caused by medical management—to the contrary, it is an inherent risk of the postpartum condition, and was until modern times among the leading causes of death of young women. Death from postpartum hemorrhage, however, is widely believed to be preventable given the methods of observation and treatment available in a modern hospital. Evidence suggests that most deaths from postpartum hemorrhage indeed occur owing to delay in recognition and treatment. Because hospitals and birthing centers can have protocols in place to prevent and manage postpartum hemorrhage, any failure to do so would be considered a medical error.

As the health care system begins to uncover all the ways in which medical errors can be prevented, there seems to be agreement that the most significant reductions in medical errors need to derive from improvements to the *system* and not from the individual players within it.

Chapter 19
Teaching Visual: Managing Postpartum Hemorrhage

Neelesh Welling MD, Deborah M. Davenport MD, and Michael Belden MD

Objective

■ Describe a coherent, sequential course of action to control postpartum hemorrhage.

Medical Knowledge

- Post-partum hemorrhage is one of the most difficult obstetric emergencies the obstetrician will encounter. Fortunately infrequent, it is important to be able to assess the severity of bleeding quickly and to make appropriate interventions.
- Examine the patient and identify the source of bleeding. Let other members of the team attend to IV access, acquire necessary blood products, contact consultants as needed, and attend to concerns for changing the mode and locale of anesthesia—as may be required.
- As soon as a source of bleeding is identified, make the appropriate interventions for repair. Vaginal and cervical lacerations should be locally repaired as patient tolerance permits.
- If placental fragments remain within the uterus, remove them.
- For uterine atony, begin massage and be sure you know the appropriate sequence of uterotonic medications.
- When uterotonic medications fail to control bleeding, be mindful of options in the operating room and be cognizant of when angiographic intervention may be appropriate.

- The details of working through this problem have been set forth in the preceding chapter. This Teaching Visual has been placed here to challenge you to review the previous material and think through an appropriate treatment algorithm.

The following exercise provides an opportunity to work through the proper sequence of maneuvers, should you be faced with postpartum hemorrhage. Though there may be subtle differences from institution to institution, the principles and general course of management of post-partum hemorrhage are reasonably standard.

First, study the ovals and rectangles below and note the following competency-based representations:

Red Rectangles = Patient Care Actions
Lavender Rectangles = Medications
Orange Oval = Practice-Based Improvement
Blue Oval = Professional Interactions
Teal Oval = Interpersonal Interactions
Green Oval = Systems-Based Interactions

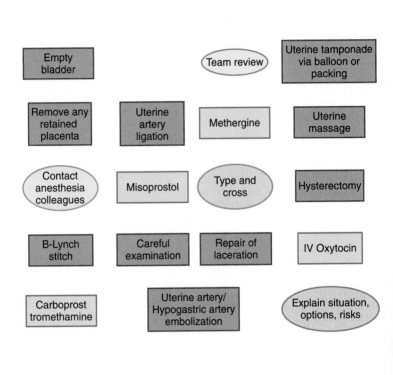

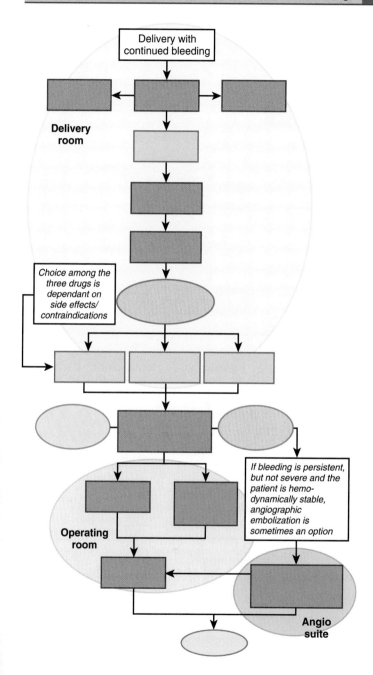

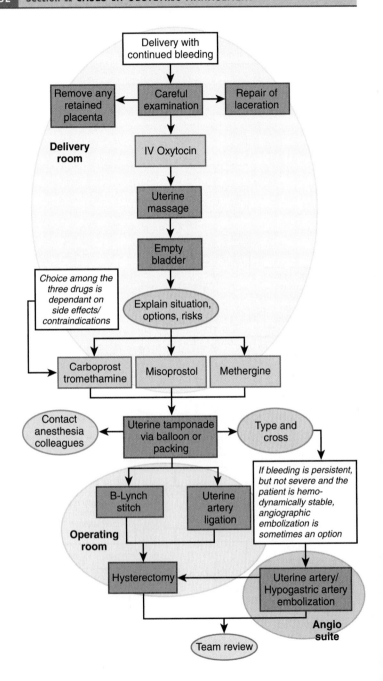

Professor's Pearls: Cases in Obstetrics Management

Consider the following clinical problems and questions posed. Then refer to the professor's discussion of these issues.

1. A 32-year-old G1P0 with a singleton intrauterine pregnancy at 39 1/7 weeks presents with chief complaints of vaginal bleeding and painful contractions. She noted that the vaginal bleeding started 1 hour ago and that her contractions started at onset of the vaginal bleeding. The patient notes good fetal movement and no leakage of fluid. The pregnancy has been uncomplicated and her group B streptococcus (GBS) test result is negative. On exam you note bloody show and decide to proceed with a cervical exam. She is 3 cm dilated, 90% effaced, and −2 station. Fetal monitoring is reassuring and she is contracting every 2 minutes. She desires natural childbirth and declines pain control. Thirty minutes later, she complains of intense pressure. You note that the perineum is covered with bloody discharge and the patient has achieved complete dilation. What is the diagnosis?

2. A 28-year-old G2P0111 with a singleton intrauterine pregnancy at 37 2/7 weeks presents with a chief complaint of leakage of fluid. One hour ago, she was voiding and "felt a pop." She has had clear continuous drainage ever since. She notes good fetal movement and no vaginal bleeding or contractions. She has had an uncomplicated pregnancy and her GBS test result is positive. Her prior delivery was at 37 weeks and the infant was delivered vaginally with no complications. On sterile speculum exam, you note that there is pooling, ferning, and Nitrazine-positive fluid. She is 3 cm dilated, 90% effaced, and −2 station. Fetal monitoring is reassuring and she is not contracting. What is your plan of management for her?

3. A 39-year-old G1P0 with a singleton intrauterine pregnancy at 40 1/7 weeks presents with complaint of painful contractions. The contractions became painful 4 hours ago. The patient notes good fetal movement, a small amount of bloody show, and no leakage of fluid. She states that she has developed gestational diabetes during this pregnancy, which was managed with insulin. She had ultrasonography 1 week ago that showed her estimated fetal weight in the 85th percentile. Her GBS test result is negative. On exam you note bloody show and decide to proceed with a cervical exam. She is 3 cm dilated, 50% effaced, and −1 station. Fetal monitoring is reassuring and she is contracting every 4 minutes. She desires an epidural. What is your approach to this patient? What factors are concerning in creating a plan for her delivery?

Discussion by Dr. Kaighn Smith, Chairman Emeritus of the Department of Obstetrics and Gynecology, The Lankenau Hospital, Wynnewood, Pennsylvania

Answer 1: Clinical Considerations: Cervical Lacerations and Placental Abruption

The sort of clinical situation described in the case is unusual for a primigravida. She has had a precipitous labor and may have a deep cervical laceration as a result. There might also be a partial placental abruption as a contributing factor. I wonder if she has had a previous D&C or D&E, which could have weakened her cervix? She should have a vaginal delivery and careful inspection of the vagina and cervix immediately after delivery.

Answer 2: Clinical Considerations: Inducing Labor

Do we have to worry about this patient? I think not. She is not yet in labor but has a "ripe," or favorable cervical exam. Because her pregnancy is full term and she has a favorable cervical exam (as well as a positive GBS screening culture), there is little to be gained with expectant or conservative management. Start oxytocin and expect an uneventful outcome.

Answer 3: Clinical Considerations: Anticipating Placental Insufficiency

This patient has "two strikes" against her from a placental function point of view. She is an older primigravida and is an insulin-dependent gestational diabetic. That she is also not hypertensive is a blessing. Fetal monitoring may be reassuring now, but as labor progresses fetal distress could easily develop. A cesarean section would then become necessary. As long as her fetal monitoring is reassuring she should be allowed to labor, but delivery could be hastened by judicious vacuum extraction or low forceps if there are any signs of trouble with the monitor strip. A prolonged second stage should be avoided. Be entirely prepared for the possibility of shoulder dystocia.

Section III
CASES IN MATERNAL/ FETAL MEDICINE

Section Editor
Gary D. Blake MD

Section Contents

Chapter 20
Early Pregnancy Loss and Miscarriage (Case 8)

Suzanne S. Nogami MD

Case: A 25-year-old G1P0 with an intrauterine pregnancy at 8 6/7 weeks based on her LMP presents to the Emergency Department with vaginal bleeding.

Differential Diagnosis

Categorization of Spontaneous Abortion		
Threatened abortion	Complete abortion	Missed abortion
Incomplete abortion	Inevitable abortion	Recurrent abortion

Other Reasons for Vaginal Bleeding in Early Pregnancy		
Postcoital bleeding	Ectopic pregnancy	Vaginal or cervical laceration
Cervicitis		Normal intrauterine pregnancy

Speaking Intelligently

When a patient of reproductive age presents to the emergency room with a gynecologic or obstetric problem or with abdominal pain, you **must** check a human chorionic gonadotropin (β-hCG) level. With a positive β-hCG and vaginal bleeding, **always** think about an ectopic pregnancy because a ruptured ectopic pregnancy can be a true emergency. In conjunction with a β-hCG, ultrasonography of the pelvis is essential. In the face of vaginal bleeding, once an ectopic pregnancy and a normal intrauterine pregnancy can be reasonably excluded, you must consider the various diagnoses listed in the preceding differential diagnosis boxes.

PATIENT CARE

Clinical Thinking
- Confirm that the patient is pregnant using the history and β-hCG
- Identify the location of the pregnancy with transvaginal ultrasonography.
- After the pregnancy and its location are confirmed, formulate a management plan.

History
- The LMP, regularity of menses, and sexual activity are paramount concerns that must be addressed in the initial history.
- As a consultant, it is almost always appropriate to ask the questions you feel are medically relevant and hear the answers from the patient yourself, regardless of what you are told by other health care providers, including emergency department physician colleagues and nurses. It is occasionally appropriate to excuse family members for this segment of the history to ensure patient truthfulness and confidentiality.
- Take a thorough obstetric and gynecologic history. Be sure to ask about vaginal bleeding, prior similar episodes, pain, cramping, history of prior miscarriages, and the passage of tissue associated with vaginal bleeding.

Physical Examination
- Vital signs are essential: is the patient hemodynamically stable?
- Do the patient's abdominal and pelvic examinations reveal the diagnosis?
- Pay particular attention to the appearance of the cervix. Assess whether the cervical os is open or closed.
- Assess the amount of bleeding; if pregnancy tissue is observed in the cervix or vagina, and
- Assess for overall uterine tenderness.

Tests for Consideration
- **Quantitative β-hCG:** Be sure to obtain this test as soon as possible. $135
- **CBC:** The hemoglobin and hematocrit can suggest intra-abdominal bleeding or hemorrhage if these levels are lower than anticipated. $35
- **Gonorrhea/chlamydial cultures:** These tests are easy to perform at the time of the examination and have a high yield. $250
- **Wet prep:** Allows you to assess for bacterial vaginitis, trichomoniasis, and candidiasis. $60

IMAGING CONSIDERATIONS

→**Pelvic and abdominal ultrasonography:** Evaluates the location of pregnancy, fetal viability, and accurately assesses estimated date of confinement and gestational age. $225

Clinical Entities	Medical Knowledge

Threatened Abortion

Pφ The pathophysiology of most first-trimester bleeding is unknown. Threatened abortions represent 25% of all pregnancies, and 50% of these progress to spontaneous abortion. A history of threatened abortion in a pregnancy increases the risk of preterm delivery, low birth weight, perinatal mortality, preterm labor, and preterm premature rupture of membranes. First-trimester bleeding is not associated with an increased risk of congenital malformation.

TP Typical presentation of threatened abortion is characterized by vaginal bleeding associated with an established intrauterine pregnancy. Abdominal pain and cramping are frequently, but not always, present. In the case of threatened abortion the cervix has not dilated, and the products of conception have not been spontaneously expelled.

Dx Diagnosis is reached using history, physical examination, quantitative β-hCG, and ultrasonography.

Tx The diagnosis of threatened abortion requires no particular intervention other than close follow-up. The patient requires reassurance and recommendations regarding the resumption of normal activities, or extended rest. Indeed, reassurance is probably the most helpful "therapy" one can provide. Pelvic rest for 2 to 3 weeks is suggested. Rho(D) immune globulin (RhoGAM) should be given if the patient is Rh negative. The patient should be instructed regarding the need for follow-up β-hCG levels and further ultrasonography, if indicated. **See Katz 16, Hacker 7.**

Incomplete Abortion

Pφ Incomplete abortion represents the partial passage of a miscarriage, with some products of conception expelled and some products still present in the uterine cavity.

TP	Typical presentation is vaginal bleeding with associated abdominal pain. Some products of conception have been expelled, and sometimes this can be observed on physical examination.
Dx	Diagnosis is made using history, physical, quantitative β-hCG, and ultrasonography if appropriate.
Tx	Therapy may be expectant or more interventional, including a D&E. RhoGAM should be given if the patient is Rh negative. **See Katz 16, Hacker 7.**

Complete Abortion

Pφ	Complete abortion represents full expulsion of the products of conception from the uterus.
TP	All products of conception are expelled from the uterine cavity with associated bleeding and cramping.
Dx	Diagnosis is made using physical examination, ultrasonography, and β-hCG levels. Following up on the pathology of products of conception can be of great value, especially if it is unclear if the patient has spontaneously passed all of the pregnancy tissue.
Tx	Monitor for bleeding and infection. RhoGAM should be given if the patient is Rh negative. **See Katz 16, Hacker 7.**

Inevitable Abortion

Pφ	Inevitable abortion is characterized by a pregnancy, viable or not, that cannot proceed onward and is destined to miscarry.
TP	Typical presentation is vaginal bleeding with abdominal pain and **cervical dilation.** Products of conception are usually expelled shortly thereafter.
Dx	Diagnosis is made by history and physical examination, along with pathology of products of conception.
Tx	Expectant management or performing a D&E are acceptable. Misoprostol can sometimes be used because it results in cervical dilation and uterine contractions. RhoGAM should be given if the patient is Rh negative. **See Katz 16, Hacker 7.**

Missed Abortion

Pφ Missed abortion usually progresses to complete abortion in 1 to 3 weeks, but this can vary by individual.

TP Typical presentation is a nonviable pregnancy diagnosed before the 20th week, but without associated bleeding, cramping, and passage of tissue.

Dx This diagnosis is almost always made using ultrasonography.

Tx Expectant management, D&E, or administration of misoprostol are acceptable. RhoGAM should be given if the patient is Rh negative. **See Katz 16, Hacker 7.**

Recurrent Abortion

Pφ Recurrent abortion occurs in approximately 1% of women of reproductive age, and in only 50% of these cases will the true etiology of this problem be diagnosed.

TP Typical presentation is three or more first-trimester pregnancy losses, usually in succession.

Dx Diagnosis is based on history of the above.

Tx The management of this problem is often handled by maternal/fetal medicine specialists or reproductive endocrinologists. Offer emotional support, sometimes with the assistance of organized support groups, and recommend genetic counseling. The following studies may be indicated in the evaluation: parental karyotyping, anti-cardiolipin antibodies (IgG, IgM), lupus anticoagulant, day 3 follicle-stimulating hormone (FSH) and estradiol, factor V Leiden, protein S, activated protein C, prothrombin G20210A, thyroid-stimulating hormone (TSH), and thyroid peroxidase antibody. Any identifiable uterine abnormality (e.g., uterine septum or uterine scarring) must be corrected. **See Katz 16, Hacker 7.**

Postcoital Bleeding

Pφ The cervix is very friable/sensitive during pregnancy.

TP The patient experiences vaginal bleeding (often after intercourse); at times there may be associated pain.

Dx Diagnosis is made by history and physical examination.

Tx Recommend pelvic rest and offer reassurance.

Ectopic Pregnancy

Pφ The history of an ectopic pregnancy increases the risk of a subsequent ectopic pregnancy. Ectopic pregnancy is the cause of 9% of all maternal deaths.

TP Severe abdominal pain sometimes associated with vaginal bleeding.

Dx Diagnosis is made by history, physical examination, blood count, β-hCG and abdominal and pelvic ultrasonography.

Tx If the patient is clinically unstable, treatment should be surgical and immediate. If the patient is stable and you can be assured of good patient compliance and follow-up, medical management with methotrexate may be considered. RhoGAM is given if the patient is Rh negative. **See Katz 17, Hacker 24.**

Vaginal/Cervical Laceration

Pφ Laceration of the cervical capillaries results in vaginal bleeding.

TP Typical presentation is vaginal bleeding.

Dx Diagnosis is made by history and physical examination.

Tx Expectant management is acceptable, with possible application of sutures or pressure. **See Katz 18, Hacker 19.**

Cervicitis

Pφ Inflammatory changes in the cervix result in bleeding.

TP Typical presentation is vaginal or cervical bleeding.

Dx History and physical examination are key to diagnosis; gonorrhea and chlamydial cultures are helpful, as is a wet prep test.

Tx Gonorrhea: ceftriaxone 125 mg IM or cefixime 400 mg PO, plus treat for assumed chlamydial coinfection (azithromycin 1 g PO). **See Katz 22, Hacker 22.**

Normal Intrauterine Pregnancy

Pφ Normal, appropriate intrauterine pregnancy.

TP Normal pregnancies can, on occasion, be associated with bleeding and painful cramps, especially in the first trimester.

Dx	The diagnosis of a normal intrauterine pregnancy can be made with appropriately rising β-hCG levels and ultrasonography.
Tx	No therapy is required for a normal intrauterine pregnancy with pain and vaginal bleeding except reassurance. **See Hacker 7.**

ZEBRA ZONE

a. **Molar pregnancy or gestational trophoblastic neoplasia:** This is an uncommon cause of heavy vaginal bleeding in early pregnancy (see Chapter 55, Gestational Trophoblastic Disease).

Practice-Based Learning and Improvement: Evidence-Based Medicine

Title
Expectant care versus surgical treatment for miscarriage

Authors
Nanda K, Peloggia A, Grimes D, et al.

Institution
Family Health International, Clinical Research Department

Reference
Cochrane Database Systematic Reviews 2006(2):CD003518

Problem
Evaluates expectant management versus surgical intervention in the treatment of miscarriage.

Intervention
Dilation and evacuation versus expectant management.

Outcome/effect
Expectant management led to a higher rate of incomplete abortion, and surgery resulted in a higher infection rate.

Historical significance/comments
This Cochrane Review demonstrates that the care for patients with miscarriage must be individualized, and the patient's preference may be used in the decision-making process. Note that Cochrane Reviews are standardized analyses of particular treatments or interventions. These Reviews typically select only the best, most highly powered studies, and carry a fair amount of evidence-based credibility.

Interpersonal and Communication Skills

Delivering Bad News

Delivering information to patients that they will perceive as "bad" requires a complex set of skills. Do not assume that all patients will value the same information in the same way. Miscarriage may have different meanings for different patients.

Miscarriage and early pregnancy loss are very common. It is important to help the patient realize that many such occurrences are due to severe chromosomal anomalies and that no medical intervention is needed. Further, by way of alleviating potential guilt, it is important for the physician to emphasize that there is almost nothing a patient can do to prevent a miscarriage.

Empathy is the ability to acknowledge the patient's emotions. Empathic statements include:

- "I can see this is very upsetting for you."
- "I know this is distressing."

When empathic statements are coupled with reassurance, the patient is likely to feel supported. Examples include:

- "Please understand that this is not your fault ... miscarriages are common and are almost always a result of embryonic chromosome abnormalities."
- "Virtually all couples have at least one or two miscarriages throughout the course of their lives ... they are far more common than many people think, and are almost never a medical emergency, so it is unlikely anything bad will happen to you as a result of this."
- "Based on experience there is an extremely good chance you will be back in the next year or so with a healthy and normal pregnancy."

These sorts of communication techniques provide empathy and encouragement while delivering bad news effectively. You should also make the point, when it is appropriate, that a single miscarriage does not predict future pregnancy loss. Only after three consecutive miscarriages is further evaluation warranted, and this is usually done in conjunction with a perinatologist or reproductive endocrinologist.

Professionalism

Principles: Social Justice and Patient Autonomy

At some time in your career, you may find a patient's personal beliefs in conflict with what you believe to be in her best interest. Consider, for example, the Jehovah's Witness who presents to the emergency department requiring emergency surgery for a ruptured ectopic pregnancy and refuses the use of blood products because of her religious beliefs. The obstetric surgeon may be placed in a difficult position. It is our professional responsibility to provide equal care to all people regardless of their religious beliefs. However, if a surgeon does not feel comfortable performing a surgery in which there may be considerable loss of blood without the option to transfuse, it may be most appropriate to arrange for transfer of care to a surgeon who would be comfortable under such circumstances. Because of the potentially disastrous consequences of waiting for surgery, however, such a transfer would be appropriate only if there were no undue delay. Otherwise, the principle of patient autonomy would apply and the surgery should be performed without transfusion. For more in depth on Jehovah's Witnesses and transfusion, see the *Journal of Medical Ethics* at http://www.ajwrb.org/physicians/jme.shtml.

Systems-Based Practice

Case Management: History, Purpose, and Utilization

In cases of early pregnancy loss and multiple miscarriages, it is important to coordinate the care provided by radiologists, subspecialists (e.g., perinatologists and reproductive endocrinologists), genetic counselors, grief counselors, and other care providers. In such situations, case managers can be especially helpful. The Case Management Society of America defines case management as "a collaborative process of assessment, planning, facilitation and advocacy for options and services to meet an individual's health needs through communication and available resources to promote quality cost-effective outcomes." Although case managers have been around for many decades, the role of case management in health care became particularly important during the rise of managed care in the 1990s. Because effective case management can both increase the quality of care as well as decrease overall costs, case managers are often used by hospitals, insurance companies, and employers, each of whom has an interest in ensuring high-quality, cost-effective care. Case managers at a hospital often focus on verifying coverage and benefits, coordinating services associated with discharge, coordinating care with other health care providers, providing patient education, and providing postcare follow-up. Case managers employed by an insurance company focus on ensuring that care fits within the patient's specified benefits, negotiating rates with providers who are not part of the plan's network, coordinating referrals to specialists, arranging for special services, and helping patients to access government and community services when available. Health plan case managers also work proactively to identify patients with potentially expensive complications and to minimize the expected costs—which often involves providing higher-quality care. For example, a health plan's case manager may proactively identify high-risk pregnancies and provide those mothers with access to prenatal care. Employers in larger companies may hire case managers to work on similar issues that are in the employer's interests, such as verifying medical reasons for employee absences, providing health education, and assisting employees with chronic illnesses.

Chapter 21
Hypertensive Disorders in Pregnancy (Case 9)

Gennady G. Miroshnichenko MD, Paul S. Robbins DO and Andrew Gerson MD

Case: An 18-year-old African-American G2P0010 presents to the labor and delivery suite at 36 and 2/7 weeks of pregnancy with complaints of severe headache, blurred vision, and epigastric pain with nausea and vomiting. The patient has noted progressive edema of her feet within the past week. She also states that she has no prenatal care with this current pregnancy. On admission, patient's blood pressure is 182/110.

Differential Diagnosis

Mild preeclampsia	Gestational hypertension	Eclampsia
Severe preeclampsia and HELLP syndrome	Chronic hypertension	Superimposed preeclampsia with chronic hypertension

Speaking Intelligently

Elevated blood pressure in pregnant patients significantly increases maternal and fetal morbidity and mortality. The overall approach to hypertensive conditions in pregnancy is to assess maternal and fetal wellbeing, by judicious use of history, physical exam, and laboratory findings, and then to decide if delivery is indicated. Understanding the spectrum of physiologic changes which occur during pregnancy is essential in choosing the right approach and medical therapy.

PATIENT CARE

Clinical Thinking

- First, determine if the patient has any risk factors for development of hypertensive disorders in pregnancy. Your considerations should be young age, advanced age, first pregnancy, advanced parity, and a history of preeclampsia with a prior pregnancy.
- Assess the severity of the condition.
- Assess maternal and fetal well-being.
- What is the most ominous condition you would encounter in this patient? Unless she is having a true eclamptic seizure, severe preeclampsia including its variant **HELLP** syndrome (**H**emolysis, **E**levated **L**iver Enzymes, and **L**ow **P**latelets) should be considered the most worrisome possibility in the differential diagnosis of pregnant patients with elevated blood pressure (BP). The two main goals of management are prevention of seizures (eclampsia) and control of hypertension. The appropriate work-up, including physical examination and laboratory work, should be undertaken simultaneously as you differentiate the acuity and severity of the hypertensive disorder.
- Is there an ultimate treatment for preeclampsia/eclampsia? Fortunately, we know that most cases of preeclampsia resolve shortly after delivery. What can complicate matters is that not all cases of preeclampsia develop after 37 weeks of gestation, when delivery of a mature infant is warranted. Remember that obstetric conditions such as this present with two patients who must be taken into consideration. Fetal well-being and the risks of prematurity must always be balanced in relation to the health of the mother.
- How do the severity of the condition and gestational age of the fetus influence the management? Women with mild disease developing at 36 weeks' gestation or later, or those who are considered

noncompliant, should undergo induction of labor. Delivery is also recommended for those with mild disease at a gestational age of 34 weeks or more in the presence of labor, rupture of membranes, or nonreassuring fetal testing results or fetal growth restriction.

- The presence of severe disease mandates immediate hospitalization. During the observation period, maternal and fetal conditions are assessed and a decision is made regarding the need for delivery. Those with gestational age of 24 to 34 weeks are given corticosteroids to accelerate fetal lung maturity. Patients with resistant severe hypertension despite maximum doses of intravenous antihypertensive medications or neurologic symptoms while on magnesium sulfate should be delivered within 24 to 48 hours regardless of fetal age. Patients with HELLP syndrome or a serum creatinine level of 2 mg/dL or more should also be delivered within 48 hours.

- Patients with a pregnancy of 24 to 34 weeks' gestation and who have severe preeclampsia are given corticosteroids and then delivered after 48 hours. Those with a gestational age below 23 weeks are offered termination of pregnancy as a choice of last resort. This is a matter of maternal well-being because severe preeclampsia can jeopardize the life of the mother if no effective treatment can be provided.

- How to choose the mode of delivery? There are no randomized trials comparing optimal methods of delivery. A plan for vaginal delivery should be attempted for all women with mild disease and for the majority of women with severe disease, particularly those beyond 30 weeks' gestation.

- The decision to perform cesarean delivery should be based on gestational age, fetal condition, presence of labor, and cervical Bishop score (Bishop score is a synthesis of cervical physical examination findings that predicts the favorability of a patient's cervix for a vaginal delivery).

- Elective cesarean delivery would be recommended for all women with severe preeclampsia below 30 weeks' gestation who are not in labor with a low Bishop score, suggesting low likelihood of a successful vaginal delivery. In addition, elective cesarean delivery would be preferable for those with severe preeclampsia and fetal growth restriction if gestational age is below 32 weeks in presence of unfavorable Bishop score.

History
- Determine the age, gravity, and the length of time the patient has had an elevated BP. Of the risk factors associated with preeclampsia, nulliparity, multifetal gestations, preeclampsia in a previous pregnancy, chronic hypertension, pregestational diabetes, vascular and connective tissue disease, nephropathy, antiphospholipid

antibody syndrome, obesity, age 35 years or older, and African-American race are among the most important.
- Thoroughly assess the patient's complaints, particularly signs and symptoms of end-organ damage, such as severe headache, visual changes, epigastric or right upper quadrant pain, nausea/vomiting, and decreased urine output. Intrauterine growth restriction is also considered end-organ damage.
- Onset of hypertension in relation to gestational age helps to distinguish between gestational and chronic hypertension.
- The gestational age at the onset of preeclampsia as well as the gestational age of the fetus at the time of delivery would predict maternal and perinatal prognosis. Early-onset preeclampsia usually carries a worse prognosis.

Physical Examination
- **General appearance:** The typical patient with severe preeclampsia will truly look ill. Many patients complain of feeling "horrible," with a sense of tiredness and crushing fatigue. The headache associated with preeclampsia is described as intolerable, the "worst headache ever." Severe preeclampsia is also characterized by visual disturbances, epigastric pain, nausea, vomiting, and oliguria, which are all signs of multiorgan involvement.
- **Vital signs:** Elevated BP of 140/90 or higher would indicate mild disease, whereas a BP elevation of 160/110 or higher indicates severe preeclampsia. Maternal tachycardia is usually explained by contraction of the intravascular space due to vasospasm and subsequent hemoconcentration.
- **Lungs:** Bibasilar rales can be appreciated in the case of pulmonary edema in patients with unrecognized severe preeclampsia, particularly after expansion of their intravascular space with vigorous fluid resuscitation.
- **Abdominal examination:** The estimated fetal weight during abdominal examination may reveal possible fetal growth restriction due to the chronic hypertensive condition associated with vascular changes of the fetoplacental unit. The palpation of a painful uterus in the state of hypertonus may raise the suspicion for placental abruption.
- **Neurologic examination:** Hyperreflexia with the presence of myoclonus will be appreciated in patients with central nervous system involvement and would immediately warrant the administration of magnesium sulfate for seizure prophylaxis.
- **Extremities:** Edema can be significant due to capillary leakage and decreased colloid oncotic pressure. This is often the first finding patients identify themselves, and is described by the patient as rapidly progressing, first involving the lower and then upper extremities, face, and abdominal wall.

Tests for Consideration

- **CBC:** Low hemoglobin due to hemolysis and thrombocytopenia (platelet count <100,000/mm^3) may occur as part of HELLP syndrome. $38
- **LDH:** Lactate dehydrogenase is present in erythrocytes in high concentrations. A disproportionate elevation of LDH in serum may be a sign of hemolysis. $42
- **Uric acid:** An elevated serum level of uric acid usually occurs with renal hypoperfusion due to vasoconstriction and hemoconcentration. However, the positive predictable value to identify high-risk patients is only 33%. $38
- **Serum creatinine:** Elevated level suggests renal hypoperfusion. $23
- **Liver enzymes:** Elevated levels of aspartate aminotransferase (AST) and alanine aminotransferase (ALT) are observed as a part of HELLP syndrome. $78
- **Peripheral blood smear:** The classic findings of microangiopathic hemolysis include an abnormal peripheral blood smear with schistocytes, burr cells, and fragmented red blood cell morphology.   Free*
- **Nonstress test or biophysical profile:** This helps to assess fetal well-being. $300

*and instructive, if you do this yourself.

IMAGING CONSIDERATIONS

→**Perinatal ultrasonography:** In the assessment of fetus, fluid, and placenta, this is an excellent tool to diagnose fetal growth restriction and oligohydramnios due to vasculopathy of the fetoplacental unit secondary to maternal hypertensive disease. $245

→**Doppler velocimetry:** Increased vascular resistance of uterine, umbilical, and fetal middle cerebral arteries can be very sensitive in diagnosis of fetal growth restriction in hypertensive disorders of pregnancy. $375

→**CT scan/MRI of brain:** Although not routine tests, these are considered if a patient experiences a change in mental status. These tests will reveal the presence of edema or infarction in the subcortical white matter and adjacent gray matter, mostly in the parieto-occipital lobes, in approximately 50% of patients with eclampsia. These tests are not essential, but indicated for differentiating between the diagnoses of eclampsia and cerebrovascular accidents, previously undiagnosed brain tumors, and metastatic gestational trophoblastic disease. $800

Clinical Entities   Medical Knowledge

Mild Preeclampsia

Pφ Preeclampsia is a disorder unique to pregnancy, characterized by poor perfusion of multiple vital organs (including the maternal brain, liver, kidneys, and fetoplacental unit) secondary to vasospasm. Preeclampsia completely reverses after delivery.

TP Preeclampsia is primarily a disease of the first pregnancy. Obesity and insulin resistance are also risk factors associated with preeclampsia. Patients usually present with elevated BP, and proteinuria with consequent peripheral edema due to loss of intravascular oncotic pressure and increased vascular permeability. This leads to third-spacing. The signs and symptoms of hypoperfusion of vital organs can be significant, leading to headache, visual changes, right upper quadrant/epigastric pain, shortness of breath, and pulmonary congestion.

Dx Elevated BP of 140/90 or higher that occurs after 20 weeks of gestation in a patient with previously normal blood pressures. Proteinuria should be 300 mg or more in a 24-hour urine collection.

Tx The ultimate treatment of preeclampsia is delivery. However, mild preeclampsia can be managed expectantly in certain select circumstances, particularly when the patient has not reached full term. Initially, the patient with suspected preeclampsia should be hospitalized and carefully monitored with frequented lab evaluations and vigilant fetal surveillance. If the patient appears stable, and the preeclampsia does not appear to be worsening, outpatient management can be an option with weekly or semi-weekly non-stress testing or biophysical profiles, and vigilant lab evaluations.

Severe Preeclampsia and HELLP Syndrome

Pφ The pathophysiologic process that causes preeclampsia is not well understood. Furthermore, it is not clear why certain patients with preeclampsia will progress to severe preeclampsia. The constellation of laboratory findings characterized by **H**emolysis, **E**levated **L**iver enzymes, and **L**ow **P**latelet count is called HELLP syndrome. HELLP syndrome is observed in about 20% of patients who have severe preeclampsia.

TP Severe preeclampsia is characterized by oliguria, severe headache and/or visual disturbances, pulmonary edema, right upper quadrant pain and/or generalized upper abdominal pain. Edema is often present. Interestingly, protienuria can sometimes be absent, but this is rare.

Dx The diagnosis of **severe preeclampsia** is made when one or more of the following criteria is met:
- BP of 160/110 or higher on two separate occasions
- Proteinuria of 5 g or higher in 24-hour urine collection
- Thrombocytopenia (usually <100,000/mm^3)
- Abnormal liver enzymes in association with persistent epigastric or right upper quadrant pain
- Multiorgan involvement such as cerebral or visual disturbances, pulmonary edema, or oliguria (<500 mL/24 hours)
- Fetal growth restriction

Tx The ultimate treatment of preeclampsia is delivery. The goals of management are prevention of seizures, control of hypertension, and a good maternal/fetal outcome. The use of magnesium sulfate is highly efficacious for the prevention of seizures. A suggested regimen of **intravenous magnesium sulfate** is a 6-g loading dose (producing serum Mg levels of 5 to 7 mg/dL) followed by 2 g/hr continuous magnesium sulfate infusion with resultant Mg levels of 4 to 8 mg/dL. Intravenous magnesium sulfate infusion continues throughout the process of labor and in most situations for at least 24 hours in the postpartum period. Antihypertensive therapy is generally recommended for systolic BP levels of 160 to 180 or higher, and diastolic BP of 105 to 110 mm Hg or higher. Labetalol and hydralazine are the two agents most commonly used:
- **Labetalol:** 20-mg IV bolus dose followed by 40 mg if not effective within 10 minutes; then, 80 mg every 10 minutes to maximum total dose of 220 mg.
- **Hydralazine:** 5- to 10-mg doses IV every 15 to 20 minutes until desired response is achieved, for maximum dose of 30 mg.
- **Nifedipine:** 10 to 20 mg orally every 30 minutes for a maximum dose of 50 mg. Recent studies have suggested that oral nifedipine is as effective as the foregoing medications, but with fewer side effects.

See Gabbe 33, Hacker 14.

Gestational Hypertension

Pφ Gestational hypertension is a disorder in which elevated BP without proteinuria develops in a woman after 20 weeks of gestation and BP levels return to normal within 12 weeks postpartum.

TP The disorder is more prevalent in healthy nulliparous women. The rate is increased in women with previous preeclampsia and in women with multiple gestations. The rate of progression to preeclampsia reaches 50% when gestational hypertension develops before 30 weeks of gestation.

Dx Diagnosis is based on a systolic BP of at least 140 mm Hg and/ or a diastolic BP of at least 90 mm Hg on at least two occasions at least 6 hours but no more than 7 days apart. **Severe gestational hypertension** is diagnosed if there is sustained elevation in systolic BP to at least 160 and/or in diastolic BP to at least 110 mm Hg for at least 6 hours.

Tx The main goal in the initial evaluation of women with gestational hypertension is to distinguish this disorder from preeclampsia. Most patients can be safely managed on an outpatient basis with twice-weekly antenatal testing. *Antihypertensive agents should be avoided, unless hypertension is severe, because medical therapy of mild hypertension has not been shown to improve neonatal outcome.* Severe hypertension is treated with antihypertensive agents to reduce the risk of potential cerebrovascular and cardiovascular complications. Generally, women with severe gestational hypertension should be managed as inpatients. **See Gabbe 33, Hacker 14.**

Chronic Hypertension

Pφ Chronic hypertension is subdivided into two categories: primary (essential) and secondary. Essential hypertension is by far the most common cause of hypertension seen in pregnancy (90%). In about 10% of cases, chronic hypertension occurs secondary to the following disorders: renal disease (glomerulonephritis, interstitial nephritis, and polycystic kidney disease), collagen vascular disease (lupus, scleroderma), and endocrine disorders (diabetes mellitus with renal involvement, Cushing disease, thyrotoxicosis, hyperaldosteronism).

TP Patients present with either a history of elevated BP before pregnancy, or a persistently elevated BP first diagnosed before 20 weeks' gestation. As much as one third of women with severe chronic hypertension may have a small-for-gestational-age (SGA) infant, and two thirds may have a preterm delivery. Placental abruption and fetal demise are among other complications.

Dx The criteria for diagnosis of chronic hypertension are as follows:
- Mild: Systolic BP ≥140 mm Hg; diastolic BP ≥90 mm Hg
- Severe: Systolic BP ≥180 mm Hg; diastolic BP ≥110 mm Hg
- Use of antihypertensive medications before pregnancy
- Onset of hypertension before 20th week of gestation
- Persistence of hypertension beyond the usual postpartum period
- No laboratory evidence of preeclampsia

Women with chronic hypertension should be evaluated for potentially reversible etiologies, preferably before pregnancy. Patients with long-standing hypertension should be evaluated for end-organ disease, including cardiomegaly, renal insufficiency, and retinopathy, preferably before pregnancy.

Tx Women with mild hypertension generally do well during pregnancy and do not, as a rule, require antihypertensive medication. It is reasonable not to start antihypertensive therapy in women with mild hypertension who become pregnant unless they have other complicating factors (e.g., cardiovascular or renal disease). In some instances it is reasonable to stop or reduce medication in women who are already taking antihypertensive therapy. Therapy should be increased or reinstituted for women with BPs exceeding 150 to 160 mm Hg systolic or 100 to 110 mm Hg diastolic. In women with severe chronic hypertension antihypertensive therapy should be initiated or continued.
- **Methyldopa and labetalol** are appropriate first-line long-term antihypertensive therapies. Methyldopa: 250 mg twice a day starting dose, maximum dose 4 g/day. Labetalol: 100 mg twice a day starting dose, maximum dose 2400 mg/day.
- **Angiotensin-converting enzyme inhibitors** are contraindicated during pregnancy and are associated with fetal and neonatal renal failure and death.
- The **beta-blocker atenolol** may be associated with growth restriction and is not recommended for use in pregnancy.

When chronic hypertension is complicated by fetal growth restriction or preeclampsia, fetal surveillance and, frequently, delivery are warranted. **See Gabbe 33, Hacker 14.**

Superimposed Preeclampsia with Chronic Hypertension

Pφ/TP The development of superimposed preeclampsia in women with chronic hypertension is relatively common and often difficult to diagnose, especially in patients with renal involvement.

Dx The presence of the following findings suggests superimposed preeclampsia:
- In women with chronic hypertension and without proteinuria early in pregnancy (<20 weeks' gestation), preeclampsia is diagnosed if there is new-onset proteinuria (≥300 mg of protein in a 24-hour specimen).
- In women with chronic hypertension and preexisting proteinuria before 20 weeks' gestation, the diagnosis is confirmed if there is a demonstrable increase in BP to the severe range in a woman whose hypertension has previously been well controlled with antihypertensive drugs. This type of progression can be associated with headaches, blurred vision, epigastric pain, a significant increase in liver enzymes, or a platelet count below 100,000/mm^3.

Tx Principles of management of severe preeclampsia apply when the diagnosis of superimposed preeclampsia is made. **See Gabbe 33, Hacker 14.**

Eclampsia

Pφ The etiologic mechanisms implicated in the pathogenesis of eclamptic convulsions have included cerebral vasoconstriction or vasospasm, cerebral edema or infarction, cerebral hemorrhage, and metabolic encephalopathy.

TP Eclampsia is a condition when new-onset grand mal seizures occur in a woman with preeclampsia. The onset of eclamptic seizures can be antepartum, intrapartum, or postpartum (most occur within 48 hours postpartum, but may occur as many as 7 days from delivery).

Dx Diagnosis is based on the presence of preeclampsia and convulsions. There is a wide spectrum of signs, ranging from severe hypertension, severe proteinuria, and generalized edema to minimal hypertension. Hypertension and proteinuria are considered the hallmarks for the diagnosis, ranging from severe to mild.

Several clinical symptoms may occur before or after the onset of convulsions, including persistent occipital or frontal headaches, blurred vision, photophobia, epigastric or right upper quadrant pain, and altered mental status.

Tx The priority is to prevent maternal injury and to support respiratory and cardiovascular functions. During or immediately after the acute convulsive episode, supportive care (elevated and padded side rails, padded tongue blade inserted between teeth, and physical restraints if needed) should be used. To minimize the risk of aspiration, the patient should lie in the left lateral decubitus position with oral suction as needed. Supplemental oxygen administration is used. Prevention of recurrent convulsions is managed with magnesium sulfate (IV loading dose of 6 g over 15 to 20 minutes, followed by a maintenance dose of 2 g/hr as a continuous IV infusion). BP should be maintained below 160 mm Hg systolic and 105 mm Hg diastolic. The presence of eclampsia is not an indication for cesarean delivery. The decision to perform cesarean delivery should be based on fetal gestational age, fetal condition, presence of labor, and cervical Bishop score. **See Gabbe 33, Hacker 14.**

ZEBRA ZONE

a. **Pheochromocytoma:** This can be a potentially lethal complication during pregnancy. The suspicion of this rare condition can arise in the presence of unexplainable fluctuating BP. The diagnosis can be made by ordering serum or urinary catecholamines.

b. **Coarctation of the aorta:** This rare condition often is diagnosed before a woman reaches reproductive age. The diagnosis can be made by detecting a difference between the radial and femoral pulses or abnormal findings on chest radiography that may include notching in the posterior thoracic ribs and indentation of the descending aortic arch. Echocardiography is usually diagnostic.

Practice Based Learning and Improvement: Evidence-Based Medicine

Title
Diagnosis and management of gestational hypertension and preeclampsia

Author
Sibai BM

Institution
Department of Obstetrics and Gynecology, University of Cincinnati College of Medicine, Cincinnati, Ohio

Reference
Obstetrics and Gynecology 2003;102:181–192

Problem
Background information and practical guidelines on diagnosis and treatment.

Intervention
Recommended management of mild/severe preeclampsia.

Comparison/control (quality of evidence)
Review article

Historical significance/comments
This is the definitive article that describes in detail current opinion on management of different groups of patients with preeclampsia, depending on severity and gestational age.

Interpersonal and Communication Skills

Communicate Frequently and Efficiently When Patients Are in Danger
The patient with a hypertensive disorder of pregnancy has a medical condition that may result in morbidity and even a fatal outcome if not managed aggressively. Although the emergent nature of severe preeclampsia may obligate the clinician to act rapidly, time should be taken to explain comprehensively to the patient what is happening and why certain measures are necessary. The clinician must remember that for most patients the well-being of their baby is the most important thing. Often a speedy explanation with reassurance that neither mother nor baby is in grave danger is all that a patient requires to help put her at ease as you proceed with vital medical tasks and decisions. Because there may be many uncertainties during this time, the clinician should communicate frequently, effectively, and efficiently to the patient and her family to keep them as informed and reassured as possible.

Professionalism

Principle: Commitment to Professional Responsibilities

A medical student working on the labor and delivery floor notices that her patient's BP has been rising. She asks whether it would be appropriate to start giving magnesium sulfate and is told only that this would not make sense right now. Later, her resident tells her that questioning the team's management of patients is unprofessional and serves only to slow down rounds. The student is left with the impression that being professional means getting along with and not questioning authority figures.

It is possible that the team's decision was incorrect, but it is also possible that the patient had gestational hypertension without proteinuria, in which case magnesium would not have been indicated. In either case, this represents a missed opportunity: ideally, the resident would have taken the time to explain the indications to treat gestational hypertension and preeclampsia and the proper roles of magnesium sulfate, antihypertensives, and eventually delivery of the infant. A culture of respect and collaboration is essential for effective medical education and for patient care. This culture can be created only if physicians who are in a teaching capacity serve as exemplars of these ideals.

Systems-Based Practice

Solving the Uninsured Crisis in America

The fundamental constraints of health care policy are often referred to as the "iron triangle" of health care: the three obvious goals of the system—**quality, access,** and **cost**—cannot all simultaneously be sought; focusing on any one of them will necessarily require sacrificing one or both of the others. Accordingly, to expand coverage (access) requires either increasing total health care costs or decreasing quality (in essence, spending less per person). Similarly, increasing the quality of care either requires raising total health care costs or providing fewer people with access to care. There is a compelling logic to this theory, and most policy experts would agree that in the larger sense it holds true.

The most important exception to this rule, however, involves the considerable waste and inefficiency that takes place in our health care system. At present, the United States spends roughly $2 trillion a year on health care, or 16% to 17% of the gross domestic product, and fails to cover some 46 million uninsured people, or about 15% of the country.

People who believe in the iron triangle concept articulated above argue that to cover the 46 million uninsured people in the United

States will either require spending significantly more on health care or giving up the quality of care that many people believe is the hallmark of the U.S. health care system.

A core tenet of the Obama administration's health care plan is that sufficient investment in health information technology will reduce unnecessary and wasteful spending by eliminating costs like extra hospital days due to medical errors or duplicative diagnostic tests ordered because the original results were not immediately available. Another core tenet is that improving prevention and the management of chronic conditions will result in not only improved quality of care but lower overall health care costs. It is thought that expanding preventive care to the uninsured, who often seek care through emergency rooms only after their conditions have progressed unnecessarily will ultimately reduce the cost of their care. Finally, the administration hopes that by increasing competition, health care costs that result from insurance and pharmaceutical company profits can be reduced.

Chapter 22
Diabetes in Pregnancy (Case 10)

Sue-Anne Toh MD and Michael Crutchlow MD

Case: You follow a 30-year-old Hispanic woman throughout her second pregnancy. At initial presentation, she is 8 weeks pregnant with her second child and feeling well. Her first child, a son, was born 5 years ago in rural Panama. The delivery was difficult because the baby was large—about 11 lbs (5000 g) at delivery. The patient has no personal history of diabetes, but her mother and several maternal aunts and uncles were diagnosed with diabetes in adulthood. She comes to all scheduled visits and is compliant with all of your recommendations.

Differential Diagnosis

This case encompasses this patient's **entire** pregnancy to permit consideration of two related, but distinct entities.

Gestational diabetes mellitus (GDM)
Pregestational diabetes mellitus type 1 or type 2

Speaking Intelligently

Diabetes during pregnancy, either preexisting or occurring as a consequence of pregnancy ("gestational diabetes"), is very common and has serious repercussions for both mother and child. Both types of diabetes are entirely treatable. Screening for these entities is straightforward, and they do not present a complex differential diagnosis. However, they are most often asymptomatic and once diagnosed add a layer of complexity to prenatal care. Therefore, the challenges presented by diabetes in pregnancy are those of effective screening and management.

You must at least consider the possibility of diabetes in pregnancy in all of your obstetric patients and screen all or nearly all of them at some point. As discussed in the following, your level of suspicion that your patient may be, or become, hyperglycemic during pregnancy will determine the timing of this screening. Once diabetes is diagnosed you must initiate effective management immediately.

PATIENT CARE

Clinical Thinking

At the first prenatal visit, the critical questions depend on whether the patient has known established diabetes mellitus.

- **No known diabetes:** "When do I screen for diabetes?"
  - Screen *promptly* if the history suggests that the patient may have previously undiagnosed diabetes.
  - Screen *at 24 to 28 weeks* if the patient is at low risk for GDM. The majority of women fall into this category.
- **Known established diabetes (type 1 or type 2):** "Is current management optimal?" The physician needs to determine if the patient is meeting glycemic targets for pregnancy (Table 22-1).
  - Is the patient taking hypoglycemic medications that present a risk to the developing fetus?
  - Is the patient at risk from diabetes-related end-organ damage—specifically, retinopathy, nephropathy, and cardiovascular disease?

Table 22-1 Goal Blood Sugars in Pregnancy

Timing of Glucose Measurement	Goal Blood Sugars (mg/dL)
Fasting	70-95
1 hr postprandial	<140
2 hr postprandial	<120
During labor	70-90

History
- **No known diabetes:**
  - Assess the risk of undiagnosed pregestational diabetes or GDM. Red flags for possible pregestational diabetes include:
    - A previous history of GDM.
    - Suspected prior GDM because of a history of a baby with macrosomia (>4000 g at delivery), congenital malformation, or an unexplained perinatal death.
    - Hyperglycemia-associated infections such as cystitis and recurrent vaginal yeast infections.
    - A strong family history of type 2 diabetes.
    - Marked obesity (body mass index [BMI] >35 kg/m^2).
    - Glycosuria at the initial visit.
  - *The presence of any of these factors suggests high risk for pregestational diabetes and should prompt immediate screening.*
- **Known established diabetes (type 1 or type 2):**
  - Assess the safety and adequacy of current treatment.
    - *Safety:* Oral hypoglycemic agents such as the sulfonylureas have been shown to be safe for the developing fetus. If one or more is used, the patient is commonly converted to an insulin regimen. Patients with diabetes are commonly prescribed other medications that do present a risk to the developing fetus. These include angiotensin-converting enzyme (ACE) inhibitors, angiotensin receptor blockers (ARBs), and statins (e.g., simvastatin). These medications need to be discontinued.
    - *Adequacy:* The adequacy of glycemic control is determined by home monitoring, which shows that glycemic targets for pregnancy (see Table 22-1) are being met.
  - Search for the presence of diabetes-induced end-organ damage that might complicate pregnancy:
    - *Retinopathy:* Is screening up to date? Is there a history of laser treatment? Does the patient have any vision problems?
    - *Nephropathy:* Is there a history of microalbuminuria or proteinuria?
    - *Cardiovascular disease:* Is there any history of atherosclerotic arterial disease or symptoms suggestive of angina or claudication?

Physical Examination
- **No known diabetes:**
  - Look for signs suggesting the presence of insulin resistance placing the patient at risk for GDM. Insulin resistance is common in subjects who are overweight (BMI >25 kg/m^2) before pregnancy, especially if fat distribution is central (baseline waist circumference >35 inches). The presence of acanthosis nigricans (dark, velvety hyperpigmentation of the skin present most

commonly in the lateral folds of the neck, axilla, and groin) is strongly suggestive of insulin resistance.
- Look for the presence of diabetic end-organ damage in subjects at high risk for undetected type 2 diabetes mellitus. Assessment of light touch and vibration sense in the feet may reveal evidence of peripheral neuropathy.
- **Known established diabetes (type 1 or type 2):**
  - Look for evidence of diabetic end-organ damage as discussed previously. Patients with known type 1 or type 2 diabetes should be evaluated at least once in the pregnancy by an ophthalmologist for an eye examination.

Tests for Consideration
- **Oral glucose tolerance testing:**
  - **The 50-g, 1-hour oral glucose tolerance test:** This is the initial screening test for diabetes in pregnancy. If the 1-hour postglucose concentration is above 130 mg/dL, a diagnostic 3-hour glucose tolerance test should be performed. $60
  - **The 100-g, 3-hour oral glucose tolerance test:** This is the diagnostic test used to confirm the results of a positive screening test (Table 22-2). $100

Table 22-2 100-Gram, 3-Hour Oral Glucose Tolerance Test Criteria for GDM*	
Timing of Glucose Measurement	**Plasma Glucose (mg/dL)**
Fasting	95
1 hr	180
2 hr	155
3 hr	140

*Results reflect upper limit of normal. Diagnosis of GDM is made if any two values are exceeded.

- **Other tests:**
  - **Hemoglobin A$_{1c}$:** Reflects long-term glycemic control in subjects with known or suspected diabetes before pregnancy. $60
  - **Urine microalbumin:** Screens for established diabetic nephropathy in subjects with known or suspected diabetes before pregnancy. $35

Clinical Entities   Medical Knowledge

Editors note: Gestational diabetes mellitus and established diabetes mellitus, along with the more common and serious fetal/neonatal and maternal complications, are discussed as Clinical Entities. A more comprehensive list of diabetes-related complications is found in Table 22-3. An overview of the management of diabetes in pregnancy is provided in Table 22-4.

Gestational Diabetes Mellitus (GDM)

Pφ Normal pregnancy is characterized by insulin resistance. This is due primarily to the secretion of human placental lactogen, free cortisol, estrogen, and progesterone by the placenta. Insulin resistance increases with the size of the placenta and is most pronounced in the third trimester. Women who are unable to appropriately increase insulin secretion develop GDM.

TP The presentation of GDM is typically silent. Therefore, proactive screening is required, as previously discussed. Severe hyperglycemia may lead to polyuria and polydipsia.

Dx The diagnosis of GDM is suggested by a positive screening test (1-hour oral glucose tolerance test) and confirmed with a 3-hour oral glucose tolerance test.

Tx Initial treatment of GDM is dietary and implemented by a trained dietician. This includes carbohydrate restriction in all patients and calorie restriction in those who are obese (BMI >30 kg/m^2). If glycemic targets (see Table 22-1) are not achieved, treatment with oral hypoglycemic agents or insulin is indicated. **See Gabbe 37, Hacker 16.**

Pregestational Diabetes Mellitus Type 1 or Type 2

Pφ This may be type 1 or type 2 diabetes. Patients with type 1 diabetes have had autoimmune destruction of their pancreatic islet cells, resulting in a complete deficiency of insulin production. In contrast, patients with type 2 diabetes have insulin resistance and inadequate insulin secretion (similar to GDM).

TP Age (<30 years), habitus (thin), and clinical presentation (ketoacidotic, acutely ill) at the time of diagnosis can suggest type 1 diabetes. Subjects with type 2 diabetes are often asymptomatic and obese and typically have a strong family history of type 2 diabetes. However, there can be substantial overlap in the presentations of type 1 and type 2 diabetes.

Dx Elevated fasting (≥126 mg/dL), random (≥200 mg/dL), or 2-hour post oral glucose challenge (≥200 mg/dL) glucose values are diagnostic of diabetes mellitus if repeated on more than one occasion.

Tx Type 1 diabetes is always treated with insulin. Type 2 diabetes may be treated with a wide array of oral agents, noninsulin injected agents, or insulin. Occasionally, patients with type 2 diabetes are converted to insulin before conception. The glycemic targets during pregnancy are the same as those for GDM (see Table 22-1). Nutritional intervention is a cornerstone of management of all diabetic patients. **See Gabbe 37, Hacker 16.**

Table 22-3 Maternal and Fetal Complications of Diabetes during Pregnancy

Maternal Complications	Fetal Complications
Obstetric complications	Macrosomia
• Spontaneous abortion	• Traumatic delivery
• Infection	• Shoulder dystocia
• Polyhydramnios	• Erb's palsy
• Postpartum hemorrhage	Metabolic
• Preeclampsia	• Hypoglycemia
Vascular and end-organ involvement	• Hypocalcemia
• Cardiac	Hematologic
• Renal—worsening nephropathy	• Hyperbilirubinemia
• Opthalmic—worsening retinopathy	• Polycythemia
Neurologic	Delayed organ maturity
• Peripheral neuropathy	• Pulmonary
• Gastroparesis	• Hepatic
Diabetic emergencies	• Neurologic
• Hypoglycemia	• Pituitary-thyroid axis
• Ketoacidosis	Congenital malformations
	• Neural tube defects
	• Cardiovascular defects
	• Caudal regression syndrome
	• Situs inversus
	• Duplex renal ureter
	• Intrauterine growth retardation
	• Intrauterine fetal death

Table 22-4 Diabetes in Pregnancy—Management at a Glance

Time	Concerns	Tests	Interventions
Preconception	• Abnormal organogenesis • Establishing habits for glycemic control • Assessing underlying maternal end-organ disease	• Hemoglobin A_{1c} • Home glucose readings • Retinal examination • Assess proteinuria • Electrocardiogram	• Optimize glycemia • Discontinue potentially teratogenic medications • Counsel regarding risks/challenges of pregnancy
First trimester	• Same as preconception • Asymptomatic bacteriuria	• Same as preconception (if not done) • Urinalysis/urine culture	• Optimize glycemia • Same as preconception (if not done) • Treat bacteriuria if present
Second trimester	• Congenital anomalies • Fetal growth • Impact of pregnancy on retinopathy/nephropathy	• Detailed ultrasonography at 18–20 wk • Hemoglobin A_{1c}/home glucose monitoring • Retinal and proteinuria surveillance as indicated	• Optimize glycemia • Counseling if congenital anomaly detected • Ophthalmologic care as indicated • Optimize blood pressure if increased proteinuria

Third trimester	• Increased potential for fetal demise • Impact of hyperglycemia on fetal growth • Impact of pregnancy on retinopathy/nephropathy • Preeclampsia	• Semiweekly antepartum testing after 32 weeks • 38-Week ultrasonography for fetal weight estimation • Hemoglobin A_{1c}/home glucose monitoring • Retinal and proteinuria surveillance as indicated	• Optimize glycemia • Ophthalmologic care as indicated • Optimize blood pressure if increased proteinuria • Labor induction at 39-40 weeks, earlier if indicated
Intra- and peripartum	• Macrosomia Neonatal hypoglycemia • Maternal ketoacidosis (if type 1 diabetes)	• Maternal and neonate glucose monitoring	• Consider cesarean delivery of a macrosomic fetus • Maternal insulin infusion for hyperglycemia • Neonate glucose infusion as needed
Postpartum	• Persistent maternal type 2 diabetes (if GDM)	• Oral glucose tolerance test 3 months postdelivery (if GDM)	• Hypoglycemic regimen as needed, taking into account breast-feeding status and plans for additional pregnancies

Items in red apply to both established diabetes mellitus and GDM. All other items are specific to established diabetes mellitus unless specifically indicated.

ZEBRA ZONE

a. **Gestational diabetes insipidus (GDI):** This condition must be considered in women presenting in the second half of pregnancy with polyuria and polydipsia that cannot be attributed to hyperglycemia. This inability to concentrate urine appropriately may be due to placental degradation of vasopressin, and can result in hypernatremia and hyperosmolarity if untreated and access to water is limited. If GDI is diagnosed, it is typically highly responsive to treatment with the vasopressin analog, desmopressin, and can be expected to resolve after delivery.

Practice-Based Learning and Improvement: Evidence-Based Medicine

Title
Effect of treatment of gestational diabetes mellitus on pregnancy outcomes

Authors
Crowther CA, Hiller JE, Moss JR, et al.

Reference
New England Journal of Medicine 2005;352:2477–2486

Problem
Does active treatment of mild gestational diabetes decrease perinatal complications?

Intervention
Active treatment was compared with no treatment. Actively treated patients were informed of GDM and prescribed diet and insulin as needed to achieve treatment targets (a fasting glucose of 63 to 99 mg/dL and a 2-hour postprandial glucose of <140 mg/dL). Untreated patients and their physicians were not informed of the diagnosis of GDM.

Comparison/control (quality of evidence)
Large, prospective, randomized, controlled clinical trial.

Outcome/effect
Serious perinatal outcomes (death, shoulder dystocia, fracture, and nerve palsy) were seen in 1% of the infants of actively treated mothers and 4% of infants of untreated mothers ($P = 0.01$).

Historical significance/comments
Although it had been known that mild GDM was associated with poor perinatal outcomes, this was the first study to demonstrate that detection and treatment of mild GDM has a clinical benefit.

Interpersonal and Communication Skills

Conveying the Serious Nature of a Problem

Although reassurance is important, one should not downplay the seriousness of diabetes in pregnancy. Although usually asymptomatic, patients should not be lulled into complacency. The clinician must convey to the patient that optimal glycemic control is very important for her own health and that of her baby. The patient should understand that she herself will be the principal manager of this condition. To meet these goals, the patient should be instructed specifically on how to follow an optimal diet, how to monitor blood glucose levels, and how to take the medications or insulin that may be prescribed. The patient must recognize that these efforts need to continue throughout pregnancy.

When it is essential that patients understand and remember the information conveyed, you can use the following skills:

- Use language that the patient understands.
- Be logical and systematic in your explanation.
- Use explicit categorization—"There are dietary and monitoring considerations. Let's discuss the dietary considerations first. ... And now the monitoring. ..."
- Use emphasis—"This is really important. ..."
- Repeat critical information.
- Check the patient's understanding—"I've told you a lot of things today. It is important that I know you understand what you have to do. Can you tell me what you think I have told you?"

This is also an opportunity to demonstrate to your patient that there will be support for her within your practice and within the community. Patient education should start with referral to a skilled dietician. One should consider referral to a physician who is highly experienced in the management of diabetes during pregnancy. Patients will have many questions as they begin to address these challenges. It is important to dedicate an appropriate amount of time to address these issues at prenatal visits.

Professionalism

Principle: Commitment to Appropriate Relations with Patients

An unexpected delivery has delayed your office hours. Going to the surgeons' lounge to change out of your scrubs will cause an additional 15-minute delay to your waiting patients. What do you do?

Wearing professional attire is a matter of showing respect for your patients. Wearing scrubs in an outpatient setting can give the impression that you are squeezing your patients in between more important activities. By not taking the time to change you are also giving the impression that you are in a rush, thus undermining your patients' ability to feel comfortable bringing up additional issues that may be important to their health. Even though you may feel that you are giving the same level of care to your patients regardless of what clothes you are wearing, we must remember that our clothes do send a message and that appropriate dress is part of a commitment to appropriate relations with patients.

Systems-Based Practice

Health Care Information Technology: PDAs, CPOE, and EHRs

It's the weekend and you are covering for three separate OB practices totaling 12 obstetricians. A pregnant patient comes in with blurry vision and dizziness, and is found to have a blood sugar of 284. She has seen a doctor for whom you cover, but she has not seen you and has not been to this emergency department before. She knows she takes some medications to keep her sugar under control, is not sure what they are, and knows little else about her condition.

There is almost nothing else in your life that is paper-based anymore. Banking, communication, and even holiday shopping are online and easily retrievable. However, when your complex OB patient arrives in the emergency department with hypertension and hyperglycemia, you have no way of retrieving her chart because all the information is in a file locked in your office or someone else's office miles away. This matter increases both costs (you redo many of the same lab tests that are already on her chart) and the chance for errors (the patient may not communicate her entire history). A patient such as this one will also likely require the careful tracking of multiple lab tests—a task that can be done on paper, but much more easily on a hand-held computer or personal digital assistant (PDA).

This scenario raises the enormous potential of information technology (IT) to affect the way in which we practice medicine. The ideal situation would allow you to access this patient's electronic health record (EHR) on your PDA, write inpatient orders wirelessly through the hospital's computerized physician order entry (CPOE) system, or even wirelessly transmit outpatient prescriptions to the patient's drugstore (with no handwriting problems!). Although for most of us this is still something of a distant vision, the widespread adoption of PDA-based software (e.g., Epocrates) by physicians suggests that this transition may be welcomed by the medical community.

Chapter 23
Pulmonary Diseases in Pregnancy (Case 11)

Leah Lande MD

Case: A 32-year-old woman, at 28 weeks' gestation, presents with a 1-week history of dyspnea at rest, which is worse with exertion and associated with an intermittent dry cough.

Differential Diagnosis

Asthma	Pulmonary embolism	Pneumonia
Pulmonary edema	Anemia	Dyspnea of pregnancy
Pulmonary hypertension	Pleural effusion	

Speaking Intelligently

When considering the cause of dyspnea in a pregnant woman, one must distinguish between a true pathologic condition and the normal dyspnea of pregnancy. Physiologic dyspnea is caused primarily by a progressive rise in progesterone levels and decreased lung capacity due to mechanical obstruction. At 28 weeks' gestation, approximately 50% of women experience dyspnea walking up hills or climbing stairs, and 20% of women have dyspnea walking on flat ground. It is very unusual, however, to experience dyspnea at rest. Pulmonary function should remain normal throughout the duration of pregnancy, except for functional residual capacity, which decreases by 10% to 20% by term. All of the disease states that cause dyspnea during pregnancy are relatively serious and, left untreated, can lead to significant maternal hypoxemia, which can lead to intrauterine growth restriction, developmental abnormalities, and preterm deliveries. Therefore, the appropriate diagnostic and treatment modalities should not be withheld; failing to properly diagnose and treat these conditions is likely to be more harmful to the fetus than the theoretical risks of the tests and therapies.

PATIENT CARE

Clinical Thinking
- The priority is to rule out the conditions that can be potentially life-threatening to the patient and in which any delay in diagnosis and treatment could be dangerous. These include pulmonary embolism (PE) and pneumonia.
- If there is a high clinical suspicion for either PE or pneumonia based on the history and physical examination, the appropriate radiographic studies should be performed immediately.
- If these problems seem unlikely, noninvasive tests can then be performed to try to distinguish between the other entities in the differential diagnosis.
- Diagnostic tests should be done sequentially, in the order of the most likely problem, based on clues from the history and physical examination.

History
- **Duration:** If symptoms have been present for more than 1 to 2 weeks, it is more likely to be asthma, pulmonary edema, pulmonary hypertension, anemia, or dyspnea of pregnancy. PE and pneumonia are more likely to have an acute or subacute presentation.
- **Onset:** Sudden (PE, pneumonia) or insidious (pulmonary hypertension, pulmonary edema, asthma, anemia).
- Do the symptoms inhibit the patient's ability to participate in normal daily activities?
- Associated symptoms for **pneumonia:** Fever, chills, sputum production, chest pain, malaise, anorexia, myalgias, headache, nausea, and vomiting.
- Associated symptoms for **PE:** Chest pain, heart racing, anxiety, sudden onset, leg swelling, recent immobility, syncope.
- Associated symptoms for **asthma:** Cough, environmental triggers, recent upper respiratory infection, wheezing, worse at night.
- Associated symptoms for **pulmonary edema** or **pulmonary hypertension:** Leg swelling, irregular or fast heart beat, orthopnea, chest pain.
- Associated symptoms for **anemia:** Pallor, tachycardia.
- Associated symptoms for **dyspnea of pregnancy:** Occurs primarily with exertion, rarely at rest; usually mild, *without* any of other associated symptoms.
- It is important to obtain the patient's preexisting medical history, including history of tobacco or drug use, and occupational history because certain work environments can increase a patient's susceptibility to lung disease.
- Has the patient ever had similar symptoms in the past?

Physical Examination

- The **vital signs** are the most important predictors of illness severity in pulmonary disease: Fever usually suggests pneumonia. Low-grade fever can be present in PE. Tachycardia can be present in any of the aforementioned conditions that cause dyspnea. Hypotension may be present in severe pneumonia or massive PE. Hypertension may be present in pulmonary edema. Manually counting the respiratory rate is an important way to evaluate the severity of illness. Pulse oximetry is an essential component of the physical examination in pulmonary disease. There can be significant arterial hypoxemia but still a normal pulse oximetry reading because the pulse oximetry percentage will drop below the 90s only if the Pa_{O_2} is less than 60.
- **General appearance:** Use of accessory muscles of respiration and inability to speak in complete sentences are markers of illness severity.
- **Neck:** The presence of elevated jugular venous pulsations indicate right heart strain, which can be present in cardiogenic pulmonary edema, PE, or pulmonary hypertension. In the third trimester of a normal pregnancy, the blood volume is increased by as much as 50%, which can also lead to mild jugular venous distention.
- **Lungs:** Clear lungs suggest PE, pulmonary hypertension, or anemia. Crackles, decreased breath sounds, or egophony suggest pneumonia, pleural effusion, or pulmonary edema. Wheezing or rhonchi suggest bronchospasm, which can occur in asthma, pulmonary edema, viral or atypical pneumonia, or, rarely, PE.
- **Heart:** In pulmonary hypertension and PE, signs of right heart strain may be present, including a loud P2, right ventricular heave, and the murmur of tricuspid regurgitation, which is a high-pitched, pansystolic murmur, heard best at the left lower sternal border, and is augmented during inspiration and decreased during Valsalva maneuver. In cardiogenic pulmonary edema, an S3 gallop may be heard. In anemia, a systolic ejection murmur may be present. Keep in mind that a benign flow murmur may be found in normal pregnancy, which is characterized by a short, soft, systolic ejection murmur. This can be distinguished from a pathologic murmur, which is more likely to be loud, pansystolic, late systolic, or diastolic.
- **Extremities:** Asymmetric lower extremity edema is worrisome for deep vein thrombosis. Bilateral symmetric lower extremity edema can be seen in 30% of normal pregnancies, but may also be found in the setting of a cardiomyopathy or pulmonary hypertension. Cyanosis indicates profound hypoxemia, and clubbing suggests chronic lung disease.

Tests for Consideration

- **Pulmonary function tests:** To distinguish between obstructive and restrictive pulmonary disease, and to better define physiologic abnormalities; can be particularly helpful in diagnosis of asthma. $560

- **Arterial blood gas:** For a true assessment of maternal Pao$_2$ and calculation of A-a gradient. $75
- **D-dimer:** D-dimer testing can help establish whether there is a high likelihood of an embolus, but cannot tell you the source of the clot. A negative value decreases clinical suspicion for PE, but does not completely rule out PE. D-dimer levels can be elevated in normal pregnancy, with levels increasing as gestation progresses (elevated in 5 % in first trimester, 10% in second trimester, 40% in third trimester). $80
- **CBC:** To diagnose anemia; elevated white blood cell count suggests possible infection. $35

IMAGING CONSIDERATIONS

→**Chest radiograph:** To rule out pneumonia, pleural effusion, pulmonary edema; remember that although in PE the CXR can be normal, a significant number of patients with PE will have atelectasis, a small pleural effusion, or infiltrate on their CXR. $130
Radiation dose to fetus = 1 mrad (average person is exposed to 360 mrad/year)

→**Ventilation-perfusion scan:** To diagnose PE; excludes PE only if entirely normal study. Overall, 14% of patients with a scan that is read as low probability still have a PE. $860
Radiation dose to fetus = 32 mrad

→**Spiral CT chest with IV contrast:** To rule out PE, with extra benefit of being able to diagnose other pulmonary, pleural, pericardial, and mediastinal abnormalities. $1330
Radiation dose to fetus = 32-66 mrad (radiation dose increases as pregnancy progresses)

→**Echocardiogram:** To diagnose cardiomyopathy, diastolic dysfunction, and pulmonary hypertension. $800

→**Lower extremity Doppler:** To diagnose a deep vein thrombosis that may have migrated to form a PE. $330

Clinical Entities   **Medical Knowledge**

Asthma

Pφ Asthma is reversible airway obstruction, characterized by inflammation, mucus secretion, and bronchospasm.

TP The patient typically experiences dyspnea, cough, wheezing, chest tightness; symptoms often are worse at night and with exercise, very hot or cold air, inhaled irritants, and other triggers. Thirty percent of patients with preexisting asthma will have worsening of symptoms during pregnancy, 30% will remain the same as they were before pregnancy, and 30% will improve.

Dx Diagnosis is based on presence of wheezing with or without rhonchi on lung examination and evidence of expiratory airflow obstruction on pulmonary function tests. A bedside peak flow measurement should be performed on presentation, and can be used to monitor a patient's progress and response to therapy.

Tx Avoid triggers; follow stepwise treatment with medications: if mild intermittent, prescribe beta-adrenergic agonist inhaler as needed; if mild persistent, low-dose inhaled corticosteroid; if moderate persistent, low- to medium-dose inhaled corticosteroid plus inhaled long-acting beta agonist; if severe persistent, high-dose inhaled corticosteroid plus long-acting inhaled beta agonist or course of systemic corticosteroids, if needed. **See Gabbe 35, Hacker 16.**

Pulmonary Embolism

Pφ Pregnancy is a relatively hypercoagulable state, resulting in an increased incidence of lower extremity deep vein thrombosis, pelvic vein thrombosis, and subsequent PEs during pregnancy. PEs can have various different hemodynamic and respiratory consequences, depending on the size, location, and acuity of the clot, as well as the patient's baseline cardiopulmonary status.

TP The typical presentation includes dyspnea, which may be acute or subacute; pleuritic chest pain, tachycardia/palpitations, lightheadedness, diaphoresis, anxiety, cough, and leg pain or swelling.

Dx If leg edema or pain is present, start with lower extremity Dopplers to assess for deep vein thrombosis; if positive, there is no need to proceed with further testing. CT of the chest with IV contrast is the test of choice. Ventilation-perfusion scan may also be performed if the patient has renal insufficiency or an allergy to IV contrast dye, but this is usually a less definitive test.

Tx Administer intravenous unfractionated heparin with monitoring of partial thromboplastin time, or subcutaneous low-molecular weight heparin with monitoring of factor Xa levels. **See Gabbe 41, Hacker 16.**

Pneumonia

Pφ Community-acquired pneumonia is caused by typical bacterial pathogens (*Streptococcus pneumoniae* is the most common), atypical bacterial pathogens (*Mycoplasma, Chlamydia, Legionella*), viruses (influenza, varicella), and, if epidemiologically at risk, tuberculosis. Aspiration pneumonia can also occur with increased frequency during pregnancy, with increased incidence of gram-negative rods and anaerobes (see Chapter 26, Pneumonia in Pregnancy).

TP Dyspnea, cough, fever, chest pain, and malaise are the typical signs and symptoms.

Dx Diagnosis is based on physical examination and CXR.

Tx Community-acquired pneumonia, mild disease in outpatients: macrolide alone (azithromycin); if hospitalized: third-generation cephalosporin (ceftriaxone) plus macrolide. Avoid quinolones, sulfa, tetracyclines. Aspiration pneumonia treatment should include coverage of gram-negative rods and anaerobes. An extended-spectrum penicillin such as ampicillin/sulbactam is a good choice for this. **See Gabbe 35.**

Pulmonary Edema

Pφ Peripartum cardiomyopathy is a rare condition that most commonly occurs in the last month of pregnancy or within 5 months after delivery, and can ultimately lead to pulmonary edema. It is a dilated cardiomyopathy of unclear etiology. Pulmonary edema can also occur in the setting of preeclampsia, thyrotoxicosis, or after the use of tocolytics, especially the combination of magnesium sulfate and terbutaline.

TP The patient presents with cough, orthopnea, paroxysmal nocturnal dyspnea, fatigue, palpitations, hemoptysis, chest pain, and rapid onset or worsening of lower extremity edema. Elevated blood pressures (systolic >140 mm Hg and/or diastolic >90 mm Hg) and hyperreflexia with clonus suggest preeclampsia.

Dx Echocardiography shows systolic dysfunction and dilated cardiac chambers in peripartum cardiomyopathy, and normal systolic function with impaired left ventricular relaxation in the diastolic dysfunction that can occur in preeclampsia. The pulmonary edema that occurs in the setting of tocolytic use or thyrotoxicosis is noncardiogenic, and the echocardiogram should be normal. The physical examination and CXR show signs of pulmonary edema.

Tx For peripartum cardiomyopathy, digoxin, loop diuretics, and afterload reduction with hydralazine and nitrates are reasonable medical interventions to consider. Uteroplacental perfusion should be maintained with inotropes if necessary. Because of a high risk for venous and arterial thrombosis, subcutaneous heparin should be instituted. In noncardiogenic forms of pulmonary edema, diuretics should be given with caution, only in the setting of volume overload, to avoid maternal hypovolemia. In preeclampsia, antihypertensive medication should be initiated if the diastolic blood pressure is greater than 105 mm Hg or the systolic blood pressure exceeds 160 mm Hg. **See Gabbe 34.**

Pulmonary Hypertension

Pφ Patients with preexisting pulmonary hypertension can undergo marked worsening of this condition during pregnancy. In addition, the process of labor and delivery can be life-threatening in the setting of severe pulmonary hypertension. Pregnancy should be discouraged in patients with preexisting moderate or severe pulmonary hypertension. Occasionally, primary pulmonary hypertension is diagnosed for the first time during pregnancy.

TP The patient typically experiences progressive dyspnea, first with exertion, then with rest. The condition can be associated with chest pain, lower extremity edema, fatigue, lightheadedness, syncope.

Dx Diagnosis is made by echocardiography or stress echocardiography, with confirmation by right heart catheterization.

Tx Prostacyclin analogs such as intravenous epoprostenol or inhaled iloprost have been used with some success during pregnancy. Delivery is usually by cesarean section, with close monitoring of maternal hemodynamics by right heart catheterization. **See Gabbe 34.**

Pleural Effusion

Pφ Most pleural effusions that occur during pregnancy are secondary to other conditions, such as PE, congestive heart failure, and pneumonia. Small pleural effusions can be seen in normal pregnancy after cesarean section. More unusual causes of pleural effusion include ovarian hyperstimulation syndrome after the use of fertility agents.

TP The patient complains of dyspnea, cough, and pleuritic chest pain.

Dx Physical examination reveals decreased breath sounds and dullness to percussion; CXR shows effusion.

Tx If moderate to large in size, unilateral, or associated with significant respiratory symptoms, a diagnostic or therapeutic thoracentesis should be performed with pleural fluid analysis. If small and bilateral, or if clearly a secondary manifestation of another primary pulmonary condition, observation is appropriate. **See Gabbe 35, 41.**

Anemia

Pφ Owing to the increase in blood volume by up to 30% to 50% during pregnancy, the concentration of red blood cells becomes hemodiluted. This usually results in a mild anemia. The most common cause of a significant anemia in pregnancy is iron deficiency, which occurs most commonly in the third trimester. Vitamin B_{12} and folate deficiency can also cause anemia, although less commonly. If severe anemia is present, sources of blood loss should be investigated.

TP The typical patient may present with dyspnea, fatigue, pallor, dizziness, and/or tachycardia.

Dx CBC and iron studies are diagnostic; rule out any active bleeding.

Tx Iron supplementation; blood transfusion only if significant active bleeding or extremely low hemoglobin. **See Gabbe 40, Hacker 6.**

Dyspnea of Pregnancy

Pφ Dyspnea can be seen in a significant percentage of normal pregnancies because of a progressive rise in progesterone levels during the course of gestation, as well as the increase in intra-abdominal pressure leading to cephalad displacement of the diaphragm. A mild respiratory alkalosis can typically be seen on arterial blood gas analysis.

TP At least 20% of women in the first trimester, 40% in the second trimester, and 50% in the third trimester experience dyspnea climbing stairs or up hills. Five percent, 10%, and 20% in the respective trimesters experience dyspnea walking on flat ground, but less than 10% experience dyspnea at rest, and when this does occur, it is almost always during the final 4 weeks of gestation.

Dx An evaluation to search for pathologic causes of dyspnea should be pursued, especially if dyspnea is acute in onset, is severe or particularly bothersome to the patient, occurs at rest, or is associated with any other symptoms, such as fever, cough, or chest pain.

Tx Reassurance of the patient and close monitoring for any new or worrisome signs or symptoms. **See Gabbe 3, Hacker 6.**

ZEBRA ZONE

a. **Amniotic fluid embolism:** A rare but potentially fatal complication. Maternal death can occur in as much as 75% of cases.

b. **Interstitial lung disease:** Uncommon; characterized by scarring of the lung interstitium.

c. **Bronchiolitis:** Inflammation of the bronchioles, most commonly caused by viral infection.

d. **α_1-Antitrypsin deficiency:** A genetic disorder that results in shortness of breath and chronic obstructive pulmonary disease secondary to an inability to produce sufficient amounts of α_1-antitrypsin, which inhibits neutrophil elastase. Increased levels of neutrophil elastase then damage the lungs.

e. **Valvular heart disease:** Can be particularly dangerous in pregnancy because of increased maternal blood volumes.

f. **Cardiac ischemia:** Rare in healthy pregnant women; can occasionally be seen in "crack" cocaine abusers.

g. **Pheochromocytoma:** An endocrine tumor that can produce increased levels of catecholamines, which then cause palpitations, shortness of breath, anxiety, and so forth.

Practice-Based Learning and Improvement: Evidence-Based Medicine

Title
Pulmonary complications of pregnancy

Authors
Pereira A, Krieger BP

Institution
Pulmonary Division, Mount Sinai Medical Center, Miami Beach, Florida

Reference
Clinics in Chest Medicine 2004;25:299–310

Problem
Pregnancy induces significant physiologic stresses on the pulmonary and cardiovascular systems that may precipitate respiratory compromise.

Comparison/control (quality of evidence)
Review of the physiologic changes that affect the pregnant woman as well as a discussion of pregnancy-related pulmonary conditions.

Outcome/effect
Suggests approaches to various disease states affecting the cardiopulmonary system during pregnancy while balancing the needs of the fetus with maternal well-being.

Interpersonal and Communication Skills

Demonstrating Sensitivity to the Patient's Underlying Concerns
Although patients with dyspnea are often quite anxious, pregnant women are usually more concerned about the health of their fetus. The pregnant patient is often quite hesitant to undergo diagnostic testing and therapies that may be theoretically harmful to the fetus. In caring for these patients, it is very helpful to acknowledge these concerns and discuss them with the patient. In particular, use appropriate language to emphasize to the patient that *the health of the fetus depends on the health of the mother*, and that necessary testing and treatments must not be withheld, although every effort will be made to minimize fetal risk.

Professionalism

Principle: Commitment to Honesty with Patients
The risks and benefits of diagnostic testing and treatments must be explained carefully to the patient, emphasizing that maternal health must be the priority. You are obligated to explain that there are possibly small risks associated with certain radiologic and diagnostic procedures that may be required when caring for a pregnant patient, but that the health and well-being of the mother probably supersedes these small risks. Open communication and discussion between the patient and the obstetrics and pulmonary teams is essential.

Chapter 24
Premature Labor, Abnormal Bleeding, and Abdominal Pain in the Second and Third Trimester (Case 12)

Patricia I. Carney MD *and Anthony C. Sciscione* DO

Case: A 26-year-old G3P0202 at 26 weeks' gestation presents to the labor and delivery suite with a 4-hour history of moderate to severe abdominal and back pain, as well as vaginal bleeding. She has had two previous preterm vaginal deliveries, at 29 and 33 weeks.

Differential Diagnosis			
Premature labor	Placental abruption	Preterm premature rupture of the membranes (PPROM)	Pyelonephritis

Speaking Intelligently

When called on to see a pregnant patient who is presenting unexpectedly and in pain, first assess if she is medically stable. Take a detailed medical and surgical history and review the circumstances surrounding the chief complaint. Inquire about the severity and location of the pain and the timing of events leading up to the patient's presentation.

Crucial to determining treatment options and disposition of the patient is establishing a reliable gestational age. If a sonogram has not previously been obtained to establish an estimated date of confinement (EDC), perform this test at the bedside to corroborate the menstrual history. Check the amniotic fluid level and placental position and look for evidence of a placental abruption. Perform a thorough cervical examination, both visual and digital, looking for cervical change. Establish large-bore intravenous access and obtain lab tests for blood count, blood type and screen, fibrinogen, prothrombin time (PT), partial thromboplastin time (PTT), and Kleihauer-Betke (a test that establishes if fetal blood is present in the maternal circulation). Depending on the gestational age, the fetal heart rate and uterine activity are monitored. If the patient has signs of uterine activity and there are no contraindications, tocolysis can be considered to prevent the progression of labor. If preterm delivery is threatened, administer antenatal corticosteroids to promote lung maturity.

PATIENT CARE

Clinical Thinking

- The most serious problem for this patient is maternal or fetal instability. Quick assessment of the status of both the mother and fetus is paramount.
- Once the mother and fetus are considered stable, the work-up for a potential cause of premature contractions can proceed.
- Often it is not possible to establish the cause of the bleeding or abdominal pain that compelled the patient to present to the hospital. Because sonography is not particularly accurate in detecting most cases of placental abruption (abruption will not be evident in as much as 75% of cases), the diagnosis of abruption is usually determined by clinical circumstance.

History

- Ensuring an accurate gestational age is critical to the proper management of preterm labor.
- Determining the timing, character, and severity of the vaginal bleeding is important to guide therapy and secure a diagnosis.

- The approach to a **nonviable** pregnancy in a woman who has vaginal bleeding is focused on **maternal** health.
- Ask about a prior history or family history of clotting abnormalities.
- A history of previous preterm births places this patient at a higher risk for a subsequent premature delivery.

Physical Examination
- **Vital signs:** Maternal tachycardia and/or hypotension suggest significant blood loss. Fever may represent an intrauterine infection with associated rupture of membranes.
- **General appearance:** Significant discomfort is worrisome and likely represents intrauterine pathology such as a placental abruption or preterm labor. Pallor likely represents significant blood loss.
- **Heart:** Many pregnant women have a midsystolic functional murmur. A holosystolic murmur, however, especially when accompanied by tachycardia, may represent significant blood loss.
- **Abdominal examination:** Signs of peritonitis such as guarding and rebound likely represent peritoneal irritation from appendicitis or a ruptured uterus. A tender abdomen and uterus suggests placental abruption.
- **Speculum examination:** The presence of blood confirms the patient's history of vaginal bleeding. In general, brown or dark blood represents older blood and bright red blood a more acute bleed. Every attempt should be made to clear the vagina of blood so that the vagina and cervix can be completely inspected for trauma or a lesion. Assess the patient for ruptured membranes.
- **Pelvic examination:** A pelvic examination should be performed only once ultrasonography has confirmed that the placenta does not overlay the cervix. Uterine tenderness or pelvic mass are both worrisome signs.

Tests for Consideration
- **CBC:** Low hemoglobin is worrisome, especially if the vaginal bleeding is copious or the patient gives a history of excessive or long-standing vaginal bleeding. A high white blood cell count is indicative of infection. Thrombocytopenia is concerning and likely represents acute hemorrhage. $35
- **PT, PTT, fibrinogen, and D-dimer level:** If there are clinical signs of heavy bleeding, disseminated intravascular coagulation (DIC) needs to be considered. $300
- **Urinalysis and urine culture:** Asymptomatic bacteriuria and urinary tract infection are associated with preterm birth. $30

- **Cervical fetal fibronectin (fFN):** Tests for a specific protein released from the chorionic–decidual interface in patients who have a higher likelihood of preterm delivery. A negative fFN level is very reassuring and the risk of a preterm birth within 2 weeks is less than 1%. Blood in the vaginal cylinder, recent intercourse, or a cervical examination would make this test less reliable, and are contraindications to performing the test. $150

IMAGING CONSIDERATIONS

→**Ultrasonography:** Ultrasonography is the most definitive tool in the evaluation of abnormal bleeding in pregnancy. Placental implantation over the cervix establishes the diagnosis of placenta previa. Visualization of a hypoechogenic area beneath the placenta suggests abruption. A sonogram should be obtained early in the evaluation of anyone who has undiagnosed vaginal bleeding. Oligohydramnios should prompt further investigation of the possibility of rupture of membranes. Estimates of fetal weight and gestational age should be determined. A measurement of cervical length is helpful and can be a potential predictor of possible premature delivery. A cervical length less than 2.5 cm is typically used as a threshold for concern regarding increased risk of preterm birth, and a normal cervical length is reassuring. $225

Clinical Entities	Medical Knowledge

Premature Labor

Pφ The etiology of premature labor is multifactorial, including infection, multiple gestation, and polyhydramnios. Many cases are idiopathic. Although controversial, underlying intrauterine infection appears to be a key component of the genesis of premature labor. A prior preterm delivery is a significant risk factor for a subsequent preterm delivery. Complaints of cramping, contractions, or abdominal pain should be given a high level of clinical consideration if a patient reports a prior preterm birth.

TP The most common presentation is rhythmic lower abdominal or back pain. This is often accompanied by scant vaginal bleeding or an increase in vaginal discharge. Pelvic pressure is a less specific patient complaint.

Dx The diagnosis of preterm labor is established by the finding of regular uterine contractions associated with documented cervical change in dilation or effacement. The addition of cervical fetal fibronectin testing has been a useful diagnostic tool to help distinguish "false labor" from true preterm labor.

Tx Tocolytic therapy (medical therapy using *magnesium sulfate, terbutaline,* or *nifedipine* targeted toward diminishing uterine contractions) is commonly used to treat documented preterm labor. Antenatal steroids have been shown to improve neonatal outcomes in premature infants and should be administered to women who are threatening to deliver between 24 and 34 weeks' gestation. In addition to these strategies, there is now convincing medical evidence that weekly progesterone injections may have a significant impact on the recurrence rate of preterm birth in patients who have had premature deliveries in the past. **See Gabbe 26, Hacker 12.**

Placental Abruption

Pφ Placental abruption is a common complication of pregnancy associated with smoking, cocaine use, trauma, and hypertension. However, in many cases, placental abruption is idiopathic.

TP The typical presentation of placental abruption is painful vaginal bleeding and uterine tenderness. There are usually signs and symptoms of preterm labor, such as associated contractions. If the abruption is severe, a nonreassuring fetal heart rate on monitoring is common.

Dx The diagnosis is usually made based on clinical presentation. Although a sonographic examination should be performed on all women presenting with vaginal bleeding, sonography will be helpful in the diagnosis of abruption only in about 25% of cases. The lack of sonographic evidence of a placental abruption does not rule out the diagnosis.

Tx A patient suspected of having a placental abruption is always admitted to the hospital for fetal and maternal surveillance. If continuous fetal heart rate monitoring, serial lab studies, and clinical parameters remain stable, the patient may ultimately be discharged for outpatient surveillance if the bleeding resolves. The use of tocolytics in women who have a placental abruption is potentially hazardous. **See Gabbe 18, Hacker 10.**

Preterm Premature Rupture of Membranes (PPROM)

Pφ The etiology of PPROM is not well understood. The condition may result from ascending vaginal infection, uterine overdistention, or idiopathic causes.

TP The most common presentation of PPROM is a mother reporting a "gush" of fluid or, less commonly, an ongoing "leak." Urinary incontinence is common in pregnancy, and incontinence must be ruled out.

Dx Diagnosis is made by a sterile speculum examination, with testing for "ferning" (crystallization of amniotic fluid seen with microscopy), "pooling" of amniotic fluid in the vaginal fornix, or pH testing of the fluid (amniotic fluid will turn Nitrazine paper purple because amniotic fluid is a base).

Tx The risks of ascending infection to the mother and the fetus must be weighed carefully against the risks of delivering a premature infant. If the mother is not in active labor, it is wise to begin antibiotic therapy. A short course of tocolytics and steroid therapy may be beneficial for the treatment of severely preterm fetuses. Once 34 weeks of gestation is reached, induction of labor is recommended. **See Gabbe 27, Hacker 12.**

Pyelonephritis

Pφ Pyelonephritis is a relatively common upper urinary tract infection during pregnancy and can present with significant abdominal and flank pain, especially if there are concurrent renal calculi, hydronephrosis, or ureteral dilation. Pyelonephritis is most often caused by gram-negative enteric pathogens. Pregnant women may be more susceptible to pyelonephritis owing to physiologic ureteral dilation and poor bladder emptying in pregnancy.

TP The most common presentation of pyelonephritis is fever and flank pain, occasionally accompanied by anorexia, nausea, and vomiting. In many instances uterine contractions are also seen. Dysuria, although a common symptom in the nonpregnant patient, is often absent.

Dx The diagnosis of pyelonephritis is suspected by the combination of physical findings including flank pain, fever, an abnormal urinalysis, and positive urine Gram stain. A positive urine culture confirms the diagnosis. Blood cultures should also be collected if you have a high suspicion of pyelonephritis.

Tx In pregnancy, pyelonephritis is usually treated as an inpatient case. Intravenous antibiotics are started empirically before culture and sensitivities return. The most commonly used first-line antibiotic is a first-generation cephalosporin. Once culture and sensitivities are returned, then treatment can be tailored to the particular pathogen and antibiotic sensitivity. (See Chapter 27.) **See Gabbe 36.**

ZEBRA ZONE

a. Uterine rupture: Uterine rupture should be considered in a woman who has a history of previous uterine surgery who presents with abdominal pain and a nonreassuring fetal heart rate tracing. (*The patient presented in the introduction of this chapter who had two previous vaginal deliveries would not be at high risk for uterine rupture.*)

b. Cervical cancer: Although this is rare during pregnancy, a speculum examination of the vagina and cervix should be performed on any patient presenting with vaginal bleeding. Unexpected findings should prompt colposcopy or biopsy.

c. Bleeding dyscrasia: Bleeding dyscrasia should be considered in any patient with a history of bleeding where the etiology of the bleeding is unclear. The most common defects would be von Willebrand disease, hemophilia, and idiopathic thrombocytic purpura.

d. Vasa previa: This rare condition occurs when an intramembranous placental vessel traverses the internal os. This unusual presentation can be diagnosed with a transvaginal sonogram using color Doppler.

e. Musculoskeletal pain: Musculoskeletal pain, specifically back pain, is common during pregnancy. This is often attributed to the progesterone-induced relaxation of joints, maternal weight gain, and exaggerated lordosis of pregnancy.

Practice-Based Learning and Improvement: Evidence-Based Medicine

Title
Management of preterm labor

Authors
American College of Obstetricians and Gynecologists Committee on Practice Bulletins, with the assistance of John M. Thorp Jr., MD

Institution
American College of Obstetricians and Gynecologists

Reference
ACOG Practice Bulletin, Number 43, May, 2003

Problem
Management of preterm labor

Intervention
Discusses various interventions and recommendations regarding the management of preterm labor.

Comparison/control (quality of evidence)
Numerous studies are cited, and subdivided into "Level A" (good and consistent scientific evidence) and "Level B" evidence (limited or inconsistent scientific evidence).

Outcome/effect
Reviews the role of tocolytic drugs, poor response to antibiotic therapy, and absence of demonstrable benefit to maintenance tocolytic therapy. This review does emphasize the clear benefit of administering antenatal steroids to facilitate fetal lung maturity.

Historical significance/comments
Definitive position statement from the American College of Obstetricians and Gynecologists regarding the management of preterm labor.

Additional articles of importance
1. ACOG Committee on Obstetric Practice: Use of progesterone to reduce preterm birth. ACOG Practice Bulletin, Number 291, November 2003. Obstetrics and Gynecology 2003;102:1115–1116.
2. ACOG Committee on Obstetric Practice: Premature rupture of membranes. ACOG Practice Bulletin, Number 80, April 2007. Obstetrics and Gynecology 2007;109:1007–1019.

Interpersonal and Communication Skills

Be Mindful That *Translation* Goes through a *Translator*
Preterm labor is always a stressful situation for the patient and her family. In some areas of the country, you may be called upon to discuss preterm labor or other serious medical situations through use of a translator. In some settings, a family member is often chosen as the translator for such purpose. Be mindful that not only may some of your nuances be "lost in translation," but, when dealing with family members as translators, you must consider the personal dynamics of the translator as well as potential family dynamics that could be operative. When beset with this situation it is wise to have the *patient* feed back to you (even, if necessary, through the

auspices of the same translator) the understanding she has gained of the situation. Your nonverbal body language, focusing on the patient rather than the translator, should be indicating to the patient that *she*, not the translator, is the real object of your concern and attention.

Professionalism

Principle: Commitment to Just Distribution of Finite Resources
An infant is born to a primigravida woman at 28 weeks' gestation and has respiratory distress syndrome. The attending physician in the neonatal intensive care unit comes to speak with the parents about treatment options for the baby.

A. The physician explains to the parents that the infant will need surfactant therapy to survive. He promises that they will monitor the infant very closely and that he will keep the parents informed as any developments take place. The parents, although frightened, agree with this plan of action.

B. The physician says that for the baby to survive it will need several costly treatment courses with surfactant. He tells the parents exactly how much this will cost and goes on to describe what the child's medical needs are likely to be in the future. The parents decide that it will be best to withhold treatment.

I have seen both of these scenarios play out; one was in a developing country. Although we may be individually unable to right the inequitable distribution of health care resources, as students, trainees, and physicians, our duty as professionals requires that we be mindful of such global issues.

Systems-Based Practice

Collaboration among Services
Management of preterm labor is best undertaken as a multidisciplinary approach. Multiple services and physician specialists are often involved to provide the patient and her fetus with optimum care. Antenatal consultation by a neonatologist and visits by neonatal intensive care unit nursing staff can be extremely helpful, especially in helping the patient to understand the complex issues of prematurity. Such an interdisciplinary approach will help patients appreciate that, even if preterm delivery cannot be prevented, the newborn will be cared for in a highly specialized neonatal environment.

Chapter 25
Twin Gestations (Case 13)

Jennifer Agrusa, Michelle M. Edwards DO,
and David Seubert MD, JD

Editor's note: Although the overall incidence of multiple gestations is increasing with the increased use of assisted reproductive technology, only twin gestations will be considered in this chapter. An extensive discussion of the management of higher-order multiple gestations is beyond the scope of this text.

Case: A patient presents to your obstetrics practice after undergoing assisted reproductive technology (in vitro fertilization after gonadotropin stimulation and oocyte harvesting). Her reproductive endocrinologist informed her that she is pregnant with a twin gestation and is currently 10 weeks' gestation. The patient is curious if these are identical (monozygotic) or fraternal (dizygotic). She has many other questions, including concerns regarding the risks associated with a twin gestation and whether she will delivery vaginally or by cesarean section.

Types of Twin Gestations and Placentation

Fraternal twins: Dizygotic twinning—arising from two separate ova

Two Fertilized Ova	Placentation
Dizygotic	Dichorionic, diamniotic

Identical twins: Monozygotic twinning—arising from a single ovum, which then further subdivides

Day of Fertilized Ovum Division	Placentation
0-3	Dichorionic, diamniotic
4-7	Monochorionic, diamniotic
8-12	Monochorionic, monoamniotic
Beyond 12	Conjoined twins

Speaking Intelligently

When I see a patient with a twin gestation or higher-level multiple gestation, it is important to determine the chorionicity of the gestation as early as possible. This can typically be determined with early ultrasonographic evaluation. Seeing two placentas with two sets of membranes in the first trimester indicates that the gestation is *dichorionic*. Later in gestation, as the placental masses merge, the two sets of membranes assume a "lambda" sign. These two sets of fused amnions and chorions are visualized as being "thick," greater than 2 mm. Although these twins are determined to be of dichorionic placentation, they may in fact be either *dizygotic* or *monozygotic*. If these twins are determined to be of different genders, it is obvious that they are dizygotic twins. If the twins are the same gender, it is difficult to discern the zygosity. Dizygotic twins account for 90% of twins and are always dichorionic. Monozygotic twins account for 10% of twins. Approximately 20% of monozygotic twins are dichorionic. Thus, if both fetuses are of the same gender, the zygosity cannot be determined with certainty using ultrasonography alone. Eighty percent of monozygotic twins are monochorionic, diamniotic. These twins present with a single placenta with a thin dividing membrane less than 2 mm in thickness. Approximately 1% of monozygotic twins are monoamniotic, presenting with a single placental mass and no separating membrane. Conjoined twins have one placenta and are fused at various parts of the body, most commonly at the thorax (i.e., thoracopagus twins).

PATIENT CARE

Clinical Thinking

- We must consider the patient's nutritional status, and be sure that her nutritional state is optimized. Consider supplementation of folic acid, calcium, and iron.
- Monitor for signs and symptoms of maternal complications such as gestational diabetes, placental abruption, gestational hypertension, and preeclampsia.
- Plan an antenatal surveillance regimen to evaluate fetal growth and well-being.
- We must be ready to manage premature rupture of membranes and preterm labor, and to decide on the safest route of delivery.
- Postdelivery complications such as postpartum hemorrhage must be anticipated.

History

- It is important to establish whether the multiple gestation was conceived using assisted reproductive technologies or through spontaneous conception. For reasons that are largely unexplained, in vitro fertilization seems to increase the likelihood of pregnancy complications such as preeclampsia and intrauterine growth restriction. This observation is still under clinical investigation.
- This patient should be asked routine antenatal visit questions, such as: Are you feeling the babies move? Have you been able to tolerate food without nausea? Do you have leaking of fluid? Do you have vaginal bleeding? Are you experiencing cramping or contractions?
- In addition, it is important to ask about signs and symptoms of prenatal complications. Questions regarding the presence of headache, blurry vision, and right upper quadrant abdominal pain can screen for gestational hypertension and preeclampsia. Diabetes screening can be reviewed to detect the presence of gestational diabetes.

Physical Examination

- Careful attention should be paid to maternal vital signs. Blood pressure, urine dipstick for protein and glucose, and maternal weight are checked at every visit.
- Fetal heart tone identification can be done by Doppler or conventional ultrasonography.
- The position of each fetus can be assessed by Leopold's maneuvers or ultrasonography.
- The length of the patient's cervix can be determined by ultrasonography or bimanual examination, depending on clinical scenario.
- Of note, the measurement of fundal height is not sensitive in determining growth abnormalities in twin gestations.

Tests for Consideration

- **Ultrasonography:** Diagnosis of twin gestation is best made by ultrasonography in the first or early second trimester. Identification of amnionicity and chorionicity are best determined at that time. Ultrasonography is also used to evaluate fetal growth. Fetal growth restriction and discordance are risk factors for increased perinatal morbidity and mortality in twin pregnancies. Serial ultrasonography is usually performed in the second and third trimester to monitor for these abnormalities. Ultrasonographic examinations can also detect the majority of major fetal malformations whose rate is higher in twin pregnancies than singletons. Fetal presentation is determined with the help of ultrasonography. This is important for planning the route of delivery. $600

- **Amniocentesis and chorionic villus sampling:** These are appropriate methods of prenatal diagnosis in the hands of experienced operators. $300
- **Nonstress testing:** Weekly or semiweekly nonstress testing can be valuable in the ongoing antenatal surveillance regimen. $125

IMAGING CONSIDERATIONS

→**Ultrasonography:** Serial ultrasonography, usually performed every 4 weeks or more frequently if needed, is used to evaluate the growth of the fetuses to establish concordance. Early sonograms can be used to address zygosity and chorionicity. $600

Clinical Considerations for Multifetal Gestations   Medical Knowledge

Maternal Physiologic Adaptations in Twin Gestations

Normal maternal adaptations seen in singleton pregnancies are exaggerated in multiple gestations. Levels of progesterone, estradiol, human placental lactogen, human chorionic gonadotropin, and alpha-fetoprotein are elevated above expected pregnancy levels in twin gestations. Maternal heart rate and stroke volumes are higher. Uterine volume and blood flow are markedly increased. Larger increases in oxygen consumption and tidal volume are noted. The glomerular filtration rate is higher in multiple gestations. **See Hacker 13.**

Maternal Nutritional Requirements in Twin Gestations

The Institute of Medicine recommends a 35- to 45-pound total weight gain at term for women carrying twins. More specific recommendations can be made based on prepregnancy body mass index. Additional folic acid, calcium, and iron should be considered.

Maternal Complications Associated with Multifetal Gestations

- **Preterm labor and delivery:** Over half of all multifetal pregnancies are delivered preterm. Preterm labor and delivery is the single leading cause of neonatal morbidity in multifetal pregnancies. Patients with multiple gestations often require prolonged periods of bed rest at home or in the hospital, administration of tocolytic agents to attempt to stop uterine contractions, and administration of antenatal corticosteroids to aid in the prevention of intraventricular hemorrhage, hyaline membrane disease and other respiratory compromise, and necrotizing enterocolitis. The mean gestational age for twins at the time of delivery is approximately 36 weeks; for triplets it is approximately 33 weeks' gestation, and shorter for higher-level multiples.
- **Hypertensive disease:** Both gestational hypertension and preeclampsia are 2.6 times more common in twin gestations compared with a singleton gestation. These conditions may warrant preterm delivery. The incidence of these conditions is further increased with each additional fetus; with multiple gestations conceived through use of assisted reproductive technologies, the incidence is increased beyond that expected for naturally conceived multiples.
- **Gestational diabetes:** This disorder complicates 3% to 6% of twin gestations. Each additional fetus increases the risk of this metabolic disturbance owing to the greater placental masses producing higher levels of human placental lactogen, which is antagonistic to insulin.
- **Intrauterine growth restriction:** Intrauterine growth restriction of one or both twins can lead to adverse obstetric outcomes, including cesarean section for nonreassuring fetal status, umbilical artery pH less than 7.1, low Apgar scores, and neonatal intensive care unit admission. It is important in multiple gestations to consider not only individual growths of the fetuses but the concordance of the growth patterns. Once the discordance of the growth of a twin gestation exceeds 20%, higher rates of morbidity are associated with the gestation. **See Gabbe 28, Hacker 13.**

Mode of Delivery in Twin Gestations

The route of delivery depends on several factors, including fetal presentations at the time of delivery, estimated fetal sizes at the time of delivery, and the experience of the operator. Typically, a non-vertex first twin is a contraindication to vaginal delivery and the twin gestation should be delivered by cesarean section. Typically, a twin gestation where both twins are cephalic in presentation and of concordant size can be allowed a trial of labor as long as there are no other obstetric contraindications to vaginal birth. If the first twin is cephalic and the second twin is noncephalic, the patient can be offered a trial of labor or cesarean section. If she chooses a trial of labor and successfully delivers the first twin vaginally, there are two options for vaginal birth for the second twin. The first option is internal podalic version with breech extraction, whereby the examiner locates the fetal feet digitally and with the aid of intraoperative sonography. The lower extremities are then delivered and the remainder of the birth completed with assisted breech extraction. Alternatively, external cephalic version aided by sonography may be used to guide the second fetus' head into the maternal pelvis so that the fetus is now cephalic in presentation. All patients attempting a vaginal birth must be aware that the successful vaginal birth of the first twin does not necessarily imply the vaginal birth of the second baby. If after the delivery of the first twin the second twin develops a nonreassuring heart rate tracing, a malpresentation refractory to maneuvers that would allow a safe delivery, or other evidence of a nonreassuring environment, cesarean section of the second twin is indicated. When this information is presented to some patients even where both twins are cephalic in presentation, the patient may rightfully elect to proceed with cesarean delivery rather than a trial of labor. **See Gabbe 28, Hacker 13.**

ZEBRA ZONE

a. **Twin-to-twin transfusion syndrome:** Twin-to-twin transfusion syndrome (TTTS) is now also commonly referred to as *polyhydramnios-oligohydramnios syndrome*. This complication is usually unique to monochorionic, monoamniotic twin gestations. Although 80% of monozygotic twins have this type of placentation, only 15% of these twins develop TTTS. Of the 15% that develop this complication, only about half require intervention. TTTS develops when a series of arteries from one twin's placenta drains into a series of veins of the other twin's placenta. The result is that one twin becomes larger with polyhydramnios and associated hyperviscosity because of an increased red blood cell and fluid volume. The other twin is growth restricted and suffers from oligohydramnios and occasionally anhydramnios, giving the appearance of a fetus wrapped in a silhouette, the so-called "stuck twin." The most common cause of mortality and morbidity with this complication is preterm delivery due to the polyhydramnios of one twin. There are several treatment options. If the size and fluid levels are minimally altered and the patient is asymptomatic, no invasive treatment is indicated except for careful surveillance. If there is polyhydramnios and the patient is suffering from contractions causing cervical change, the patient may benefit from serial amnioreduction (AR), whereby amniotic fluid is withdrawn from the polyhydramniotic sac. In severe cases in which there are extreme differentials in size and fluid levels, the patient may benefit from an invasive procedure known as *selective fetoscopic laser photocoagulation* (SFLP). SFLP, first described by De Lia and colleagues,[1,2] is an intrauterine endoscopic procedure in which the aberrant arteriovenous communications in the monochorionic placenta are obliterated, essentially creating a de novo dichorionic placentation. Although some authorities believe laser surgery improves short- and long-term perinatal outcomes by reducing the hemodynamic stresses,[3] a large, prospective, randomized, multicenter trial of AR versus SFLP for the treatment of severe TTTS did not show a statistically significant advantage of either procedure for the donor or recipient twin.[4]

b. **Higher-order multiple gestations:** Triplet and quadruplet pregnancies are virtually always managed at tertiary care centers by skilled perinatologists.

Practice-Based Learning and Improvement: Evidence-Based Medicine

Title

A trial of 17 alpha-hydroxyprogesterone caproate to prevent prematurity in twins

Authors

Rouse DJ, Caritis SN, Peaceman AM, et al; National Institute of Child Health and Human Development Maternal-Fetal Medicine Units Network

Institution

Multi-institutional

Reference

New England Journal of Medicine 2007;357:454–461

Problem

Preterm birth is responsible for a substantial portion of infant mortality. More than half of twin gestations result in preterm birth. This study hoped to address the possible advantage of the use of weekly 17 alpha-hydroxyprogesterone caproate injections to prevent premature delivery in twin gestations.

Intervention

Weekly injections of 17 alpha-hydroxyprogesterone caproate from weeks 16 to 20 through week 35 in asymptomatic women with twin gestations.

Comparison/control (quality of evidence)
This study was a randomized, double-blind, placebo-controlled trial conducted at 14 centers.

Outcome/effect
Treatment with progesterone injections did not reduce the rate of preterm birth in women with twin gestations.

Historical significance/comments
In a previous landmark study, weekly injections of 17 alpha-hydroxyprogesterone caproate were shown to lower the risk of recurrent preterm birth in women who had had a previous preterm delivery. This encouraging finding shaped our management of women with history of preterm delivery. Because of the study findings summarized here, extension of treatment to women with twin gestations cannot be supported.

Interpersonal and Communication Skills

Communicate Effectively with Appropriate Consultants
Patients with twin pregnancies potentially face more risks and complications than patients with a singleton gestation. It is important to convey to the patient at the beginning of a twin pregnancy or multiple gestation that the risks to the patient and the babies are real, especially the risks of premature delivery. You must further explain that a whole team of health care professionals may be called upon to help optimally manage a twin or higher-order multiple gestation.

First, you may need to contact the reproductive endocrinologist who helped achieve the pregnancy for the couple to obtain subtle details of the first trimester, if you feel this is necessary or if the patient is a poor historian. Second, you must be willing to refer to perinatologists when needed, particularly to make a plan regarding antenatal chromosomal diagnosis (if the couple desires this) as well as second- and third-trimester surveillance for sonography, cervical length determination, and general antenatal surveillance. Third, at the time of delivery, make the members of the neonatology staff aware that the delivery of premature infants may be on the horizon. Be sure to discuss any complications the mother may have had, or any other concerns regarding fetal status.

It is also important to be proactive and discuss plans for surveillance and delivery with the patient and family. One of the keys to the management of such complex cases is effective communication with the perinatologists, neonatologists, and other specialists and consultants who become involved in the patient's care. Of course, the patient needs to be involved with these consultations and decisions as well.

Professionalism

Principle: Commitment to Scientific Knowledge and Professional Competence

Improving the quality of care we provide to patients by improving our knowledge is an important aspect of professionalism. Modern obstetrics has advanced dramatically over the span of the last 30 to 50 years, and this is quite evident in the way we provide care for patients with multiple gestations. What we do and the care we provide should be derived from evidence-based medicine. Evidence-based medicine would suggest that twin gestations are at much greater risk for preterm delivery, and vigilance in this regard is justified. Also, evidence-based medicine suggests that in many cases, especially when the second twin is not vertex (head-down), there may be benefit to offering a cesarean section rather than a trial of labor. Keeping up with the literature of our profession keeps us current and assists in the evidence-based decision making that is part of our professional responsibility.

Systems-Based Practice

Billing and Reimbursement

A systems-based approach is used when caring for a patient with a multifetal gestation. Typically, the obstetrician and perinatologist engage the assistance of other health care providers to best care for the patient. Such personnel typically include ultrasonographers to evaluate fetal growth throughout gestation; dieticians to educate the patient about nutritional needs during and after the pregnancy; neonatologists and neonatal intensive care unit staff, as well as pharmacists, radiologists, and respiratory therapists, to care for the infants after delivery.

Billing and reimbursement policies for multifetal gestational services are variable and have no national standard. For all billing and reimbursement issues, the practitioner must become familiar with each carrier's specific rules and requirements. Most insurance carriers make this type of information available through their websites, provider manuals, or the provider "call center."

References

1. De Lia JE, Cruikshank DP, Kaye WR: Fetoscopic neodymium: YAG laser occlusion of placental vessels in severe twin-twin transfusion syndrome. Obstet Gynecol 1990;75:1046–1053.
2. De Lia JE, Kuhlmann RS, Harstad TW, Cruikshank DP: Fetoscopic laser ablation of placental vessels in severe twin-twin transfusion syndrome. Am J Obstet Gynecol 1995;172:1202–1211.
3. Chmait RH, Quintero RA: Operative fetoscopy in complicated monochorionic twins: Current status and future directions. Curr Opin Obstet Gynecol 2008;20;169–174.
4. Crombleholme TM, Shera D, Lee H, et al: A prospective, randomized, multicenter trial of amnioreduction vs selective fetoscopic laser photocoagulation for the treatment of severe twin-twin transfusion syndrome. Am J Obstet Gynecol 2007;197:396.e1–396.e9.

Professor's Pearls: Cases in Maternal/Fetal Medicine

Consider the following clinical problems and questions posed. Then refer to the professor's discussion of these issues.

1. You see a 25-year-old G0 with a 10-year history of poorly controlled type 1 diabetes for preconception counseling. She is recently married and desires pregnancy as soon as possible. She currently uses insulin glargine (Lantus) for basal glycemic control and insulin aspart (NovoLog) with each meal to control postprandial glycemic elevations. Six months ago her hemoglobin A_{1c} was 9%. She reports that she had no evidence of diabetic retinopathy at her last ophthalmologic examination, which was 3 years ago. Her mild hypertension is well controlled (120/75 mm Hg) with lisinopril. What steps should be taken before conception?

2. A 17-year-old G2P0010 at 32 weeks presents by EMS with a 2-hour history of severe abdominal pain and bright red bleeding per vagina. Her history is significant for cocaine abuse. On physical examination, her abdomen is gravid, very firm, and tender.

3. A 39-year-old G6P2042 with known history of antiphospholipid antibody syndrome (APS) and chronic hypertension for the last 8 years (well controlled with hydrochlorothiazide [HCTZ] and recently started enalapril) visits your office for a preconception visit. She got remarried 6 months ago and expresses strong desire to become pregnant. Her concern is that her medical conditions might potentially cause complications in her pregnancy.

Discussion by Dr. Nancy S. Roberts, Chairman, Department of Obstetrics and Gynecology, Main Line Health, Wynnewood, Pennsylvania

Answer 1: Clinical Considerations: Preconception Counseling and Diabetes

Preconception counseling is essential for a White class C (duration of 10 years) insulin-dependent diabetic patient such as this. Careful glycemic surveillance and control are vital to improve her chances of a successful pregnancy outcome. The following issues should be discussed:

■ **Harmful effects of hyperglycemia:** As suggested by her hemoglobin A_{1c} of 9% from 6 months ago, she should not even consider a pregnancy until she achieves good enough glycemic control to bring the glycosylated hemoglobin level down to a normal range (<6%). Elevated blood glucose levels in the first trimester place the fetus at increased risk of anomalies (of 2 to 6 times the baseline risk of 3%) as well as fetal macrosomia. Anomalies of the heart, CNS, and skeletal system are most common.

- **Evaluation for end-organ disease:** This should include an ophthalmologic examination within the last 6 months, evaluation of renal function with a urinalysis including microalbuminuria, creatinine clearance, and serum creatinine, and evaluation of cardiac health with a lipid profile and electrocardiogram. If she proves to have end-organ disease she may be reclassified as having more advanced diabetes than Class C, and this would increase her pregnancy risk.

- **Evaluation of current medications and a plan for the upcoming pregnancy:** This patient would need to stop her lisinopril because it is an angiotensin-converting enzyme (ACE) inhibitor and this class of antihypertensive has been shown to cause renal dysplasia or dysfunction in the fetus. This results in anuria and eventual oligohydramnios, creating the fetal risks of lung hypoplasia, limb abnormalities, and craniofacial abnormalities. Her antihypertensive therapy should include either alpha methyldopa (Aldomet), a beta blocker such as labetalol (Normodyne), or a calcium channel blocker such as nifedipine (Procardia) for control of hypertension. She would need to change from Lantus to NPH Humulin insulin because there is no prior clinical experience using Lantus in pregnant women. This patient may need an insulin pump to achieve rigid glycemic control. She may continue the NovoLog because this has been used in pregnancy and has a shorter duration of action than regular insulin.

- **Nutritional consultation:** I would ensure that the patient consumes the proper balance of food groups. I would write a prescription to begin folic acid 4 mg daily for at least 1 month before conception and to continue for the first 3 months of the pregnancy to reduce the risk of a neural tube defect. The benefits of breast-feeding, including the possibility of a protective effect against type 1 diabetes, should be reinforced. Also, I would take a complete history to ensure that adverse behaviors such as smoking or alcohol consumption are stopped before the pregnancy.

- **Family history review:** The patient should be evaluated for inherited disorders such as cystic fibrosis, sickle cell anemia, the thalassemias, or the recessive disorders found in the Jewish population (if these tests are indicated).

- **Routine testing:** This would include HIV status, cytomegalovirus, parvovirus, and toxoplasmosis antibodies, and immunization status including rubella, varicella, tetanus, and hepatitis B vaccination, with preconception vaccination if possible.

- **Counseling about the pregnancy risks:** The patient should understand that the pregnancy may worsen her existing diabetic retinopathy and that the diabetes could place her pregnancy at an increased risk of miscarriage, congenital anomalies, preeclampsia, prematurity from preterm labor, premature rupture of the membranes, or iatrogenic prematurity, cesarean section, stillbirth, growth aberration including small-for-gestational-age (SGA) or large-for-gestational-age (LGA) fetus, and delivery problems including shoulder dystocia.

Answer 2: Clinical Consideration: Placental Abruption

A patient who arrives by EMS with a 2-hour history of severe abdominal pain and vaginal bleeding and a history of cocaine use is considered to have a placental abruption until proven otherwise. Up to 10% of women in the third trimester who are using cocaine will have a placental abruption. The abdominal pain, uterine tenderness, and bleeding with the association of cocaine is the trio that suggests placental abruption. Other causes of third-trimester bleeding are less likely, such as cervical dilation, cervical erosion, placenta previa, or maternal coagulopathy. The classic findings of acute abruption include vaginal bleeding in over 80% of cases and abdominal pain in over 50% of cases. Uterine tenderness presumably results from the blood extravasating into the uterine myometrium. The amount of vaginal bleeding does not correlate well with the extent of maternal hemorrhage.

In this scenario, we have to consider two patients—the woman and her baby. We should balance the fetal risks of prematurity versus the maternal risks of continuing the pregnancy, including hemorrhage and a coagulopathy, and potential maternal death. A disseminated intravascular coagulopathy is less common without fetal death. At 32 weeks' gestation, I would administer corticosteroids to accelerate lung maturity because a preterm delivery is highly likely to occur. I would not use tocolytic agents to stop any contractions. I would obtain clotting studies, including a fibrinogen; type and crossmatch the patient for at least 2 units of blood; and monitor the baby closely with electronic fetal monitoring and obtain a sonogram. Only about 25% of cases of abruption have sonographic findings that confirm this diagnosis. If the vaginal bleeding continues, or there are signs of a nonreassuring fetal heart rate pattern or evidence of an early maternal coagulopathy, I would deliver the patient. Cesarean section would probably be the safest route because this is the patient's first baby and a prolonged labor may result in a poor outcome for mother or baby, or both.

Answer 3: Clinical Considerations: Antiphospholipid Antibody Syndrome and Chronic Hypertension

This is a 39-year-old multiparous woman with a history of APS and an 8-year history of chronic hypertension. She presents for a prenatal consultation to discuss the pregnancy risks associated with her medical conditions. The risks are threefold: her advanced maternal age, APS, and, last, chronic hypertension. Her advanced maternal age places her at risk of infertility, first-trimester miscarriage, dizygotic twinning, abnormal fetal chromosomes, placenta previa, prematurity, aberration of fetal growth of babies that are too large or too small, stillbirth, cesarean section, and postpartum hemorrhage. The prematurity is usually iatrogenic if the older mother requires a preterm delivery for age-related pregnancy complications. Further, the higher frequency of cesarean section is likely related to several factors, including more frequent inductions of labor, increased malpresentations, increased labor abnormalities (such as uterine dysfunction or fetal intolerance of labor), and more women who are having repeat cesarean sections.

In APS, there are moderate to high levels of circulating antiphospholipid antibodies. Several adverse pregnancy outcomes have been attributed to the presence of these antibodies, including recurrent pregnancy loss, preterm delivery, and stillbirth. Some studies suggest that preeclampsia, fetal growth restriction, early severe preeclampsia or eclampsia, unexplained fetal death after 10 weeks' gestation, and potentially fatal maternal thromboembolic disease of venous or arterial origin are also associated problems. The treatment for APS includes aspirin alone, or aspirin and unfractionated or low–molecular-weight heparin daily in prophylactic doses. The risks of heparin in pregnancy include bleeding, osteoporosis, and thrombocytopenia.

Chronic or preexisting hypertension poses further risk to this patient and her fetus, including a threefold increase in perinatal mortality. Because this patient was initially treated with only a diuretic and has recently been placed on an antihypertensive agent, I would categorize her as a mild chronic hypertensive. As discussed in case no. 1, the patient's enalapril, an ACE inhibitor, will have to be changed to a different medication because the ACE inhibitors are contraindicated in pregnancy due to teratogenicity. The HCTZ may be continued because it was initiated before pregnancy, but this is controversial. HCTZ may deplete maternal electrolytes and there are rare maternal side effects of thrombocytopenia and hemorrhagic pancreatitis and neonatal thrombocytopenia. Although there is a decrease in the incidence of severe maternal hypertension, antihypertensive medications have not resulted in improved perinatal outcomes. The beneficial effects of treatment of chronic hypertension appear to be limited to prevention of maternal morbidity and continuation of treatment should depend on the severity of maternal hypertension because antihypertensives may result in impaired fetal growth.

In this mildly hypertensive patient, other pregnancy complications include a 15% to 25% risk of superimposed preeclampsia, possibly resulting in iatrogenic prematurity, a 0.7% to 1.5% risk of placental abruption, a 12% to 34% risk of prematurity, and an 8% to 16% risk of fetal growth restriction. The maternal risks include increased likelihood of cesarean section, retinopathy, cerebrovascular accident or congestive heart failure, acute renal failure, and even death.

Section IV
CASES IN INFECTION DURING PREGNANCY

Section Editors
Katherine A. Belden MD and Alan Tunkel MD

Section Contents

Section IV
CASES IN INFECTION

Chapter 26
Pneumonia in Pregnancy (Case 14)

Katherine A. Belden MD

Case: A 32-year-old woman at 27 weeks' gestation presents to the office with complaints of fever, cough, and myalgias. She is healthy and has had an uncomplicated pregnancy thus far. She was in her usual state of health until 2 days ago, when her symptoms began abruptly. On examination, she is diaphoretic and in moderate distress. Her temperature is 101.1° F, heart rate 122 beats/min, blood pressure 100/50 mm Hg, and respiratory rate 34/min. Her lung examination reveals crackles at the right base and her lower extremities are cool and mottled.

Differential Diagnosis
Etiologies Associated with Pneumonia in Pregnancy

Bacterial pneumonia: community acquired	Viral pneumonia	Pneumonia in human immunodeficiency virus (HIV)–infected women	Mycobacterium tuberculosis

Speaking Intelligently

The woman described in the case above is clearly in distress. When I am asked to treat a pregnant woman with respiratory symptoms, it is important first to evaluate the patient's stability. Once the woman's vital signs are obtained and an examination is performed, I can better assess the acuity of her presentation. The differential diagnosis for a pregnant woman with respiratory symptoms should always include pneumonia, especially if fever is present. Other important considerations include thromboembolic disease, reactive airways disease, aspiration pneumonitis, and pulmonary edema. (This differential in the pregnant patient is considered in Chapter 23, Pulmonary Diseases in Pregnancy.) Timely initiation of antimicrobial therapy is crucial in managing pneumonia in pregnancy, and it is important to be aggressive in the diagnosis and treatment of this serious condition.

PATIENT CARE

Clinical Thinking

- Although pneumonia is not more common in pregnant than nonpregnant women, it can result in increased maternal and fetal morbidity and mortality because of the physiologic changes of pregnancy, which include a diminished pulmonary functional residual capacity and altered cell-mediated immunity. Pneumonia can complicate pregnancy at any time during gestation.
- Risk factors for pneumonia in pregnancy include asthma, other chronic respiratory diseases, anemia, HIV infection/acquired immunodeficiency syndrome, smoking, and drug use.
- Maternal complications of pneumonia in pregnancy include higher rates of disseminated infection, hospitalization, mechanical ventilation, empyema, and pneumothorax. Fetal complications include an increased risk of preterm delivery and infant low birth weight.
- With the availability of antimicrobial therapy and modern medical management, the majority of pregnant women with pneumonia are successfully treated. Nevertheless, pneumonia remains the third leading cause of death in pregnant women and is the most common nonobstetric infectious cause of mortality during pregnancy and the puerperium.[1-3]

History

- When evaluating a pregnant woman with pneumonia, it is important to consider the recent history of the pregnancy as well as past events.
- **Past medical history:** What is her underlying health status? Does she have medical conditions that require management or put her at risk for pneumonia or other infections?
- What is her **gestational age** and has her pregnancy been complicated in any way thus far?
- **Social history:** Does she use tobacco, drink alcohol, or have a history of illicit drug use? Does she have any unusual travel history or animal exposures? Has she been tested for HIV infection? Where was she born and raised?
- What are her **symptoms?** The clinical presentation of pneumonia frequently includes fever, cough, dyspnea, and pleuritic chest pain. Rigors or chills may be associated with bacteremia, which complicates from 2% to 16% of cases of community-acquired pneumonia. It is important to establish the duration of symptoms because an abrupt onset of illness is more suggestive of typical bacterial or viral infection than is a more indolent time course.
- Does she have known **drug allergies?**

Physical Examination

- What is the woman's **general appearance?** Is she in visible distress, pale, or cyanotic? Is she using accessory muscles of respiration to breathe?
- Are her **vital signs** stable?
- Does her **chest examination** reveal crackles, rhonchi, wheezes, or absent breath sounds? Check for the presence of a pleural friction rub, dullness to percussion, and egophony.
- Are the results of her **cardiac examination** within normal limits? Is she tachycardic or is a murmur or rub detected?
- Are findings on **abdominal and fundal examination** appropriate for gestational age?
- Is the woman awake and alert? Are there any gross abnormalities on **neurologic examination?**
- Always check for the presence of a **rash.**

Tests for Consideration

- **Complete blood count:** Leukocytosis, especially with a "left shift," suggests a bacterial infection. Leukopenia, anemia, and thrombocytopenia can be associated with sepsis and raise concern for a more severe infection or underlying disease process. $35
- **Electrolytes, creatinine, and glucose testing.** $35
- **Pulse oximetry** is a fast and easy way to assess the woman's oxygenation.
- **Arterial blood gas sampling:** Should be performed if the woman appears in any distress or is sick enough to require hospital admission. This test will determine her true oxygenation status and acid-base condition. $100
- **Sputum Gram stain and culture:** Helpful if the woman has a productive cough and can provide an adequate specimen. $250
- **Blood cultures:** Important for pathogen identification and should be obtained before the administration of antimicrobial therapy. $250
- **Urine antigen testing** for *Legionella* (only detects *Legionella pneumophila* serogroup 1) or *Streptococcus pneumoniae*: Negative tests do not exclude these organisms as the etiology of pneumonia. $350
- **Fetal monitoring** as appropriate for gestational age. $130

IMAGING CONSIDERATIONS

→**Posteroanterior chest radiograph:** This is safe in pregnancy, but should be done using a "shielded" technique. A chest radiograph is important in confirming the diagnosis of pneumonia and distinguishing pneumonia from acute bronchitis. $50

→**CT scan of chest,** with possible spiral CT if indicated: This test can help to evaluate for pneumonia or pulmonary embolism. $1800

→**Ventilation and perfusion scan** if indicated. $1600

| Clinical Entities | Medical Knowledge |

Bacterial Pneumonia: Community-Acquired Pneumonia in Pregnancy

Pφ Community-acquired pneumonia is the most common form of pneumonia seen in pregnancy and *S. pneumoniae* is the most common pathogen identified. Less frequent bacterial pathogens include *Haemophilus influenzae*, *Staphylococcus aureus*, *Klebsiella pneumoniae*, and other gram-negative pathogens. Atypical bacterial pathogens include *Mycoplasma pneumoniae*, *L. pneumophila*, and *Chlamydophila pneumoniae*.

  ■ In 40% to 60% of cases no etiologic agent is identified.[1]

TP Typical bacterial pneumonia in the pregnant woman, regardless of etiology, usually presents with the acute onset of fever, chills, and productive cough with lobar infiltrates seen on chest radiograph. Atypical pneumonia is associated with a more indolent presentation of lower fever, dry cough, and patchy or interstitial infiltrates on chest radiograph. *Legionella* pneumonia, however, can present with a more acute illness, mimicking typical bacterial pneumonia.

Dx An accurate history and thorough physical examination are most important in establishing the diagnosis of pneumonia in a pregnant woman. Chest radiograph findings offer additional information. Sputum culture, blood cultures, and urine antigen testing for *Legionella* and *S. pneumoniae* (in some settings) can help to identify bacterial pathogens. Pathogen identification is important in guiding therapy and monitoring the patient for clinical improvement.

Tx Mild cases of community-acquired pneumonia in pregnancy can be managed in the outpatient setting with oral antimicrobial therapy. Given the risks of pneumonia in pregnancy to both the mother and fetus, however, hospital admission should be seriously considered in all patients. Empiric antimicrobial therapy for moderate to severe infection should include a third-generation cephalosporin such as ceftriaxone (U.S. Food and Drug Administration [FDA] pregnancy category B), which provides coverage for the majority of pathogens causing community-acquired pneumonia as well as penicillin-resistant *S. pneumoniae*. A macrolide such as azithromycin (FDA pregnancy category B) should be added for atypical coverage. If the patient has a history of severe penicillin allergy, vancomycin (FDA pregnancy category C) plus azithromycin is appropriate empiric treatment.[2,3] It is important to note that if the woman has risk factors for hospital-acquired, aspiration, or methicillin-resistant *S. aureus* (MRSA) pneumonia, antimicrobial coverage should be broadened accordingly. Antimicrobial therapy should be continued for 7 to 14 days in uncomplicated cases with appropriate clinical response. **See Gabbe 35.**

Viral Pneumonia in Pregnancy

Pφ The most important causes of viral pneumonia in pregnancy are influenza and varicella-zoster virus (VZV).

TP **Influenza:** Influenza infection is seasonal, with most infections occurring in late fall through the winter months. It is associated with a 1- to 4-day incubation period, followed by the onset of fever, dry cough, headache, and malaise. If symptoms persist for more than 5 days, complications should be suspected. Both primary influenza pneumonia and secondary bacterial pneumonia can cause significant respiratory and systemic illness. Pregnancy increases the risk of severe infection. Chest radiographic findings range from clear to diffuse bilateral infiltrates.[3,4] Of note, at the time of this publication a global pandemic of novel H1N1 influenza A (referred to early on as "swine flu") is underway. There have been case reports of more serious illness and death in some pregnant women infected with H1N1 influenza. A vaccine for H1N1 influenza is now available.

VZV infection: Up to 10% of cases of primary VZV infection (chickenpox) traditionally occur after the age of 15 years, although this percentage may decrease within the vaccinated population. Primary VZV infection is associated with an incubation period of 10 to 14 days followed by a vesicular rash, fever, and constitutional symptoms. VZV pneumonia, which complicates 1 in 400 cases of primary infection in adults, typically presents 2 to 5 days after the onset of rash and is characterized by dyspnea, dry cough, chest pain, and hemoptysis. The course of VZV pneumonia ranges from a mild respiratory illness to fulminant pneumonitis and respiratory failure. Chest radiographic findings in severe cases include diffuse miliary or nodular infiltrates. Pregnancy may increase the risk of developing VZV pneumonia and this infection can be life-threatening, especially during the second or third trimester.[3]

Maternal VZV infection can have significant effects on the fetus, including preterm birth and the congenital varicella syndrome. The congenital varicella syndrome occurs in 1.2% to 2% of primary infections in pregnancy and includes fetal dermatomal scarring, limb abnormalities, microcephaly, cataracts, and chorioretinitis. Perinatal VZV infection occurring 5 days before delivery through 48 hours postpartum is associated with a high infant mortality rate.[3,5]

| **Dx** | **Influenza** is usually a clinical diagnosis. Rapid nasal or throat swab testing by immunofluorescence or immunoassay can provide a same-day diagnosis, but is not as sensitive as viral culture, which is also available.

VZV infection is also usually a clinical diagnosis made by history and physical examination. Skin lesions can be scraped and sent for a Tzanck smear or direct fluorescent antibody. Chest radiographic abnormalities support the diagnosis of pneumonia in the setting of primary VZV infection. |

| **Tx** | **Influenza:** All women who will be pregnant during the influenza season should receive influenza vaccination! Inactivated influenza vaccination can be performed safely during any trimester of pregnancy. Hand washing and other secondary prevention techniques are also important to remember during the influenza season.

There are a number of antiviral medications approved for the prevention and treatment of influenza infection. All are FDA pregnancy category C and should be taken when the benefits are thought to outweigh the risks to the woman and fetus. The adamantane derivatives, amantadine and rimantadine, traditionally have had activity against influenza A (the most common cause of epidemic infections). The neuraminidase inhibitors, including oseltamivir, traditionally have had activity against both influenza A and B. Of note, resistance has been reported to both of these classes of antiviral agents and their use should be guided by regional influenza resistance information.

Because secondary bacterial pneumonia is a serious complication of influenza infection, antimicrobial therapy directed against *S. pneumoniae*, *S. aureus*, *H. influenzae*, and |

other gram-negative pathogens should be started in addition to antiviral therapy in serious cases.[3,4]

■ Remember to place any hospitalized patients with known or suspected influenza infection in droplet isolation.

VZV infection: The currently available VZV vaccine is a live-attenuated vaccine and is contraindicated in pregnancy. VZV immunoglobulin can prevent or attenuate infection in susceptible pregnant women if given within 96 hours of exposure to VZV. Pregnant women with primary VZV infection and pneumonia should be treated with acyclovir 5 to 10 mg/kg IV every 8 hours (FDA pregnancy category B).[3,5]

■ All patients with known or suspected VZV pneumonia should be placed in airborne isolation if hospitalized.[3,5]

See Gabbe 35, Hacker 16.

Tuberculosis in Pregnancy

Pφ *Mycobacterium tuberculosis* causes millions of infections worldwide each year. In spite of a decline in the number of cases occurring in the United States in recent years, tuberculosis remains a source of concern, especially in foreign-born individuals and those with HIV infection. Multidrug-resistant strains are often difficult to treat. *M. tuberculosis* infection in pregnancy requires treatment and close monitoring of both the mother and fetus.

TP/Dx **Latent tuberculosis:** Pregnant women at high risk for tuberculosis exposure should be screened for latent infection with subcutaneous intermediate-strength purified protein derivative (PPD) testing. This tuberculin skin test is safe in pregnancy. Most patients with a positive PPD are asymptomatic, and all should be evaluated for active tuberculosis with a thorough history and physical examination as well as a chest radiograph.

Active tuberculosis: Pregnant (and nonpregnant) women with active tuberculosis typically present with cough, hemoptysis, fever, sweats, weight loss, and fatigue. Chest radiographic findings include multinodular infiltrates, cavitation, adenopathy, loss of volume in the upper lobes, and effusions.

Sputum samples should be examined for acid-fast bacilli (AFB) and sent for culture. Polymerase chain reaction testing can be performed on AFB-positive sputum. If the woman cannot produce sputum, a diagnostic bronchoscopy should be performed.

Extrapulmonary tuberculosis occurs in 10% to 20% of active infections in the United States. Higher rates are described in HIV-infected patients. Sites of extrapulmonary infection include lymph nodes, bone, central nervous system, and kidneys. Pregnancy does not increase the risk of extrapulmonary tuberculosis, but extrapulmonary disease may adversely affect pregnancy outcome.[3]

Tx **Latent tuberculosis:** Pregnant women with a positive PPD and no evidence of active tuberculosis should be evaluated for prophylaxis with isoniazid (INH; FDA pregnancy category C) 300 mg daily plus vitamin B_6 50 mg daily. Because the greatest risk for progression to active disease is within the first 2 years after exposure, pregnant women with a known recent exposure should undergo prophylaxis with INH plus vitamin B_6 starting after the first trimester for 9 months. Pregnant women with an unknown or prolonged history of a positive PPD should start prophylaxis after delivery.

Active tuberculosis: Pregnant women with active tuberculosis should be treated. Initial therapy should include INH 300 mg daily plus vitamin B_6, rifampin 600 mg daily (FDA pregnancy category C), and ethambutol 25 mg/kg daily (FDA pregnancy category B). If resistant disease is anticipated a fourth agent may be required. After culture and sensitivity results are known and 2 months of therapy have been completed, treatment can be reduced to INH/B_6 + rifampin to finish 9 months of total therapy. Resistant infections, however, require a longer course of therapy.

- All patients with known or suspected active tuberculosis should be placed in airborne isolation if hospitalized.
- All pregnant women receiving antimycobacterial therapy should be monitored closely for side effects, which include, among others, hepatitis, peripheral neuropathy, rash, and optic neuritis. Pregnancy increases the risk of drug-related hepatotoxicity.
- Mothers who are being treated with antimycobacterial agents may breast-feed. Their infants should undergo PPD testing at birth and at 3 months of age. Infants born to women with active tuberculosis at the time of delivery should receive INH + B_6 prophylaxis until maternal disease is inactive. Active tuberculosis in the neonate should be treated with combination therapy.[3,6]

See Gabbe 35, Hacker 16.

Pneumonia in HIV-Infected Pregnant Women

Pφ Pneumonia in HIV-infected pregnant women with a CD4+ cell count greater than 200 cells/μL will be caused by pathogens similar to those causing pneumonia in non–HIV-infected pregnant women. These include bacterial, viral, fungal, and *M. tuberculosis* infection, with bacterial pathogens, in particular *S. pneumoniae*, being the most common.

Pneumonia in HIV-infected pregnant women with a CD4+ cell count less than 200 cells/μL can be caused by a variety of pathogens, including those mentioned previously as well as *Pneumocystis jirovecii* pneumonia (PCP), atypical mycobacteria, and *Toxoplasma gondii*. These women are at risk for more severe pneumonia with all pathogens given their degree of immune suppression.

M. tuberculosis and lymphoma should be considered in any HIV-infected pregnant woman with pulmonary disease regardless of her CD4+ cell count. Kaposi sarcoma can present with pulmonary symptoms in HIV-infected persons with a CD4+ cell count less than 100 cells/μL.

TP Women with a low CD4+ cell count are at greater risk for opportunistic infection and may have a more indolent presentation of pneumonia because of their inability to mount an inflammatory response. Therefore, they may be more seriously ill than their presentation suggests.

PCP typically presents with the insidious onset of dry cough and dyspnea with or without fever progressing over 2 to 4 weeks. Patients are often hypoxic. Chest radiographic findings range from minimal, if any, abnormalities to diffuse interstitial infiltrates. Lobar and asymmetric infiltrates, cavities, and nodules, however, have been described, and any HIV-infected pregnant woman with a low CD4+ cell count and respiratory symptoms should be evaluated for PCP.[7]

PCP in pregnancy carries significant risk to both the mother and fetus with higher reported rates of respiratory failure, maternal morbidity and mortality, and preterm delivery.[7]

Dx Evaluation of the pregnant woman with HIV infection and pneumonia is the same as for a non–HIV-infected pregnant woman, with consideration given to the possibility of opportunistic infection if her CD4+ cell count is less than 200 cells/μL.

A definite diagnosis of PCP requires visualization of organisms in pulmonary secretions or tissues. Induced sputum may be adequate for diagnosis, but bronchoalveolar lavage is the procedure of choice in the diagnosis. The sensitivity of this test is close to 95% when performed correctly.

In severely immunocompromised patients, more than one active infection may be present at the same time. A diagnostic bronchoscopy with or without lung biopsy looking for bacteria, mycobacteria, and fungi may be indicated in management.

Tx The initial management of pneumonia in the HIV-infected pregnant woman should be similar to that in the non–HIV-infected pregnant woman. Initial therapy should include antimicrobial agents targeting bacterial pathogens, including *S. pneumoniae*. Depending on the clinical presentation and immune status of the woman, therapy directed at viral, fungal, mycobacterial, or other opportunistic pathogens may be required. In treating pneumonia in this setting, it is important to be aware of the potential for drug interactions with antiretroviral medications.

Trimethoprim-sulfamethoxazole (TMP/SMX; pregnancy risk category C) is the drug of choice in the treatment of PCP. If the woman is stable, oral therapy with TMP/SMX-DS two tablets by mouth three times daily for 21 days is appropriate. If the woman is acutely ill or oral therapy is not feasible, intravenous TMP/SMX 15 mg/kg/day should be administered. For a Pao_2 less than 70 mm Hg, corticosteroid therapy should be added. Alternative agents include clindamycin and primaquine and atovaquone.

Pregnant women with a CD4+ cell count less than 200 cells/μL or who have had PCP should be maintained on oral TMP/SMX prophylaxis.[2,7]

Influenza and pneumococcal vaccinations are safe in pregnancy and should be given to HIV-infected pregnant women. **See Gabbe 35, Hacker 16.**

ZEBRA ZONE

a. **Fungal pneumonia in pregnancy:** Very rare in an immunocompetent population. The most common pathogens are *Cryptococcus neoformans*, as well as the dimorphic fungi *Histoplasma capsulatum*, *Blastomyces dermatitidis*, and *Coccidioides immitis*. *Aspergillus* infection has also been reported in pregnant women.[8]

Practice-Based Learning and Improvement: Evidence-Based Medicine

Title
Infectious Diseases Society of America/American Thoracic Society consensus guidelines on the management of community-acquired pneumonia in adults

Authors
Mandell LA, Wunderink RG, Anzueto A, et al.

Institution
Infectious Diseases Society of America; American Thoracic Society

Reference
Clinical Infectious Diseases 2007;44(Suppl. 2):S27–S72.

Problem
Describes general guidelines for evaluation and treatment of pneumonia in adults.

Quality of evidence
Level I, as well as expert opinion, Level III.

Historical significance/comments
Ongoing guidelines, updated as needed. This is a clinical problem; although pregnancy is a consideration, following general treatment guidelines for best treatment of the mother is recommended.

Interpersonal and Communication Skills

Communicating about Risks: Candor and Follow-up
Infections during pregnancy such as pneumonia often require diagnostic studies, radiologic imaging, and therapeutic drugs. The question will be asked by the patient: "Is it safe for the baby?"

Part of the obstetrician's job is to acquire the knowledge base of what *is* and *is not* safe for the pregnant patient and the unborn child. As your fund of knowledge and skills permit, be sure to let the patient know that what you are doing is safe, in her own best interest, and in the best interest of her unborn baby. When you are not sure whether a test or therapy is safe, be candid and say so. Then go to the literature or a knowledgeable mentor, find out, and report back, closing the loop. This basic communication skill of *candor* and *follow-up* is greatly appreciated by patients.

Professionalism

Principle: Commitment to Appropriate Relations with Patients
There is a distinct possibility that patients known to a medical student from the community in the environs of the hospital will present for care when the student is working. Although there is something to learn from all patients and the management of their illnesses, the medical student must remember that there may be personal aspects of this patient's history or physical examination that will make the student's presence uncomfortable for both student and patient. As nonessential medical personnel, it is appropriate for the student to recuse himself or herself from the medical care of the patient and remain in a supportive role, if that is in keeping with the nature of the previous relationship. It is also important to be open and honest with your colleagues about your personal relationships with patients. To avoid patients' expectations being falsely elevated, you must clarify your role with them as well.

Systems-Based Practice

Using the Critical Care Team and the Intensive Care Unit
On occasion, women who present with pneumonia in pregnancy can be extraordinarily ill, sometimes requiring mechanical ventilation and intensive care unit treatment. In these instances it is vital to have all members of the team apprised of the patient's status and involved early in the case. Often it is appropriate to coordinate consultants from a variety of services including Critical Care, Infectious Diseases, Maternal/Fetal Medicine, Radiology, Nursing, Neonatology, Pharmacy, and Respiratory Therapy. Taking extra time to speak *directly* with consultants as well as the microbiology laboratory will allow for immediate changes to the care plan if necessary. Attention to detail, as well as meticulous medical management, is sometimes the only way to get mother and baby through this very serious clinical situation.

References

1. Pereira A, Kreiger B: Pulmonary complications of pregnancy. Clin Chest Med 2004;25(2):1–15.
2. Goodnight WH, Soper D: Pneumonia in pregnancy. Crit Care Med 2005;33(10 Suppl):1–10.
3. Whitty JE, Dombrowski MP: Respiratory diseases in pregnancy. In Gabbe SG, Niebyl JR, Simpson JL (eds): Obstetrics: Normal and Problem Pregnancies, 5th ed. Philadelphia, Elsevier Churchill Livingstone, 2007.

4. Laibl VR, Sheffield JS: Influenza and pneumonia in pregnancy. Clin Perinatol 2005;32(3):1–10.
5. Whitley R: Varicella-zoster virus. In Mandell GL, Bennett JE, Dolin R (eds): Mandell, Douglas and Bennett's Principles and Practice of Infectious Diseases, 6th ed. Philadelphia, Elsevier Churchill Livingstone, 2005, pp 1780–1786.
6. Fitzgerald D, Haas D: *Mycobacterium tuberculosis*. In Mandell GL, Bennett JE, Dolin R (eds): Mandell, Douglas and Bennett's Principles and Practice of Infectious Diseases, 6th ed. Philadelphia, Elsevier Churchill Livingstone, 2005, pp 2852–2886.
7. Masur H: Pneumocystosis. In Dolin R, Masur H, Saag MS (eds): AIDS Therapy. Philadelphia, Elsevier Churchill Livingstone, 2003, pp 403–416.
8. Galgiani J: *Coccidioides*. In Mandell GL, Bennett JE, Dolin R (eds): Mandell, Douglas and Bennett's Principles and Practice of Infectious Diseases, 6th ed. Philadelphia, Elsevier Churchill Livingstone, 2005, pp 3040–3051.

Chapter 27
Acute Pyelonephritis in Pregnancy (Case 15)

Randi Silibovski MD, FACP

Case: A 25-year-old G3P2 at 21 weeks' gestation presents with dysuria for 3 days, followed by fever, chills, nausea, vomiting, and right flank and abdominal pain for 1 day before her presentation.

Differential Diagnosis

Acute pyelonephritis	Acute cystitis	Appendicitis

Speaking Intelligently

When a pregnant woman presents with urinary symptoms and fever, I almost always admit the patient to the hospital. Pregnant women may become quite ill and are at risk for both medical and obstetric complications. My history focuses on location of specific symptoms (flank vs. abdominal pain) as well as on the patient's past history of urinary tract infections. My physical examination focuses on location of tenderness, possible peritoneal findings, costovertebral angle tenderness, and presence of vaginal discharge or bleeding. A urinalysis is essential to exclude genitourinary (GU) tract disease (including nephrolithiasis), and a white blood cell count helps to gauge an infectious process. If GU tract disease is not likely or uncertain based on the results of these tests and findings, I order an imaging study searching for appendicitis. I also consider abdominal pregnancy-related problems, such as chorioamnionitis or placental abruption.

PATIENT CARE

Clinical Thinking

- A past medical history of urinary tract infections should increase your suspicion of this diagnosis.
- Outpatient screening for asymptomatic bacteriuria is standard practice at the first prenatal visit.
- If urinalysis reveals marked pyuria, a GU tract infection should become your leading diagnosis in the differential.
- **Cystitis** is an infection in the bladder (lower urinary tract). **Pyelonephritis** is an infection in the kidney (upper urinary tract). Distinguishing between these two entities is important in terms of management and potential complications. High fever, elevated white blood cell count, and flank tenderness are more suggestive of upper tract disease.
- If the urinalysis is normal or shows only a few white blood cells, GU infection becomes less likely.
- Appendicitis may be diagnosed by ultrasonography in the pregnant patient, although CT scanning is rapidly becoming the standard of care to reach this diagnosis.
- An obstetric sonogram becomes more valuable if the other diagnostic tests and studies yield equivocal results.

History

- Prior history of urinary tract infections, especially during pregnancy, increases the probability of a urologic infection.

- It is important to remember that urinary tract infections can present for the first time during pregnancy, especially during the second or third trimester.
- Obtain a history of prior pregnancies and outcomes with specific attention to premature births, low birth weight, or poor obstetric outcomes. Bacteriuria is associated with all of these adverse outcomes.
- Diabetes is a well-established risk factor for urinary tract infections in both pregnant and nonpregnant women.
- Attention to specific symptoms of abdominal pain versus flank pain and vaginal discharge (bloody or purulent) can raise the possibility of chorioamnionitis.
- Gross hematuria points to the presence of bladder or kidney stones.
- A prior history of sexually transmitted diseases should raise your suspicion for pelvic inflammatory disease (PID).
- Right lower quadrant abdominal pain (as opposed to right flank pain) is more suggestive of appendicitis. Vaginal discharge may suggest PID, but keep in mind that PID is unusual in pregnancy because of changes in the consistency and permeability of cervical mucus.

Physical Examination
- **Vital signs:** Fever, hypotension, or tachycardia suggest infection and sepsis. All of the aforementioned clinical syndromes may present with fever. Hypotension and tachycardia are suggestive of severe systemic illness.
- **General appearance:** An ill-appearing, fatigued, and "washed out" appearance suggests systemic disease, but does not pinpoint the site of infection.
- **Lungs** are usually clear.
- **Abdominal examination:** It is important to distinguish between abdominal versus flank tenderness. Peritoneal signs (tenderness, guarding, and rebound) suggest appendicitis or (less likely) PID. Uterine contractions suggest preterm labor, or a serious complication such as placental abruption.
- **Pelvic examination:** Purulent vaginal discharge suggests PID. Cervical motion tenderness is a nonspecific finding suggesting PID or pelvic peritoneal irritation. Palpation of a mass suggests abscess. Cultures should be obtained as part of the physical examination.

Tests for Consideration
- **CBC:** High white blood cell count suggests infection and low hemoglobin suggests bleeding. Neither pinpoints the site of infection. $35
- **Urinalysis:** Significant pyuria, hematuria, or both suggest GU tract pathology. $38

- **Urine, blood, and vaginal cultures:** Used to make a specific microbiologic diagnosis and to guide therapeutic decisions, especially antimicrobial therapy. $500 total
- **Chem 7 (basic metabolic profile):** Assesses renal function and helps identify acid-base disturbances during sepsis. $27

IMAGING CONSIDERATIONS

→**Graded compression ultrasonography:** A viable diagnostic imaging option to evaluate the appendix in pregnancy. $560

→**MRI:** To avoid exposure to ionizing radiation. $1500

→**CT:** Can be used judiciously with modifications to limit fetal radiation exposure. This test would be performed only if the diagnosis of pyelonephritis appeared unlikely. $800

→**Renal ultrasonography:** Helpful to evaluate for renal obstruction (hydronephrosis) or renal abscess. $350

→**Pelvic ultrasonography:** Can be helpful to help establish a diagnosis of PID or tubo-ovarian abscess. $250

Clinical Entities	Medical Knowledge

Acute Cystitis

Pφ Cystitis is an infection of the bladder.

TP Typical presentation is characterized by dysuria, urinary hesitancy, frequency, and urgency. Some patients describe a foul odor to the urine. Less commonly, hematuria is present.

Dx Initial diagnosis is made by urinalysis, which reveals white blood cells and bacteria. Urine culture confirms infection, identifies the specific agent, and defines antimicrobial sensitivities.

Tx Cystitis is treated with appropriate antimicrobials based on sensitivities from urine culture and principles of antimicrobial safety in pregnancy. Oral regimens are preferred if the patient can tolerate them and if compliance is not considered to be an issue. Ampicillin or nitrofurantoin is often considered first-line therapy. Patients are generally treated for 7 days or longer because urinary tract infections in pregnancy are considered "complicated." **See Gabbe 36, Hacker 16.**

Acute Pyelonephritis

Pφ Pyelonephritis is an upper urinary tract infection involving the kidney. Bacteriuria in pregnancy has a greater propensity to progress to pyelonephritis than in nonpregnant women. During pregnancy, the ascent of bacteria from the bladder to the kidney is facilitated by a reduction in the concentrating ability of the kidney, anatomic changes in the urinary tract (pressure on the bladder from the uterus), and ureteral dilation due to smooth muscle relaxation.

TP Typical presentation is characterized by high fever, dysuria, flank and abdominal pain, nausea, and vomiting.

Dx Diagnosis is made by physical examination, urinalysis, and urine culture. Blood cultures should be obtained. Renal ultrasonography is performed if ureteral obstruction or renal abscess is thought likely based on abnormal renal function or slow clinical response.

Tx Treatment is initially with intravenous fluids and antimicrobial agents. Once the patient has improved and can tolerate oral antimicrobials, a switch can be made based on sensitivities from cultures. Again, antimicrobials considered to be safe in pregnancy should be used and consideration should be given to the likelihood of patient compliance with oral agents when discharged. Ten to 14 days of therapy is appropriate. **See Gabbe 36, Hacker 16.**

Appendicitis

Pφ Appendicitis is usually brought about by occlusion of the appendiceal lumen by a fecalith, leading to inflammation of the appendiceal wall and eventual perforation if diagnosis and treatment are delayed.

TP Initially, the patient develops vague abdominal pain in the periumbilical region. Within the next 24 to 36 hours, the pain typically migrates to the right lower quadrant. Associated symptoms may include nausea, vomiting, and constipation.

Dx Clinical history and the judicious use of CT scanning routinely establish the diagnosis of appendicitis in pregnancy. Graded compression ultrasonography and MRI are alternative imaging studies that avoid fetal exposure to ionizing radiation, but are not used commonly. A markedly elevated white blood cell count, temperature greater than 101° F, or wider distribution of peritoneal findings may suggest perforated appendicitis.

Tx Appendicitis is a surgical emergency and, once the diagnosis is established, antimicrobial agents are administered and the patient proceeds to the operating room for a laparoscopic or open appendectomy. In the hands of a skilled surgeon, laparoscopic appendectomy should be considered, especially in the first or early second trimester. Later in pregnancy, the variable location of the appendix can make a laparoscopic approach too risky, and an open, exploratory approach would be a better choice. **See Gabbe 23, Hacker 16.**

ZEBRA ZONE

a. **"Round ligament pain":** A benign condition characterized by stretching of the round ligaments as the uterus grows. This classic finding is usually seen at about 20 weeks' gestation.

b. **Pubic symphysis separation pain:** A well-recognized weakening of the ligament that comprises the pubic symphysis.

c. **Pelvic inflammatory disease and tubo-ovarian abscess:** Relatively rare in pregnancy, and typically caused by ascending pelvic infection, most commonly gonorrhea and chlamydia. However, some cases of PID can be polymicrobial, reflecting enteric flora.

Practice-Based Learning and Improvement: Evidence-Based Medicine

Title
Guidelines for antimicrobial treatment of uncomplicated acute bacterial cystitis and acute pyelonephritis in women

Authors
Warren JW, Abrutyn E, Hebel JR, et al.

Institution
Infectious Diseases Society of America

Reference
Clinical Infectious Diseases 1999;29:745–758

Problem
Urinary tract infections, including bacterial cystitis and pyelonephritis.

Intervention
Addresses various antimicrobial therapeutic options.

Comparison/control (quality of evidence)
Recommendations based on numerous well-controlled studies, but still expert opinion, so considered Level III evidence.

Outcome/effect
Therapeutic options for pyelonephritis.

Historical significance/comments
These are evidence-based recommendations from the Infectious Diseases Society of America regarding a very common infection in women and in pregnancy.

Interpersonal and Communication Skills

Avoiding Desensitization, Considering Patient Perspective

As physicians dealing with illnesses every day, we often come to consider certain diagnoses as "routine." Remember that "routine" diagnoses may not be routine during pregnancy. Pyelonephritis, for example, may be regarded in the practice of an internist, nephrologist, or urologist as a routine problem. During pregnancy, however, pyelonephritis is an anxiety-producing condition that puts the patient at risk for sepsis, perinephric abscess, and premature delivery. To prevent yourself from becoming desensitized to issues you will ultimately learn to consider routine, ask yourself throughout the day: "Am I considering this matter from my patient's perspective?" Then, if necessary, consider spending a little extra time with your patient to be appropriately reassuring.

To check that you are considering patients' perspectives, after consultations ask yourself the following questions:

- Do I know more about this patient now?
- Do I know what matters to this patient?
- Did I really hear what the patient was telling me?
- To what extent did I tailor the information I gave to the individual patient?
- Did I check that the management plan was understood and is practical for this patient?

Professionalism

Principle: Maintaining Trust by Managing Conflicts of Interest

When treating pyelonephritis, one must, of course, choose an appropriate antibiotic. Important considerations should include sensitivity of the infectious organism to the antibiotic and its cost. Exposure to the influence of pharmaceutical companies begins at the earliest stages of medical training. Even for medical students and residents, pharmaceutical companies often pay for lunches and provide pens and other omnipresent objects, which offer a constant reminder to us of some medicines and not others. The lines of ethical involvement can be blurred. As individuals we must make decisions about what constitutes private gain versus best patient care in our interactions with these companies.

Systems-Based Practice

Calculating Cost of Oral Antibiotic Therapy

Pyelonephritis, like many bacterial infections, can be managed effectively with oral agents rather than parenteral (IV or injection) therapy, often significantly reducing the total treatment costs. Comparing the *baseline treatment cost*, which is the cost of the full course of antibiotics (cost/dose × doses/day × days of treatment), is usually straightforward. It is more difficult, however, to determine the *overall expected treatment cost* because this figure needs to factor in probabilities such as the likelihood that the therapy will be effective, safe, and complete. As a simplified example, an oral antibiotic might cost $5 per dose and require a 10-day course of 4 doses per day—for a baseline treatment cost of $200. This might be much less expensive than a parenteral drug, which might cost $25 per dose and require a 10-day course of twice-daily therapy—for a baseline treatment cost of $500. If, however, 25% of patients on the oral antibiotic fail the therapy and go on to require parenteral drugs, the expected total cost per treatment of the oral antibiotics is actually $325 ($200 + [25% × $500]). This simplified calculation does not factor in other complicating issues, such as the cost of delivering outpatient IV therapy, the likelihood of developing resistance, tolerability of the different drug options, complexity of dosage regimens, and the potential for drug–drug interactions. The point is not to fully calculate the cost of therapy exactly for every case, but rather to be aware of these factors so that you can consider them when making clinical decisions about antibiotic therapy.

As a general rule, newer antibiotics are often better tolerated and less likely to produce adverse reactions, resulting in better patient compliance, greater efficacy, and often lower overall cost of antimicrobial therapy. However, because they are new, they are often still available only as brand name drugs, and are therefore more expensive. Furthermore, it is important to be aware of new drugs that are merely "me too" drugs—drugs that offer little or no therapeutic advantage over previously available drugs, but are brought to the market by pharmaceutical companies hoping to share in lucrative treatment areas.

Chapter 28
Chorioamnionitis and Endometritis (Case 16)

Dionissios Neofytos MD

Case: A 23-year-old G1P0 at 38 weeks' gestation presents to the labor and delivery suite with fever of 101.5° F. She is in labor. She is treated with antibiotics and acetaminophen and her obstetrician delivers the baby by cesarean section because of an arrest of the active phase of labor. She is subsequently discharged to her home. Six days later, she presents to the emergency department with chills, a fever of 102.7° F, lower abdominal pain, and foul-smelling vaginal fluid.

Differential Diagnosis

Chorioamnionitis	Urinary tract infection	Pyelonephritis	Postpartum pelvic abscess
Endometritis		Appendicitis	Viral syndrome

Speaking Intelligently

When I am called to evaluate a pregnant patient who presents with a high fever, my first concern is always to rule out a diagnosis of chorioamnionitis. If the patient has been recently delivered, my chief concern then turns to the possibility of endometritis. Patients with chorioamnionitis may present with fever alone, but may also have premature rupture of membranes, lower abdominal tenderness, or signs of preterm labor. Prompt diagnosis is important to avoid serious maternal and fetal complications. Similarly, a diagnosis of endometritis (an inflammation of the endometrium, the inner lining of the uterus) should be strongly considered in women presenting with postpartum fever (particularly after cesarean section or prolonged labor/rupture of membranes). Chorioamnionitis is a clinical entity that occurs before delivery, whereas endometritis is typically seen within 1 week (but can occur up to 6 weeks) postpartum. Clinical entities, such as viral, urinary tract, or respiratory tract infections, are also included in my differential diagnosis. I always take a detailed history, perform a thorough clinical examination, and carefully review the pertinent laboratory tests (e.g., CBC), which are usually adequate to establish the diagnosis of chorioamnionitis or endometritis. A high clinical suspicion for chorioamnionitis or endometritis should lead to the right therapeutic approach. I make sure appropriate antimicrobial therapy is promptly initiated and communicate my diagnosis to the patient and the entire health care team.

PATIENT CARE

Clinical Thinking

- A diagnosis of chorioamnionitis in a pregnant woman is suggested by a temperature >100.4° F and may include the following additional findings: leukocytosis (>15,000 white blood cells/mm^3), maternal tachycardia (>100 beats/min), uterine tenderness, foul odor of the amniotic fluid, and fetal tachycardia (>160 beats/min).
- Endometritis should always be suspected when a patient presents within 1 week postpartum with chills, fever, foul-smelling vaginal discharge, lower abdominal tenderness, and no other accompanying symptoms.
- Although the diagnosis of chorioamnionitis is most frequently clinical, amniocentesis is sometimes warranted to establish a definitive diagnosis. Amniotic fluid should be sent for white blood cell count, glucose, and Gram stain and culture.
- Chorioamnionitis and endometritis are most frequently polymicrobial infections. The most commonly retrieved pathogens include the following: group B beta-hemolytic *Streptococcus*, *Escherichia coli*, *Mycoplasma hominis*, *Ureaplasma urealyticum*, and anaerobes (e.g., *Peptostreptococcus* spp., *Bacteroides* spp., and *Fusobacterium* spp.).
- Chorioamnionitis has been associated with maternal bacteremia, hemorrhage, labor abnormalities, and need for cesarean section. Fetal complications include higher risk of fetal infection, perinatal asphyxia, neurodevelopmental delay, and cerebral palsy.
- Prompt initiation of appropriate antimicrobial therapy is important. Currently, the recommended regimen for treatment of chorioamnionitis is broad-spectrum antimicrobial therapy, such as combination of appropriate dosages of ampicillin and gentamicin, until the time of delivery. In case of cesarean section, clindamycin or metronidazole should be added to that regimen for 24 hours postdelivery to broaden the coverage for anaerobic organisms. Clindamycin and gentamicin are the recommended agents for the treatment of endometritis. Other appropriate regimens for both entities include ampicillin-sulbactam, ticarcillin-clavulanic acid, and piperacillin-tazobactam.

- Immediate delivery has not been shown to improve the clinical outcome in cases of chorioamnionitis. However, appropriate planning regarding the possibility of delivery is always prudent. There is no evidence that cesarean section should be performed in uncomplicated cases of chorioamnionitis.

History

- High fever without localizing symptoms in a pregnant patient should prompt a work-up for chorioamnionitis.
- Amniotic membranes may or may not be ruptured in cases of chorioamnionitis.
- A past history of a positive screen for group B beta-hemolytic *Streptococcus* should raise the possibility of chorioamnionitis. Other risk factors associated with chorioamnionitis include bacterial vaginosis, sexually transmitted diseases, multiple digital vaginal examinations in women with ruptured membranes, nulliparity, preterm labor, young age, and low socioeconomic status.
- Risk factors associated with endometritis include uterine and cervical manipulation due to prolonged rupture of membranes, foreign bodies (e.g., sutures), infection or necrosis at the suture line, and formation of seromas or hematomas.
- A detailed history of the patient's drug allergies should be obtained before initiation of antimicrobial therapy.
- Fever associated with urinary symptoms or flank pain should raise suspicion for pyelonephritis.
- Fever with localized or generalized abdominal tenderness should raise the possibility of any intra-abdominal process, such as appendicitis.
- Fever with upper respiratory symptoms (e.g., cough, shortness of breath) should raise the possibility of viral upper respiratory infection, bronchitis, or pneumonia.
- Persistent fever despite appropriate antimicrobial management in a postpartum patient should raise suspicions for drug-resistant pathogens or development of a pelvic abscess or septic pelvic thrombophlebitis.

Physical Examination

- **Vital signs:** Fever is almost always present. Tachycardia of the mother and the fetus may also be present.
- **General appearance:** Patients with chorioamnionitis do not always appear extremely ill. Patients with endometritis may appear severely ill and occasionally become systemically septic.
- **Lungs:** Should be clear bilaterally.
- **Abdominal examination:** Should be benign, except for the uterus. Bowel sounds should be normal. Occasionally, there may be mild lower abdominal tenderness.
- **Pelvic examination:** Mild to moderate uterine tenderness may be present. When membranes are ruptured, purulent vaginal discharge (occasionally foul smelling) is suggestive of chorioamnionitis.

Tests for Consideration

- **CBC:** Elevated white blood cell count suggests infection or inflammation. Patients with chorioamnionitis and endometritis usually have high white blood cell counts. $35
- **Urinalysis** and **urine culture:** To check for a urinary tract infection. $250
- **Blood cultures:** Always obtain in patients with high fever, preferably before initiation of antimicrobial therapy. Only 10% to 15% of patients with chorioamnionitis or endometritis are bacteremic, most commonly with group B beta-hemolytic *Streptococcus* or *E. coli.* $250
- **Amniocentesis:** The gold standard diagnostic test for chorioamnionitis. It can be performed only in patients without membrane rupture. Amniotic fluid should be sent for white blood cell analysis, glucose and leukocyte esterase concentrations, Gram stain, and culture. When clinical suspicion for chorioamnionitis is high, therapy should be initiated as soon as possible without delay while awaiting further invasive diagnostic testing. $225

IMAGING CONSIDERATIONS

→**CT scan of abdomen and pelvis:** Should be performed in cases where there is clinical suspicion for an intra-abdominal source of infection (e.g., appendicitis). A CT scan is not, however, indicated in the case of chorioamnionitis. In cases of suspected endometritis, a CT scan can be used to rule out a pelvic abscess. $800

Clinical Entities   Medical Knowledge

Chorioamnionitis

Pφ Chorioamnionitis is the clinical manifestation of an inflammatory reaction occurring in the pregnant uterus, most often as a result of a bacterial infection.

TP Chorioamnionitis can occur as a result of either a blood-borne pathogen or ascending infection from the vagina, or occurs during the labor process, either as a result of prolonged rupture of membranes or prolonged labor.

Dx A high level of suspicion is the key to diagnosis. Maternal fever and tachycardia are not seen in every case. Although common, maternal leukocytosis is not always present. An amniocentesis revealing numerous white blood cells and a low glucose concentration in the amniotic fluid is sometimes the only definitive way to diagnose chorioamnionitis. Amniotic fluid should always be sent for culture and sensitivity.

Tx Because these infections are often polymicrobial, broad-spectrum antimicrobial agents to include coverage for group B *Streptococcus*, anaerobes, and *E. coli* are almost always the short-term answer. When a specific bacterial pathogen and its antimicrobial sensitivities have been identified, therapy can be tailored appropriately. **See Gabbe 49, Hacker 12.**

Endometritis

Pφ Endometritis is an infection of the decidua and myometrium after delivery.

TP The most common presentation is fever of 100.4° F or greater (typically on two separate occasions) in the immediate postpartum period, usually on day 2 or 3. There is a significantly increased likelihood that endometritis will occur after a cesarean delivery. Findings include an exquisitely tender uterus, leukocytosis, and a foul-smelling or purulent vaginal discharge. Other sources of infection, particularly urinary tract infection, pyelonephritis, pneumonia, and wound infection (in the case of prior cesarean section), must also be excluded.

Dx The correct diagnosis can be reached by physical examination findings, blood cultures, and possibly a CT scan of the abdomen and pelvis, which may reveal an inflammatory reaction involving the uterus.

Tx Therapy initially involves broad-spectrum antimicrobial agents to treat the likely infecting pathogens. Infection with pathogens resistant to the most commonly administered antimicrobial agents (e.g., ampicillin-resistant enterococci, methicillin-resistant *Staphylococcus aureus* [MRSA], extended-spectrum beta-lactamase [ESBL]–producing organisms) should be treated accordingly. Suspect resistant organisms if symptoms do not improve after 48 to 72 hours of appropriate antimicrobial therapy; repeat blood cultures and consider endometrial cultures. Adjust the patient's antimicrobial therapy based on culture results. On very rare occasions, when the patient fails antimicrobial therapy, a total abdominal hysterectomy and bilateral salpingo-oophorectomy may be required. **See Gabbe 49, Hacker 10.**

Urinary Tract Infection

Pφ A urinary tract infection represents an infection of the lower urinary tract (i.e., cystitis). (See also Chapter 27)

TP It typically presents with dysuria, urinary frequency, and occasionally low-grade fever.

Dx Urinalysis and urine culture are the tests to establish the diagnosis. In patients with a compatible clinical syndrome, urine culture is not cost effective or always necessary before initiation of therapy.

Tx Therapy is oral antimicrobials for 7 days. The therapy chosen should take into consideration whether the patient is breast-feeding, and the patient's drug allergies or sensitivities if this is relevant. Nitrofurantoin, trimethoprim-sulfamethoxazole, ampicillin, amoxicillin-clavulanate, and cephalexin are all acceptable and generally well tolerated choices. **See Gabbe 36, 49.**

Pyelonephritis

Pφ Pyelonephritis is an infection of the upper urinary tract (see also Chapter 27).

TP Patients with pyelonephritis are usually very ill and in major discomfort, and present with shaking chills, high fever, and flank tenderness.

Dx The definitive diagnostic test is renal ultrasonography or CT scan to detect local signs of inflammation, although imaging studies are not always required. Physical examination along with urinalysis (+ white blood cells, + bacteria, + leukocyte esterase), and urine and blood cultures are helpful diagnostic tools.

Tx Therapy consists of intravenous or systemically absorbed oral antimicrobial agents for 10 to 14 days. Notably, patients with pyelonephritis may remain ill appearing with high fever for several days after initiation of appropriate therapy. **See Gabbe 36, 49.**

Appendicitis

Pφ Appendicitis is an inflammatory process of the appendix.

TP Appendicitis typically presents with right lower quadrant tenderness, mild gastrointestinal complaints, low- to moderate-grade fever, and a characteristic prodrome of vague central abdominal pain that later localizes to the right lower quadrant. In late presentations of perforated appendicitis, patients may present with acute, severe, generalized peritonitis. Because of altered pelvic anatomy in pregnancy, appendicitis may be a difficult diagnosis to establish.

Dx An abdominal CT should help make the diagnosis. CT is safe in pregnancy, and one should not hesitate to use it if clinical suspicion of appendicitis is high. Compression ultrasonography is also useful. The CBC will show an elevated white blood cell count.

Tx Therapy consists of antimicrobial therapy and prompt surgical intervention. **See Gabbe 23, Hacker 16.**

Viral Syndrome

Pφ A viral syndrome is characterized by acute illness as a result of infection with any number of common and uncommon viruses that can be acquired in the community.

TP Typically, the patient presents with low- to moderate-grade fever and nonspecific symptoms such as nausea, vomiting, upper respiratory symptoms, or diarrhea.

Dx The diagnosis is usually clinical. The CBC may show a lymphocytic predominance.

Tx Treatment is primarily supportive. Reassurance of the patient is very important. **See Gabbe 48.**

Postpartum Pelvic Abscess

Pφ Pelvic abscess occurs in rare instances when infection in the pelvis does not respond to antimicrobial therapy. Areas of infection become "walled-off" and fill with a collection of infected exudate. This condition is rare before delivery, but can be seen after a cesarean section.

TP A patient with a pelvic abscess presents with persistent weakness and fever, despite appropriate antimicrobial therapy. Suspect if symptoms do not improve after 48 to 72 hours of treatment.

> **Dx** Pelvic ultrasonography and CT scan are the diagnostic tests of choice. CBC and blood cultures are important adjuncts.
>
> **Tx** Treatment consists of initiation of appropriate antibacterial therapy and surgical intervention for drainage. **See Gabbe 49; Hacker 10.**

ZEBRA ZONE

William Short, MD

Septic pelvic thrombophlebitis is an uncommon condition that has been estimated to occur in approximately 1 of every 2000 pregnancies. This condition has been classically associated with pregnancy but can be seen in other settings such as pelvic infections, endometriosis, gynecologic surgeries, and hypercoagulable states.

Pathophysiology: The pathophysiology of septic pelvic thrombophlebitis involves three factors (Virchow's triad):

1. Damage to the endothelium of the pelvic veins
2. Alteration in blood flow
3. Hypercoagulability of the blood

The venous drainage of the pelvic organs tends to flow in a left-to-right fashion through the right ovarian vein. Venous stasis in these dilated veins in the setting of a bacterial infection can lead to septic thrombosis. Sequelae include microembolization through the inferior vena cava to the lungs or other organs of the body.

Diagnosis: One needs to have a high index of suspicion and consider the diagnosis of septic pelvic thrombophlebitis in a patient in whom no etiology can be found for fever, abdominal pain, and leukocytosis despite broad-spectrum antibiotics in the appropriate setting. The diagnosis is often confused with acute appendicitis, pelvic abscess, nephrolithiasis, or adnexal torsion. Clinically, the patient may be asymptomatic, present with persistent fevers, or present with a palpable, tender mass representing the right uterine vein.

CT and MRI are useful in the prompt diagnosis of this condition once it is clinically suspected.

Management: Prompt recognition is necessary to avoid potentially life-threatening complications such as septic shock and pulmonary embolism. Treatment includes broad-spectrum antibiotics, heparin, and long-term oral anticoagulation. For very rare patients who are refractory to medical treatment, surgical intervention in the form of bilateral ovarian vein and inferior vena cava ligation may be necessary.

Practice-Based Learning and Improvement: Evidence-Based Medicine

Title
The Maternal-Fetal Medicine Units cesarean registry: Chorioamnionitis at term and its duration—relationship to outcomes

Authors
Rouse DJ, Landon M, Leveno KJ, et al.

Institution
Department of Obstetrics and Gynecology, Center for Research in Women's Health, University of Alabama at Birmingham

Reference
American Journal of Obstetrics and Gynecology 2004;191:211–216.

Problem
Is there a relationship between chorioamnionitis and its duration to adverse maternal, fetal, and neonatal outcomes?

Intervention
Cesarean section.

Quality of evidence
Level II-2.

Outcome/effect
Chorioamnionitis was associated with increased rates of morbidity after cesarean section at term. The duration of chorioamnionitis was not related to most measures of adverse maternal or fetal–neonatal outcome.

Historical significance/comments
This study showed that cesarean section should not be routinely performed in cases of chorioamnionitis because the duration of the infection was not associated with adverse outcome for the mother and fetus.

Interpersonal and Communication Skills

Choosing the Right Words to Explain Risk

A diagnosis of a serious infection toward the end of a pregnancy is obviously very stressful for the patient. It is important to communicate the suspected diagnosis and, once confirmed, explain all associated risks pertinent to both the mother and the baby. It can be a challenge to choose the "right" words when discussing problems as potentially devastating as fetal complications related to intrauterine infection. One must be truthful, but gentle.

There is a significant body of research by health communications experts seeking methods for optimal delivery of risk information. However, there appears to be no strong evidence for any one approach because singular or standardized approaches lack the flexibility necessary to deal with diverse patient groups and the variety of personal circumstances.

In general, risk can be conveyed in verbal descriptors, "The risk of this infection to your baby is very low" or it can be conveyed numerically as a ratio, "The risk is one in ten thousand." Assess how the patient you are dealing with might receive this information. Although standardized verbal risk scales have been developed (e.g., high risk >1:100, moderate risk 1:100-1:1000, etc.), there is little evidence to support their meaningful use.

As you conclude your discussion, try to emphasize positives: for example, a good outcome may result when the infection is treated promptly. Reassurance (when possible and honest) is a key factor when taking care of pregnant women, particularly when a complication arises.

Professionalism

Principle: Commitment to Professional Competence

A commitment to competence is the keystone of professionalism. It is also important to remember that competence is dynamic. A clinician must be up to date on the latest guidelines and interventions in the management of problems he or she routinely manages. Clinicians must also be prepared to practice infrequently used skills and learn new ones as they emerge. One must also be prepared to request consultation in those cases encountered infrequently. Chorioamnionitis, with its potentially morbid and mortal ramifications for both mother and fetus, is one such infrequently encountered condition. As such, to optimize care and clinical outcome, consultation with an infectious diseases specialist should almost always be obtained. In anticipation of delivery of the fetus, coordination of the appropriate nursing, medical, and neonatal intensive care unit personnel should be optimized for a successful outcome.

Systems-Based Practice

Appropriate Documentation

Best obstetric management, especially in clinically challenging cases such as chorioamnionitis, often calls for delivery of the fetus, even in the face of severe prematurity, where the likelihood of the fetus's survival is significantly reduced. We are often faced with this decision when the mother shows signs of overwhelming sepsis. This raises an important issue that—although not common—will rise from time to time in the care of obstetric patients: what are we supposed to do when the mother or parents do not agree with our clinical recommendation? In the case of inducing premature delivery, parents are tragically torn between the health of the mother and the health of the fetus—a situation that presents a delicate balance of risks and benefits. You as the clinician may be adamant in your opinion that a specific procedure or intervention should be carried out; but your patient, after being informed of the risks and benefits and knowing your opinion, may decide against your recommendation. In such cases you ultimately need to respect the patient's decision, and assure her that you will continue to do your best to achieve the best outcome possible while respecting her wishes. At the same time, it is important to document the situation carefully in the patient's chart. Document that you have explained the risks involved in the different options to the patient, and that you have explained your clinical opinion and your reason for believing it. Then document the fact that after understanding this, the patient decided to choose a different course. If there is any question of the patient's competency, document how it was determined that the patient was competent to make this decision. The patient's well-being is your first and primary concern, but when situations arise that force you to treat a patient differently than you believe is best, it is important to protect yourself by documenting the specifics of the situation.

Chapter 29
HIV and Pregnancy (Case 17)

Katherine A. Belden MD and Kathleen E. Squires MD

Editor's Note: The management of HIV has become its own "specialty within a specialty," and has a unique vocabulary. Accordingly, an introductory **Medical Knowledge** glossary is presented containing the language of HIV concepts to facilitate reading this chapter.

Glossary of Commonly Used Terms

Concept	Definition
HIV	Human immunodeficiency virus, a human retrovirus.
AIDS	The acquired immunodeficiency syndrome results from HIV-induced immune suppression and is manifested by opportunistic disease.
Opportunistic disease	Disease that typically occurs in individuals with underlying cellular immunodeficiency. Examples include *Pneumocystis (carinii) jirovecii* (PCP) pneumonia, *Mycobacterium avium* complex (MAC) infection, toxoplasmosis (*Toxoplasma gondii*), and Kaposi sarcoma.
CD4+ T-lymphocyte count	A quantitative measurement of the status of the cell-mediated immune system. The CD4+ cell count is used to predict the probability of an HIV-infected person developing an opportunistic disease.
HIV RNA viral load	A quantitative measurement of circulating HIV. HIV replication can be suppressed with antiretroviral therapy.
Highly active antiretroviral therapy (HAART)	Combination antiretroviral therapy usually includes at least three medications selected from a number of classes of antiretroviral agents. The goal of HAART is the suppression of HIV replication with a subsequent improvement in immune function.
Antiretroviral drug resistance testing	Genotype testing detects changes in the DNA sequence of relevant HIV genes that are associated with drug resistance. Phenotype testing directly assesses the ability of HIV to grow in different concentrations of antiretroviral drugs. Resistance tests are used to guide antiretroviral therapy.

Cases

Patient A	A 24-year old woman, living in suburban Philadelphia, is diagnosed with HIV infection during prenatal testing at 10 weeks' gestation.
Patient B	A 31-year-old woman from Chicago presents in labor with a full-term pregnancy. She is an active injection drug user and has received no prenatal care. She is found to be HIV positive on a rapid screening test.
Patient C	A 22-year-old pregnant woman living in sub-Saharan Africa presents for the first time to a local care clinic at 29 weeks' gestation. She is diagnosed with HIV infection on a screening test.

Speaking Intelligently

The majority of women with HIV infection are in their reproductive years. An estimated 6000 HIV-infected women give birth annually in the United States; in the developing world, this number is much greater.[1]

HIV infection can be transmitted from mother to child in utero, during labor, or with breast-feeding. Risk factors for perinatal HIV transmission include low birth weight, prematurity, a high maternal HIV viral load, advanced maternal HIV infection, prolonged duration of ruptured membranes, breast-feeding, and mastitis.[1,2]

Public health efforts undertaken in developed countries over the past two decades have decreased rates of perinatal HIV transmission from 25% to less than 3% with the following interventions:

- Universal HIV testing of pregnant women
- The use of highly active antiretroviral therapy (HAART) during pregnancy
- Intravenous zidovudine (ZDV) therapy during labor and delivery
- Elective cesarean section delivery for women with an HIV RNA viral load >1000 copies/mL
- Formula feeding[3]

PATIENT CARE

Clinical Thinking

- A clear association between maternal HIV viral load and the risk of mother-to-child transmission has been established. In February 1994, the Pediatric AIDS Clinical Trial Group (PACTG) Protocol 076 demonstrated that three-part ZDV prophylaxis could reduce perinatal HIV transmission by 70%.[4,5] The Public Health Service Task Force guidelines now recommend antiretroviral therapy for all HIV-infected pregnant women regardless of CD4+ cell count or HIV RNA viral load. Antiretroviral therapy should be started for the health of the mother, if indicated, or solely for prophylaxis against perinatal HIV transmission.[5,6]
- Combination antiretroviral therapy with three antiretroviral drugs is the current standard treatment for **nonpregnant** HIV-infected adults. This usually includes two nucleoside analog reverse transcriptase inhibitors and one protease inhibitor or non-nucleoside reverse transcriptase inhibitor.[7]
- Guidelines for the use of antiretroviral therapy during pregnancy are generally the same as those for nonpregnant HIV-infected adults, with the following considerations:
  - Drug pharmacokinetics are altered because of the physiologic changes of pregnancy.
  - Potential adverse effects of drug exposure on the fetus and newborn must be taken into account (most antiretroviral agents are U.S. Food and Drug Administration [FDA] pregnancy class B or C).

- There is the potential for future maternal antiretroviral drug resistance because of exposure to antiretroviral agents during pregnancy.
- ZDV should be included in all antiretroviral regimens given to pregnant women because it rapidly crosses the placenta and has been shown to reduce perinatal transmission independent of maternal HIV RNA viral load.
- HIV genotype resistance testing should be used to guide antiretroviral therapy in all HIV-infected pregnant women.[3,5,6]
- Several antiretroviral medications should *not* be used during pregnancy:
  - Exposure to **efavirenz** has been associated with neural tube defects.
  - The combination of **d4T/ddI** has been associated with severe lactic acidosis in pregnant women.
  - **Nevirapine** can cause severe hepatotoxicity. This side effect is more common in women than in men and in those with a CD4+ cell count >250 cells/mm³. Nevirapine should be used only in patients (especially women) with a CD4+ cell count <250 cells/mm³.
  - **Zalcitabine (ddC)** and **delavirdine** are associated with possible birth defects and inferior potency. They should be used in pregnancy only if alternative medications are unavailable.
  - **Hydroxyurea** and the liquid form of **amprenavir** (because of the propylene glycol component) are also contraindicated in pregnancy.[1-6]
- Antiretroviral therapy can be delayed until the end of the first trimester and completion of organogenesis, if desired and safe for the mother's health.
- As for nonpregnant HIV-infected adults, pregnant women with HIV infection and a low CD4+ cell count should be offered **prophylaxis** against some **opportunistic infections**.
  - For a CD4+ cell count <200 cells/mm³, patients should receive prophylaxis for *P. (carinii) jirovecii* pneumonia (PCP) with trimethoprim-sulfamethoxazole (TMP-SMZ) or dapsone. Both are FDA pregnancy class C. If TMP-SMZ is administered to a pregnant woman, her newborn should be monitored for kernicterus after delivery.
  - For a CD4+ cell count <50 cells/mm³, patients should be offered prophylaxis for *M. avium* complex (MAC) with azithromycin (FDA pregnancy class B).
  - If the patient is seropositive for *T. gondii*, TMP-SMZ will provide prophylaxis.
  - Routine prophylaxis for fungal infections is *not* recommended during pregnancy.
  - Prophylaxis for cytomegalovirus (CMV) infection is also *not* recommended during pregnancy.
  - Pneumococcal, hepatitis B, and influenza vaccinations are safe in pregnancy.[1,2]

History: Cases A, B, and C

- It is important to consider where patients A, B, and C are in the course of their HIV infection. Have they ever had an opportunistic infection such as oral candidiasis (thrush) or pneumonia? A history of opportunistic infection suggests a suppressed immune system with a low CD4+ cell count.
- How did patients A, B, and C acquire HIV infection? High-risk heterosexual contact is the most common mode of HIV transmission in women. Injection drug use is another possible mode of transmission and active substance abuse can affect compliance with medications and pregnancy outcome.[8]
- Have these patients had other sexually transmitted diseases, such as infection with herpes simplex virus (HSV), *Neisseria gonorrhoeae*, *Chlamydia trachomatis*, or *Treponema pallidum* (syphilis), that would benefit from treatment at this time?

Physical Examination

- For each patient, consider the following:
  - What is her general appearance?
  - Does she appear well nourished and comfortable?
  - Are her vital signs stable and weight appropriate for gestational age?
  - Does she have oral candidiasis or a rash?
  - Are findings on her heart, lung, abdominal, and fundal examinations within normal limits?

Tests for Consideration

- All HIV-positive patients, including those who are pregnant, will need laboratory tests performed. All pregnant women with HIV infection should undergo genotype resistance testing to optimize treatment during pregnancy.
- **CD4+ T-lymphocyte count:** A quantitative measurement of the status of the cell-mediated immune system. $128
- **HIV RNA viral load:** A quantitative measurement of circulating HIV. $118
- **Antiretroviral drug resistance testing with a genotype assay:** Genotype testing will detect changes in the DNA sequence of relevant HIV genes that are associated with drug resistance. $478.58
- **Phenotype assay:** A phenotype assay directly assesses the ability of HIV to grow in different concentrations of antiretroviral drugs. It is not used as commonly as genotype testing. $873.56
- **Screening for hepatitis A, B, and C** $263
- **Screening for *T. gondii*** $48
- **Screening for syphilis** $56
- **Purified protein derivative (PPD) skin testing:** Tests for latent tuberculosis infection. $15

Clinical Considerations for HIV and Pregnancy
Medical Knowledge

Patient A	
Laboratory testing	Patient A's CD4+ cell count is 180 cells/mm³. Her HIV RNA viral load is 67,000 copies/mL. Genotype testing reveals no baseline antiretroviral drug resistance. She has negative screening tests for hepatitis A, B, and C, as well as a negative PPD skin test and negative *T. gondii* serology.
Management during pregnancy	Patient A is started on lamivudine/zidovudine (3TC/ZDV) one tablet twice daily and lopinavir/ritonavir (LPV/r) two tablets twice daily. She also starts PCP prophylaxis with TMP-SMZ because her CD4+ cell count is <200 cells/mm³. She notes some diarrhea after starting therapy that resolves within 2 weeks. Within 6 weeks, her HIV RNA viral load is suppressed to <50 copies/mL and her CD4+ cell count increases to 205 cells/mm³. Patient A does very well throughout her pregnancy and her HIV RNA viral load remains undetectable at 37 weeks' gestation.
Management during labor	Patient A presents to the hospital in labor at 38 weeks' gestation. Because her HIV viral load is <1000 copies/mL, her risk of perinatal transmission with a vaginal delivery and limited duration of ruptured membranes is low. She is treated with intravenous ZDV therapy (2 mg/kg bolus followed by continuous infusion at 1 mg/kg/hr) during labor and through delivery.[3] She delivers a 6.7-pound male infant, with a duration of ruptured membranes less than 4 hours.
Management of the neonate	Patient A's neonate should be monitored for kernicterus because of in utero exposure to TMP-SMZ. He will undergo HIV DNA polymerase chain reaction (PCR) testing within 48 hours of delivery, at 6 weeks, 3 months, 6 months, and 1 year of age. (Antibody testing is not reliable during the first year of life because maternal antibodies may be present in the baby without true infection.) He should receive 6 weeks of ZDV therapy after birth, with close monitoring for anemia. After the completion of ZDV therapy, PCP prophylaxis with TMP-SMZ should be initiated and continued until the baby's HIV status is confirmed. Patient A's baby should be

	monitored throughout childhood for possible long-term side effects of in utero exposure to antiretroviral medications.[1,3]
Postpartum issues	Patient A will need to continue antiretroviral therapy for HIV infection given her low baseline CD4+ cell count. She should not breast-feed her infant and should receive contraceptive and psychosocial counseling as needed.

Patient B	
Laboratory testing	Patient B is presenting in active labor and her CD4+ cell count, HIV viral load, and genotype testing will be unavailable before delivery. Immediate intervention, however, can still reduce the risk of mother-to-child HIV transmission to between 9% and 12%.
Management during labor	Intravenous ZDV therapy (2 mg/kg bolus followed by 1 mg/kg/hr infusion) should be started immediately and continued through delivery. ZDV rapidly crosses the placenta and will offer some protection to the baby. (**Most perinatal HIV transmission occurs during labor and delivery.**) Patient B is counseled that because her HIV viral load is unknown and may be high, a cesarean section delivery will reduce the risk of HIV transmission to her infant, especially if done before membrane rupture.[3,5] She elects this mode of delivery and delivers a 4-pound female infant.
Management of the neonate	Patient B's neonate should be monitored for possible withdrawal symptoms given her mother's active substance abuse. She will undergo HIV DNA PCR testing and receive ZDV therapy and TMP-SMZ therapy on the same schedule as Patient A's infant.
Postpartum issues	Patient B will need a baseline CD4+ cell count, HIV viral load, and genotype resistance testing performed to assess the status of her HIV infection and need for antiretroviral therapy. She will need substance abuse and contraceptive counseling and should not breast-feed her infant.

Patient C	
Background	Over one half of HIV-infected women older than 15 years of age live in sub-Saharan Africa.[8] HIV infection is managed very differently in developing countries because of a lack of resources and infrastructure to deliver care. HIV testing for pregnant women is not universal. Patients often receive no prenatal care and frequently present in labor with an unknown HIV status.[9,10] As noted with patient B, however, intervention at the time of delivery is still beneficial in reducing transmission.
Laboratory testing	Laboratory tests, including CD4+ cell count, HIV viral load, and genotype testing, are unavailable in many parts of the developing world. Patient C does not have these tests performed.
Management during pregnancy	Antiretroviral therapy is often not started before labor and delivery. Patient C does not start treatment before presenting in labor.
Management during delivery	Patient C presents in labor at 32 weeks' gestation. Options for intervention at the time of labor and delivery in resource-poor settings include the following: 1. A single dose of nevirapine (sdNVP) can be given to mother in labor and baby after birth. Of note, exposure to sdNVP has been associated with decreased maternal response to future NVP-containing regimens, likely secondary to drug resistance. 2. An ultrashort course of ZDV can be given to mother in labor and baby for 3 days. 3. Combined therapy with NVP + ZDV or ZDV + lamivudine is an option in some settings. 4. Cesarean section delivery is often not available.[9-11] Patient C receives treatment with sdNVP and delivers a 3-pound female infant.
Management of the neonate	Patient C's infant is also treated with sdNVP after birth. Establishing the HIV status of the newborn is difficult in resource-poor settings as DNA testing is often not available and antibody testing is unreliable prior to one year of age.[1]

Postpartum management	Patient C elects to breast-feed her infant, as is common in sub-Saharan Africa. Alternative sources of nutrition are often unavailable and breast-feeding is socially expected in many parts of the developing world. Although breast-feeding can transmit HIV infection and should be avoided if possible, exclusive breast-feeding may be associated with a lower risk of transmission than combined breast-feeding with formula or solid food feeding.[12]
	Patient C may need continued antiretroviral therapy. The cost and availability of laboratory testing and medications, however, are obstacles to her further care. Patient C and her infant are lost to follow-up.

Practice-Based Learning and Improvement: Evidence-Based Medicine

Title
U.S. Public Health Service Task Force recommendations for use of antiretroviral drugs in pregnant HIV-1–infected women for maternal health and interventions to reduce perinatal HIV-1 transmission in the United States

Authors
Prepared by Lynne M. Mofensen, MD

Institution
Center for Research for Mothers and Children, National Institute of Child Health and Human Development, National Institutes of Health, Bethesda, Maryland

Reference
Morbidity and Mortality Weekly Reports 2002;51(RR18):1–51

Problem
The risk of perinatal HIV-1 transmission is approximately 25% with no intervention.

Intervention
Treatment with HAART during pregnancy and labor and the use of elective cesarean delivery for women with an HIV-1 RNA viral load >1000 copies/mL are known interventions that can reduce the risk of perinatal HIV-1 transmission.

Quality of evidence
Level I

Outcome/effect
This report provides management strategy for a variety of HIV-1–positive pregnant women that can be applied to clinical practice.

Historical significance/comments
These Public Health Service Task Force Recommendations have helped to reduce perinatal HIV-1 transmission in the United States.

Interpersonal and Communication Skills

Talking to Your Patients
The pregnant woman with HIV infection is likely to have many concerns. Pregnancy, in and of itself, can be stressful; pregnancy for the HIV-positive woman is additionally confounded by the challenges of dealing with chronic disease, potentially fatal infection, and heightened family and financial pressures. The patient may also have feelings of guilt and despair. From the very first visit, convey sensitivity and compassion. Give information and encouragement. See your patient more frequently than you might see your routine obstetric patient. Physician–patient relationships built on continuous open communication and trust will improve patient morale, adherence to therapy, and clinical outcome.

Professionalism

Principle: Commitment to Patient Confidentiality
Confidentiality is crucial in all patient–physician relationships and its importance has been legislated in the form of the Health Information Portability and Accountability Act (HIPAA). HIPAA regulations restrict access to health records and patient information.

When a physician is caring for a pregnant woman with HIV infection, her privacy should be respected at all times. Medical care or related issues should be discussed only with the patient directly or with friends or family members at her request. The patient should feel comfortable in knowing that her health information is confidential and that her caregivers are committed to its protection.

Systems-Based Practice

Access to Care and the Uninsured
Access to care is critical for pregnant women with HIV infection. Because patients with HIV are disproportionately of low-income status, lack of health care insurance looms as one of the major challenges in achieving optimal treatment for these patients. Even first-line HAART costs an average of $1000 to $2000 per month—or up to $24,000 a year—so the vast majority of patients will not have the means to pay for treatment without some form of health insurance. Accordingly, it is especially important to involve social work services in the care of these patients as early as possible to optimize the chances of their receiving adequate and timely care.

In the United States, federally funded public resources cover a significant portion of HIV/AIDS care. Many patients are eligible for Medicaid (the federally funded and state-managed program for the poor) and a small percentage may be eligible for Medicare. Depending on the state, however, Medicaid often places limits on the number of prescriptions an individual can fill each month. Because HAART therapy averages 4.8 prescriptions per month, this limit can present a barrier to complete HAART therapy and may hinder the adequate treatment of opportunistic infections requiring additional drugs. Not surprisingly, research has demonstrated that individuals with private health insurance are more likely to use HAART than individuals with public health insurance coverage or no coverage.[13]

To address this problem, the Ryan White Comprehensive AIDS Resources Emergency (CARE) Act was passed in 1990 to provide funding for the poorest patients with HIV infection who have either no insurance or inadequate insurance, and insufficient resources to cover the costs of their care. The program is not intended to cover the majority of HIV care in the United States; rather, it is intended to be a payer of last resort for patients with no other means of covering the enormously high cost of HIV care.[7]

References

1. Watts D, Minkoff H: Managing pregnant patients. In Dolin R, Masur H, Saag M (eds): AIDS Therapy. Philadelphia, Elsevier, 2003, pp 381–399.
2. Bernstein H: Maternal and perinatal infection—Viral. In Gabbe SG, Niebyl JR, Simpson JL (eds): Obstetrics: Normal and Problem Pregnancies, 5th ed. New York, Elsevier-Churchill Livingstone, 2007, pp 1204–1213.
3. Mofensen LM, preparer: Public Health Service Task Force recommendations for the use of antiretroviral drugs in pregnant women infected with HIV-1 for maternal health and for reducing perinatal HIV-1 transmission in the United States. MMWR Morb Mortal Wkly Rep 2002;51(RR18):1–38.
4. Watts DH: Management of human immunodeficiency virus infection in pregnancy. N Engl J Med 2002;346:1879–1891.
5. Clark RA, Squires KE: Gender-specific considerations in the antiretroviral management of HIV-infected women. Expert Rev Anti Infect Ther 2005;3:213–227.
6. Currier J: HIV infection in women: An update. 2003. Available at http://www.clinicaloptions.com/HIV/Annual%20Updates/2003%20Annual%20Update/Modules/ccohiv2003_currier.aspx.

7. Panel on Antiretroviral Guidelines for Adults and Adolescents: Guidelines for the use of antiretroviral agents in HIV-1-infected adults and adolescents. Department of Health and Human Services. November 3, 2008. Available at http://www.aidsinfo.nih.gov/ContentFiles/AdultandAdolescentGL.pdf.

8. Beyrer C: HIV epidemiology update and transmission factors: Risks and risk contexts: 16th International AIDS Conference epidemiology plenary. Clin Infect Dis 2007;44:981–987.

9. Taha TE, Kumwenda NI, Hoover DR, et al: Nevirapine and zidovudine at birth to reduce perinatal transmission of HIV in an African setting: A randomized controlled trial. JAMA 2004;292:202–209.

10. Rollins NC, Coovadia HM, Bland RM, et al: Pregnancy outcomes in HIV-infected and uninfected women in rural and urban South Africa. J Acquir Immune Defic Syndr 2007;44:321–328.

11. Lockman S, Shapiro RL, Smeaton LM, et al: Response to antiretroviral therapy after a single, peripartum dose of nevirapine. N Engl J Med 2007;356:135–147.

12. Coovadia HM, Rollins NC, Bland RM, et al: Mother-to-child transmission of HIV-1 infection during exclusive breastfeeding in the first 6 months of life: An intervention cohort study. Lancet 2007;369:1107–1116.

13. Bernell SL, Shinogle JA: The relationship between HAART use and employment for HIV-positive individuals: An empirical analysis and policy outlook. Health Policy 2005;71:255–264.

Chapter 30
Syphilis in Pregnancy

William R. Short MD and Katherine A. Belden MD

Medical Knowledge

Syphilis is a sexually transmitted disease caused by the spirochete *Treponema pallidum*. Syphilis can have serious sequelae if left untreated, especially in pregnant women. Transmission from an infected mother to her infant can occur at any time during pregnancy or delivery. Mother-to-child transmission is most likely to occur in the early stages of infection, but it is uncommon before 16 weeks' gestation. Complications of untreated syphilis in pregnancy include spontaneous abortion, intrauterine growth restriction, stillbirth, and congenital syphilis.

Speaking Intelligently

Although direct examination for spirochetes with a darkfield examination or immunofluorescence staining of mucocutaneous lesions can establish the diagnosis of syphilis, serologic testing is more commonly used for screening. The Centers for Disease Control and Prevention (CDC) recommends a serologic test for syphilis for all pregnant women at their first prenatal visit. Repeat screening in the third trimester and at the time of delivery should be performed for high-risk patients, those previously untested, or those who had a positive serology in the first trimester. The CDC also recommends that all newborns should not be discharged from the hospital without maternal serologic status being determined at least one time during pregnancy.

PATIENT CARE

Tests for Consideration: Serologic Testing for Syphilis

- Screening and diagnosis of syphilis involves the use of two types of tests, a nontreponemal test and a treponeme-specific test.
  - The nontreponemal tests that are approved by the U.S. Food and Drug Administration (FDA) are the Venereal Disease Research Laboratory **(VDRL)** and the rapid plasma reagin **(RPR).** $50
  - VDRL or RPR is initially sent and, if the result is positive, a second treponeme-specific test, such as fluorescent treponemal antibody absorbed **(FTA-ABS)** or *T. palladium* particle agglutination **(TP-PA),** must be sent for confirmation. $135
- The use of nontreponemal serologic testing is insufficient to make a diagnosis. False-positive nontreponemal tests are associated with various medical conditions such as human immunodeficiency virus (HIV) infection, Lyme disease, systemic lupus erythematosus, pneumonia, and malaria. All pregnant women should be routinely tested for infection with HIV. Syphilis in the HIV-infected pregnant woman may be more difficult to manage.

Treatment of the Pregnant Woman with Syphilis

- Penicillin (FDA pregnancy risk category B) remains the drug of choice in the treatment of syphilis.
- Recommendations for pregnant women are the same as for nonpregnant individuals, although penicillin G is the only therapy with documented efficacy in pregnancy.
- Women with penicillin allergy should be desensitized if necessary.
- The dosing and route of penicillin administration will vary by the stage of infection (Table 30-1).

Table 30-1 Treatment Recommendations for Syphilis

Type of Syphilis	Treatment
Early syphilis (primary, secondary, or latent infection <1 year)	Benzathine penicillin G 2.4 million units IM for one to three doses weekly; at least two doses are recommended for those in the third trimester or for secondary syphilis.
Latent syphilis (infection >1 year or an indeterminate duration)	Benzathine penicillin G 2.4 million units IM weekly for three doses
Neurosyphilis (including ocular syphilis; CSF examination for cell count, protein, and VDRL should be performed)	Penicillin G 3-4 million units IV every 4 hr for 10 to 14 days

Congenital Syphilis

Congenital syphilis occurs when a child is born to a mother with secondary or tertiary syphilis. Most fetuses infected with syphilis die shortly before or after birth. Clinical characteristics of children born with congenital syphilis are manifested by two syndromes: early congenital syphilis and late congenital syphilis, with the latter diagnosed after 2 years of age. Table 30-2 lists the characteristics frequently observed in each of the syndromes.

Table 30-2 Clinical Manifestations of Early and Late Congenital Syphilis

Early Congenital Syphilis
Prematurity, low birth weight, hepatosplenomegaly, vesicular or bullous skin lesions that progress to superficial crusted lesions, involvement of mucous membranes of nose and pharynx leading to increased mucous production and discharge, referred to as "the snuffles," hemolytic anemia

Late Congenital Syphilis
Interstitial keratitis, Hutchinson teeth, Mulberry or Moon molars, eighth nerve deafness, neurosyphilis, sclerotic bone lesions producing saber shins and frontal bossing, lytic bone lesions with destruction most frequently of the nasal septum (saddle nose deformity), perforated palate, cardiovascular lesions

Management of Congenital Syphilis
Infants born to mothers with syphilis should be carefully examined for evidence of congenital syphilis. A cerebrospinal fluid (CSF)

examination for cell count, protein, and VDRL; a complete blood count; and long bone radiographs should be considered in all cases of congenital syphilis. Infants with congenital syphilis should receive treatment with aqueous crystalline penicillin G 50,000 U/kg/dose intravenously every 12 hours during the first 7 days of life, and then every 8 hours for a total of 10 days, *or* procaine penicillin G 50,000 U/kg/dose intramuscularly (IM) in a single daily dose for 10 days.

If the mother is adequately treated for syphilis during pregnancy, shows appropriate serologic response at least 1 month before delivery, and has no evidence of reinfection or relapse, the risk of infection for the infant is low. Such infants should receive benzathine penicillin G 50,000 U/kg/dose IM as a single dose.

Infants with a penicillin allergy should be desensitized to penicillin.

All infants with congenital syphilis should receive close follow-up and serologic testing. Those with an abnormal initial CSF examination should undergo a repeat lumbar puncture every 6 months until the results are normal.

Older infants and children with reactive serology testing for syphilis should undergo full evaluation, including CSF examination. Treatment with aqueous penicillin G 50,000 U/kg/dose every 4 to 6 hours for 10 days should be administered. If CSF and physical examinations are normal, three weekly doses of benzathine penicillin G 50,000 U/kg IM can be considered with close follow-up.

References

1. Centers for Disease Control and Prevention: Sexually transmitted diseases treatment guidelines, 2006. MMWR Morb Mortal Wkly Rep 2006;55:22–33. Available at http://www.cdc.gov/std/treatment.
2. Lumbiganon P, Piaggio G, Villar J, et al: The epidemiology of syphilis in pregnancy. Int J STD AIDS 2002;13:486–494.
3. O'Connor MO, Kleinman S, Goff M: Syphilis in pregnancy. J Midwifery Womens Health 2008;53;3:e17–e21.
4. Tramont EC : *Treponema pallidum* (syphilis). In Mandell GL, Bennett JE, Dolin R (eds): Mandell, Douglas and Bennett's Principles and Practice of Infectious Diseases, 6th ed. Philadelphia, Elsevier Churchill Livingstone, 2005, pp 2768–2784.

Professor's Pearls: Cases in Infections in Pregnancy

Consider the following clinical problems and questions posed. Then refer to the professor's discussion of these issues.

1. A 34-year-old G3P2 patient who states she is human immunodeficiency virus (HIV) positive presents to the hospital at about 36 weeks' gestation by her report. She has had occasional prenatal visits throughout her pregnancy but can give no real details of her care. She had a sonogram at about 20 weeks at a nearby hospital's emergency department, which confirmed her due date. She has no records in hand. She presents with some contractions, but is not in labor. Her fetal status is reassuring. What are the necessary steps to provide this patient and her baby with optimal care?

2. A 25-year-old G1P1 patient presents to the hospital 6 days postpartum after a cesarean section for an arrest of dilation. She feels extremely ill and lethargic, and has a fever of 103.6° F. During her course of labor she stopped dilating at 6 cm, and describes a very long labor with numerous vaginal examinations. Her cesarean section went without incident, but she had a fever to 100.3° F on postoperative day 1. She received a single 1-g dose of perioperative cefazolin. What is the course of action?

3. A 40-year-old G1P0 patient at 30 weeks' gestation presents with excruciating back pain, nausea, fever of 102.1° F, and blood-tinged urine. She is not having contractions, but because of the fever a fetal tachycardia is noted with a baseline of 170 beats/min with moderate variability. How should we proceed?

4. A 30-year-old G2P1 physician at 16 weeks' gestation is seen in labor in delivery because of increasing lethargy, shortness of breath, and a fever of 104.0° F. Her pulse oximetry shows a value of 86% on 100% oxygen by face mask. What must be done to evaluate and treat this patient?

Discussion by Drs. Jennifer Aldrich, Mark Ingerman, Brett Gilbert, and Lawrence Livornese, all of the Lankenau Hospital, Division of Infectious Diseases, Wynnewood, Pennsylvania

Answer 1: Clinical Considerations: Management of an HIV-Positive Patient at Full Term by Dr. Jennifer Aldrich
One of the greatest successes in the management of HIV infection has been the ability to significantly reduce the risk of vertical HIV transmission. Before the antiretroviral era, the incidence of mother-to-child transmission was 21% in the United States. With the advent of zidovudine monotherapy use in pregnancy in 1995, that rate

dropped to 11%. Today, with the use of highly effective antiretroviral therapy (HAART), elective cesarean section when appropriate, and formula feeding, the risk of perinatal transmission may be less than 1%.

This patient presents late in her pregnancy, with a history of inconsistent prenatal care and no recent antiretroviral therapy by her report. Although this is far from an ideal situation, there is still an opportunity to dramatically reduce the risk that her infant will contract HIV. This patient should be counseled accordingly. Her care should be coordinated with an experienced HIV specialist provider, and the choice of medications should be optimized for both the mother's and the infant's health. If she has taken prior antiretroviral therapy or if she has any known genotypic resistance to any HIV therapies, that information may be helpful in choosing a regimen. A pretreatment assessment of her immunologic status with a CD4+ count, an HIV viral load, and an HIV genotypic resistance profile can be obtained, but therapy in this case should not be delayed pending those results. Unless there is a clear contraindication to doing so, zidovudine (AZT) should be included in the antiretroviral regimen because it is thought to confer protection to the fetus beyond its effects on the HIV viral load. Medication adherence counseling is vital because adherence and reduction of viral load are directly correlated. Because this patient is presenting late in pregnancy and may not achieve a viral load less than 1000 prior to delivery, she should be offered a scheduled cesarean section at 38 weeks. Elective cesarean section, performed with minimal exchange of maternal and fetal blood and before the onset of labor, has been shown to significantly reduce HIV transmission when the maternal HIV viral load is less than 1000. Furthermore, the patient should receive intravenous (IV) AZT during delivery and be counseled to avoid breast-feeding. A 6-week course of oral AZT is recommended for the infant, and both the mother and the baby should be referred to appropriate HIV specialists for follow-up care and testing.

Answer 2: Clinical Considerations: Fever in the Postpartum Patient by Dr. Mark Ingerman

The differential diagnosis for this 25-year-old G1P1 patient presenting 6 days postpartum after a cesarean section is broad. You are forced to consider endometritis, intra-abdominal or pelvic abscess, and septic pelvic thrombophlebitis. The latter diagnosis is the most elusive because it may occur immediately postoperatively after a cesarean section, or several days or even weeks later. Septic pelvic thrombophlebitis can be accompanied by fevers, shortness of breath, and signs and symptoms of sepsis.

Another possibility that needs to be considered is septicemia secondary to a genitourinary source, because a Foley catheter probably was used for this patient at some time during her hospital stay. The diagnosis of pseudomembranous colitis caused by *Clostridium difficile* must always be considered in a postoperative patient who has received antibiotics, even though only a single dose may have been administered. Owing to a biostrain of these bacteria now seen in North America (which may produce increased amounts of toxin), patients sometimes become extremely ill with high fever even before the onset of diarrhea symptoms.

This patient requires laboratory studies, including a CBC with differential, as well as a comprehensive metabolic panel. A urinalysis and a chest radiograph are also required. Two sets of blood cultures should be drawn before beginning antibiotic therapy. After these blood tests are done, antibiotic therapy should be started on an empiric basis. The organisms that should be covered with your therapy include enteric gram-negative aerobes as well as intra-abdominal anaerobes. Various combinations of antibiotics can be considered. Combinations such as ampicillin-sulbactam (Unasyn) with gentamicin, or a single agent, such as piperacillin/tazobactam (Zosyn), would be appropriate. These antibiotic regimens cover aerobic Enterobacteriaceae as well as anaerobic pathogens, along with enterococci. In a penicillin-allergic patient, other combinations should be considered.

In addition to the aforementioned laboratory studies and antibiotic therapy, a CT scan of the abdomen and pelvis with oral and IV contrast should be obtained immediately. If the diagnosis is not secure after evaluating all laboratory and radiologic studies, the next step would be magnetic resonance venography. Empiric heparin should be considered to treat septic pelvic thrombophlebitis if there is no clear diagnosis after initial testing is completed, and the patient continues to show signs of infection.

Blood and urine cultures, as well as repeat radiologic studies (if indicated), should be evaluated at 24 and 48 hours. The antibiotics should be modified to treat the appropriate pathogens.

Answer 3: Clinical Consideration: Treatment of Pyelonephritis in Pregnancy by Dr. Brett Gilbert

This patient likely has an upper tract urinary infection. Her symptoms are compatible with pregnancy-associated pyelonephritis. She should be admitted to an antepartum unit where the fetus can be appropriately monitored. The next step would be to perform basic laboratory testing to include a CBC, Chem-7, urinalysis and culture, blood cultures, and liver function studies. I would also administer IV fluids.

From an infectious diseases perspective, the microbiology of urinary tract infections in pregnancy is similar to that of nonpregnant women. *Escherichia coli* is one of the most common pathogens. I would therefore start ceftriaxone at 1 g IV daily after the appropriate cultures are obtained. Renal ultrasonography is not necessary initially but could be performed later, especially if the patient fails to defervesce. The antibiotics should be adjusted based on the culture results. Usually the patient can be discharged on an oral beta-lactam antibiotic.

Answer 4: Clinical Considerations: Diagnosis and Treatment of Pneumonia in Pregnancy by Dr. Lawrence Livornese

This patient is markedly hypoxemic and will likely require BiPAP or mechanical ventilation. A rapid, but complete, history and physical examination are required. Key points in the history will be the duration and nature of onset of symptoms, potential exposures from travel, animals, ill contacts, children, and her employment, and recent medical interventions and antibiotic usage. Knowledge of local epidemiology is vital. The physical examination must include a complete examination of the skin and lymph nodes. A key question to be addressed early on is whether the symptoms are due to pneumonia or a systemic illness.

A shielded chest radiograph is necessary. If pneumonia is present the differential includes *Streptococcus pneumoniae*, *Mycoplasma pneumoniae*, *Haemophilus influenzae*, and *Legionella pneumoniae*. Influenza A and B with or without a secondary bacterial infection should be added to the differential during the influenza season. Although *Mycoplasma* is well known to cause "walking pneumonia," it can occasionally present with acute respiratory distress syndrome in young adults and lead to respiratory failure. *Legionella* is more common in pregnancy because of T-cell suppression. Although no single clue is pathognomonic, there are some clues to the presence of *Legionella*, including high fever, a white blood cell count greater than 20 cells/μL, bradycardia relative to temperature elevation, and the early development of pleural effusions. The work-up of the patient with pneumonia includes sputum Gram stain, cultures of the blood and sputum, *Legionella* and pneumococcal urinary antigens, nasopharyngeal swab for influenza antigens, serology for *Legionella* and *Mycoplasma*, as well as a CBC, comprehensive metabolic panel, urinalysis, and an arterial blood gas measurement. The antibiotic choices will be determined by the history, physical examination, and laboratory studies. The antibiotics will generally be limited to U.S. Food and Drug Administration (FDA) pregnancy category B and C drugs. There are no category A antibiotics, and category D and X antibiotics should be avoided.

In the critically ill patient, you must not attribute an abnormal chest radiograph only to infection. There are numerous mimickers, including hypersensitivity pneumonitis, pulmonary embolism, septic emboli, bronchiolitis organizing pneumonia, and vasculitis. Two important causes of septic embolic are endocarditis and Lemierre disease. Right-sided endocarditis is usually caused by *Staphylococcus aureus* and most commonly occurs in IV drug users.

In Lemierre disease, *Fusobacterium necrophorum* infects the jugular vein, leading to septic thrombophlebitis and often with metastatic infection to the lung and other sites. It often follows an episode of exudative pharyngitis or tonsillitis, but the upper respiratory symptoms may have resolved by the time the patient presents. Some patients have neck pain; some present only with nonlocalizing sepsis. Lemierre disease is most common in adolescents and young adults. This disease must always be considered in a young adult with nonlocalizing sepsis. In the appropriate setting, imaging of the neck by ultrasonography or CT can be life-saving. Treatment consists of directed antibiotics such as ampicillin-sulbactam. Ligation of the jugular vein is often necessary.

If the chest radiograph is clear and pneumonia is not a concern, then consideration must turn to extrapulmonary diseases. Processes involving the skin and urinary tract are most likely in this setting, although meningitis and gastrointestinal infections are still possibilities. Because of the T-cell suppression of pregnancy, the incidence of *Listeria monocytogenes* infection is increased. This gram-positive rod is found in soil and water and often contaminates meats and unpasteurized dairy products. Soft cheeses, deli meats, hot dogs, and raw vegetables have been implicated in human infections. Pregnancy imparts a 20-fold increased risk of infection and accounts for one third of all cases; this can occur at any point in a pregnancy but is most common in the third trimester. *Listeria* can cause septic abortion, sepsis syndromes, meningoencephalitis, rhombencephalitis, and focal infections. In the patient with sepsis, the only specific test for *Listeria* is the blood culture. The mainstay of treatment is intravenous ampicillin or penicillin. In the penicillin-allergic patient, trimethoprim-sulfamethoxazole is the drug of choice.

Section V
CASES IN GYNECOLOGY

Section Editor
Caren M. Stalburg MD, MA

Section Contents

Chapter 31
Teaching Visual: The Menstrual Cycle

Michael Belden MD, Neelesh Welling MD,
and Deborah M. Davenport MD

OBJECTIVE

To form a simple framework for understanding the physiology of the menstrual cycle.

The physiology of the menstrual cycle is complex and is described in sophisticated detail in the next chapter (Chapter 32). The intent of this Teaching Visual is to offer a very simplified step-by-step introduction to menstrual physiology that can be used as a framework upon which to integrate the greater complexities offered in the next chapter.

The challenge of describing menstrual physiology is to consider physiologic changes occurring in five places simultaneously: the hypothalamus, anterior pituitary, ovary, follicle, and endometrium.

The menstrual cycle is generally discussed as having a follicular phase and a luteal phase.

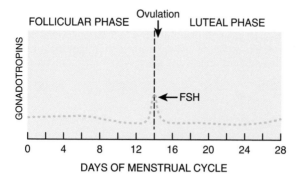

A. Complete the dashed line above representing FSH (Follicle Stimulating Hormone) secretion in the anterior pituitary.

B. Below complete the dashed lines and color in the follicles that become mature under the stimulus of FSH. A dominant follicle is usually selected by day 7.

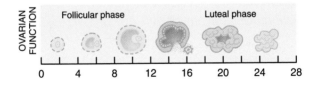

C. Now complete the dotted line representing LH (Luteinizing Hormone) secretion in the anterior pituitary. Note that the LH surge is mid-cycle.

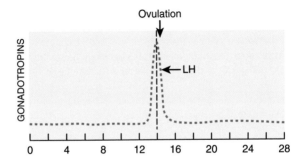

D. Note that LH surge you have graphed in C above governs the rupture of the dominant follicle and the maturation of the corpus luteum. Color the ruptured follicle and the developing corpus luteum seen below.

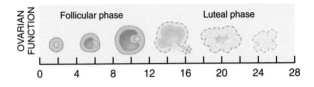

E. Connect the "e"s below representing the level of estradiol, the majority of which is secreted from the granulosa cells of the dominant follicle, then shade in the proliferative aspect of the endometrial lining. Estradiol causes the lining to thicken by increasing the number of glands.

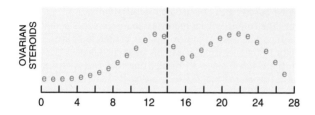

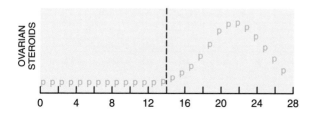

F. Now connect the "p"s demonstrating the levels of progesterone secretion from the theca and granulosa cells of the corpus luteum. Next shade in the secretory phase of the endometrium, which is under the influence of progesterone.

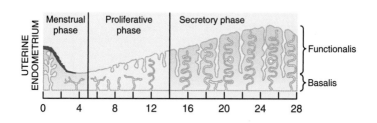

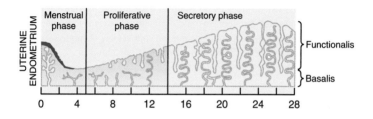

G. If the released oocyte does not undergo fertilization and implantation, the corpus luteum regresses and results in sloughing of the endometrium (menses) owing to the loss of steroid hormone support. Color in the menstrual phase of the cycle. Connect the "e"s and "p"s in the diagram below it, recognizing that menses is brought about when estradiol and progesterone are at their lowest levels.

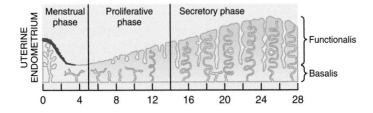

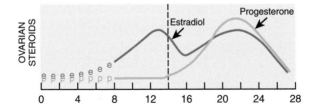

You have now developed step-by-step the classical diagram of the menstrual cycle which includes gonadotropin secretion, ovarian steroid production, follicular development and endometrial maturation. The combined graphics are presented below for your review. A more comprehensive review of the menstrual cycle is presented in Chapter 32.

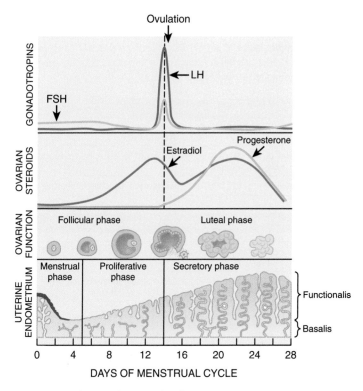

Figure 31-1 The normal menstrual cycle.

Chapter 32
The Menstrual Cycle (Case 18)

Carey Keiter DO, *Deborah M. Davenport* MD, *and Maureen Basha* PhD

An understanding of the physiology of the menstrual cycle and ovulation is essential for intelligent management of many gynecologic conditions and disorders, including contraception, fertility enhancement, abnormal bleeding, etc. In this chapter the complex interaction between the hypothalamus, pituitary, ovary, and uterus that constitutes the Menstrual Cycle will be discussed in considerable detail. This foundation of knowledge will support and enhance your clinical experience in gynecology.

Case: A 16 year-old G0 presents to the office with her mother. The patient has normal periods every 28 days which cause no significant pain or discomfort, and the patient describes normal menstrual bleeding. The patient's mother has been struggling in her attempt to describe menstrual physiology to her daughter. They ask for your help.

Phases of the Menstrual Cycle

Ovarian Cycle	Uterine Cycle
Follicular: Onset of menses to day of luteinizing hormone (LH) surge	**Proliferative:** Estrogen dependent
Luteal: LH surge to onset of menses	**Secretory:** Progesterone dependent

Hormones of the Hypothalamic-Pituitary-Ovarian Axis

Hormones	Location of Production	Action
GnRH (gonadotropin-releasing hormone)	Hypothalamus	Pulsatile secretion stimulates pulsatile release of FSH and LH from the anterior pituitary gland.
FSH (follicle-stimulating hormone)	Anterior pituitary	Binds to receptors on granulosa cells in ovarian follicles, stimulating aromatase activity, which promotes the conversion of androgens from theca cells to estrogen. Induces LH receptors in dominant follicle, priming it for ovulation.
LH (luteinizing hormone)	Anterior pituitary	Binds to receptors on theca cells in the dominant ovarian follicle, increasing androgen production. Androgens are converted to estrogens by the enzymatic action of aromatase in granulosa cells. After ovulation, luteinized theca and granulosa cells of the corpus luteum secrete progesterone.
Inhibins A and B	Ovarian follicles and corpus luteum	Inhibin B is generally produced in the follicular phase and switches to inhibin A in the luteal phase. Inhibin inhibits pituitary FSH production and secretion.
Activin (FSH "helper")	Many cell types	Increases FSH receptor expression in granulosa cells. Augments FSH stimulation of LH receptors on theca cells, aromatization, and inhibin and activin production. Stimulates GnRH in the pituitary.

Hormones	Location of Production	Action
Estradiol	Granulosa cells in ovarian follicles	Increases FSH receptors on granulosa cells, making them more responsive to FSH. Feeds back centrally to inhibit hypothalamic secretion of GnRH and pituitary secretion of FSH and LH throughout most of the follicular phase. Switches to positive feedback during late follicular phase. Creates proliferative endometrium.
Progesterone	Corpus luteum in luteal phase	Augments positive feedback of estrogen on hypothalamus and pituitary during the late follicular phase, resulting in the LH surge. Exerts negative feedback on hypothalamus and pituitary during the luteal phase. Produces secretory endometrium.

Embryology and Oocytes   Medical Knowledge

When considering the menstrual cycle, it is important to remember the embryologic origin of oocytes. Primordial germ cells originate in the endoderm of the yolk sac, allantois, and hindgut. Germ cells migrate to the genital ridge at 5 to 6 weeks' gestation, undergo rapid mitoses from 6 to 8 weeks, and **reach maximal number of 6 to 7 million oocytes by 16 to 20 weeks' gestation.** At this time, two additional processes are initiated: meiosis and atresia. Oocytes that begin meiosis I are arrested in the **diplotene stage** of **meiotic prophase. Meiosis I will not go to completion until ovulation, when the oocyte will begin meiosis II. Meiosis II will go to completion if the oocyte is eventually fertilized.** Primordial germ cells are subject to ongoing **atresia** (even during pregnancy and anovulatory cycles) from intrauterine life until menopause. The rate of decrease in oocytes is proportional to the total number of primordial germ cells present. Therefore, the most rapid decrease in the number of oocytes occurs before birth. At birth, 1 to 2 million oocytes remain. During the course of each cycle, a cohort of follicles is recruited near the end of the previous luteal phase from a larger group of follicles that have already been developing. This cohort of follicles further develops during the follicular phase under the influence of FSH. Usually, only one follicle becomes the dominant follicle and releases an oocyte in response to the LH surge. The remaining follicles that did not ovulate undergo atresia. Taking an average age of puberty of 12.5 years and an average age of menopause of 51.5 years (with only one follicle ovulating each month), only 400 to 500 follicles of the several million that were present in the embryonic stage will ovulate during a woman's reproductive years.

Hormones in Context   Medical Knowledge

Early Follicular Phase

Under pulsatile stimulation of GnRH, the anterior pituitary increases its production of FSH, which stimulates the development of a cohort of follicles.

- Early in the follicular phase GnRH and activin stimulate the release of FSH from the anterior pituitary and augment FSH action in granulosa cells by increasing FSH receptor expression and increasing aromatase activity.
- Day 1 of the menstrual cycle is the first day of menses.
- The ovary is least hormonally active (with the lowest levels of estradiol and progesterone production) during this time of the menstrual cycle.
- The endometrium is thinnest at the end of menses. **See Katz 4, Hacker 4.**

Mid-Follicular Phase

Follicular development proceeds, a dominant follicle is selected, and estradiol production increases.

- FSH continues to stimulate folliculogenesis and aromatization of androgens to estradiol in the ovarian follicles.
- The selected cohort of follicles grows to the antral stage. Antral follicles are small, fluid-filled, nondominant follicles that can be seen with ultrasonography.
- Increased estradiol inhibits GnRH release from the hypothalamus by negative feedback, which leads to a decrease in serum FSH. The decrease in FSH is also a result of rising inhibin levels. A dominant follicle (usually one) is selected at approximately day 7 of the cycle. The dominant follicle out-competes the rest of the cohort for a limited FSH supply. Estradiol production increasingly comes from the dominant follicle. The rest of the cohort will undergo atresia throughout the remainder of the follicular phase.
- Estradiol release continues to increase from the granulosa cells of the dominant follicle, and this stimulates the proliferation of uterine endometrium, increasing the number of glands. This is known as the **proliferative phase** of the uterine cycle. The thickened endometrial pattern can be seen with ultrasonography. **See Katz 4, Hacker 4.**

Late Follicular Phase

Rising estradiol production by the dominant follicle results in a switch to positive feedback that causes the LH surge and ovulation of an oocyte from the dominant follicle.

- A sustained rise of estradiol production from the dominant follicle leads to a temporary switch from negative to positive feedback of estradiol on the hypothalamus and pituitary, with rising estradiol levels now increasing LH production rather than inhibiting it. Late in the follicular phase FSH induces LH receptors in the granulosa cells, which stimulates progesterone production. This rise in progesterone production and secretion augments the positive feedback effect of estradiol.
- The positive feedback of estrogen and progesterone results in the mid-cycle **LH surge,** the critical event for ovulation.
- FSH induces LH receptors in the ovary and increased ovarian secretion of intrauterine growth factors such as insulin-like growth factor-1 (IGF-1).
- Estradiol peaks approximately 1 day before ovulation and increases endometrial thickening. The cervical mucus becomes watery and increases in volume, facilitating sperm transport. **See Katz 4, Hacker 4.**

Early Luteal Phase (Including Mid-Cycle LH Surge)

The mid-cycle LH surge causes the dominant follicle to ovulate and converts the dominant follicle into the corpus luteum.

- The LH surge occurs approximately 24 to 36 hours after the estradiol peak and stimulates:
  - Ovulation. LH stimulates an increase in local secretion of plasminogen activator, which converts plasminogen to plasmin. The LH surge also causes increased activity of collagenase to disrupt the follicular wall and allow for release of the oocyte surrounded by its cumulus oophorus. The release of an oocyte from the ovary into the abdominal cavity occurs approximately 12 hours after the peak of the LH surge. Upon ovulation, the oocyte in the dominant follicle completes its first meiotic division. The released oocyte is swept up by the fimbriated ends of the fallopian tube, and travels down the fallopian tube to the uterine cavity over the next week.
  - Conversion of the dominant follicle (now emptied of its oocyte) into a corpus luteum. Granulosa cells surrounding the dominant follicle become granulosa-lutein cells. Granulosa-lutein cells are well vascularized, grow larger during the first 3 days after

ovulation, and develop a vacuolated appearance because of the accumulation of cholesterol droplets derived from blood. The surrounding theca cells differentiate into theca-lutein cells of the corpus luteum.

- Production of prostaglandins and progesterone by granulosa cells. Plasma progesterone levels rise to levels 10-fold greater than in the follicular phase of the cycle.
- Rising progesterone production stimulates the formation of a secretory endometrium. This is the **secretory phase** of the uterine cycle.
- The actions of progesterone on the endometrium require endometrial exposure to estradiol during the follicular phase. This allows the development of progesterone receptors on endometrial cells. Secretory endometrium appears more uniformly bright on ultrasonography, in contrast to the surrounding myometrium.
  See Katz 4, Hacker 4.

Middle Luteal Phase

Progesterone produced by the corpus luteum stimulates the endometrium to develop.

- Gradual increase in progesterone leads to slowing of LH pulses.
- The transformation of the dominant follicle to the corpus luteum involves structural changes that result in an increase in the vascularity of the corpus luteum. This leads to an increased availability of cholesterol as a precursor for steroid hormone production: serum progesterone levels increase.
- The corpus luteum produces inhibin A (peaks in mid-luteal phase).
  See Katz 4, Hacker 4.

Late Luteal Phase

Under progesterone control, the endometrium continues to mature. If the released oocyte does not undergo fertilization and implantation, the corpus luteum regresses, which results in sloughing of the endometrium (menses) owing to the loss of steroid hormone support. Another cycle then begins. The approximate life span of the corpus luteum is 14 days.

- The gradual decrease in LH leads to a gradual decrease in progesterone and estrogen production by the corpus luteum (in the absence of a fertilized oocyte).

- If the oocyte is fertilized, it implants in the endometrium and the embryo synthesizes and secretes human chorionic gonadotropin (hCG), which maintains the corpus luteum and its progesterone production. Progesterone from the corpus luteum sustains pregnancy during the first trimester of pregnancy until the placenta takes over progesterone production (the luteal–placental shift).
- If the oocyte is not fertilized, decreased estrogen and progesterone secretion from the corpus luteum leads to loss of endometrial blood supply, endometrial sloughing, and the onset of menses 14 days after the LH surge.
- Via negative feedback the decrease in estradiol, progesterone, and inhibin A levels stimulates the hypothalamic-pituitary axis and FSH levels slowly increase near the end of the luteal phase. This rise in FSH is responsible for recruitment of a cohort of follicles to undergo further development during the next cycle. (See Figure 32-1 for an illustration of the menstrual cycle.) **See Katz 4, Hacker 4.**

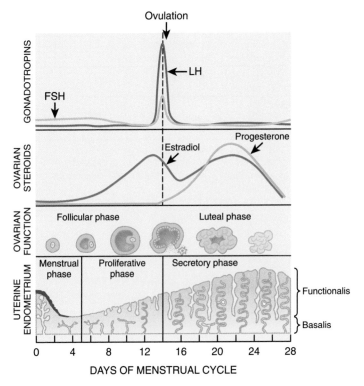

Figure 32-1 The normal menstrual cycle.

Practice-Based Learning and Improvement: Evidence-Based Medicine

Title
Menstruation in girls and adolescents: Using the menstrual cycle as a vital sign

Authors
Diaz A, Laufer MR, Breech LL

Institution
American Academy of Pediatrics Committee on Adolescence; American College of Obstetricians and Gynecologists Committee on Adolescent Health Care

Reference
Pediatrics 2006;118:2245–2250

Problem
Addresses normal variants in adolescent menstruation, in an attempt to help identify normal development and exclude pathologic conditions.

Intervention
Careful history taking, with a comprehensive knowledge of the etiology and implications of menstrual irregularities.

Comparison/control (quality of evidence)
Level III expert opinion

Outcome/effect
Identification of those adolescents with possible systemic illness by evaluating the menstrual cycle.

Historical significance/comments
This important article postulates that normal menses can be interpreted as a "vital sign," reflecting the general physiologic well-being of the patient.

Chapter 33
Contraception (Case 19)

Joan A. Keegan DO, Mehdi Parva MD, Camilo A. Ruiz DO, and Joanne Kakaty-Monzo DO

Case: A 27-year-old G0 with essentially normal menstrual cycles presents for an annual examination and to discuss her options for birth control. She had been on oral contraceptives in the past, and did well. She wants to know what else is available, and what are the advantages and risks of the various options.

Contraceptive Options

Hormonal
Combination oral contraception
Progesterone-only oral contraception
Intramuscular injection: depo-medroxyprogesterone
Transdermal patch
Contraceptive vaginal ring
Levonorgestrel-releasing intrauterine device (IUD)
Etonogestrel subdermal implant

Nonhormonal
Nonhormonal copper IUD
Barrier methods: condom and diaphragm

Permanent
Bilateral tubal ligation
Hysteroscopic sterilization (Essure)

Speaking Intelligently

Helping a patient choose a method of birth control can be a challenge. It is important to be knowledgeable about all of the options in order to offer a method that best fits your patient's needs, lifestyle, future fertility options, and medical history. To ensure a successful and reliable choice, one must consider efficacy, convenience, duration of action, reversibility, side effects, and protection against sexually transmitted infections (STIs). In addition, one must consider a patient's coexisting medical problems and social habits when choosing birth control. The most important aspect to consider when discussing options with your patient is to find a contraceptive choice with the highest rate of compliance.

PATIENT CARE

Clinical Thinking
- To be successful in the prevention of unintended pregnancy, the following factors regarding the different methods of contraception should be considered:
  - Effectiveness
  - Convenience
  - Side effects and effect on uterine bleeding
  - Duration of action
  - Reversibility
  - Contraceptive cost
  - Protection against STIs
- To date, there is no single perfect method of contraception available. A clinician should be able to fully inform the patient of the advantages and disadvantages of each method, so the patient can choose the method best suited to her needs.
- The following are the most frequently used methods of contraception, and the approximate percentage of patients who typically choose each method. Keep in mind that patient choices vary by region, age, and parity:
  - Oral contraceptive pill (OCP) (19%)
  - Female sterilization (17%)
  - Male condom (11%)
  - Male sterilization (6%)
  - Medroxyprogesterone acetate injections (3%)
- Failure rates with the first year use for the aforementioned methods are 0.3% to 8%, 0.5%, 2% to 15%, 0.1% to 0.15%, and 0.3% to 3%, respectively.
- Clinicians should also inform their patients about long-term failure rates and increases in the incidence of ectopic pregnancy when using female sterilization, IUDs, and progestin-only oral contraceptives.

History

- A complete past medical, surgical, obstetric, gynecologic, social, and family history (including medications and allergies) should be obtained from the patient. Smoking history and age should also be considered because of the rare risks of thromboembolic complications associated with several of the hormonal options.
- A variety of factors guide appropriate contraceptive choices. For example, a nulliparous woman in a mutually monogamous relationship may choose an easily reversible form of hormonal contraception because she may be interested in preserving fertility. Alternatively, a multiparous woman who has completed her childbearing may prefer a nonreversible option such as surgical sterilization.
- Remember that hormonal contraceptives may be used for other medical reasons. For example, dysfunctional uterine bleeding, menorrhagia, and chronic pelvic pain are all gynecologic problems that can effectively be treated to some degree with various contraceptive choices.
- You may find patients who have used OCPs for a prolonged period and may wish to consider other forms of contraception owing to ease of administration and the convenience of newer options.

Physical Examination

- A thorough physical examination should be performed annually throughout the treatment course. A patient may have a subclinical condition (e.g., vaginitis, pelvic inflammatory disease, cervical neoplasia) that requires immediate treatment.
- Pelvic examination includes inspection of the vagina and cervix, Pap test with human papillomavirus serotyping (if indicated), collection of cervical or discharge samples if necessary, and cultures for gonorrhea and chlamydia if the patient consents to being tested. Patients younger than 26 years of age should be offered this testing as a matter of routine.
- Bimanual examination for position, consistency, and mobility of uterus/adnexa should be included as part of the physical examination.
- The examination should also include heart, lungs, breasts, abdomen, and extremities because many young patients rely on their obstetrician/gynecologist to act as their primary care provider as well.

Tests for Consideration

- **Urine pregnancy test:** This is reasonable to perform if there is any chance a patient could be pregnant before beginning a birth control regimen. $20

Contraceptive Choices and Considerations   Medical Knowledge

Key:
M: Mechanism of action
A: Advantages
D: Disadvantages
FR: Failure rates
C: Cost

Hormonal

Combination Oral Contraception

M Combination hormonal oral contraceptive pills inhibit ovulation through a negative feedback mechanism on the hypothalamus, which alters the normal pattern of gonadotropin secretion of follicle-stimulating hormone and luteinizing hormone by the anterior pituitary. The follicular phase, follicle-stimulating hormone, and the mid-cycle surge of gonadotropins are inhibited. In addition, combination hormonal contraceptives cause changes in the genital tract, including alterations in cervical mucus, rendering it unfavorable for sperm penetration even if ovulation occurs. Changes in the endometrium may also occur, producing an unfavorable environment for implantation. Combination hormonal contraceptives may alter tubal transport of the ova through the fallopian tubes.

The most common OCP formulations include the following:

- **Monophasic extended cycle:** 84 days estrogen/progestin combination (30 µg ethinyl estradiol [EE]/0.15 mg levonorgestrel)
- **Monophasic:** 20 to 50 µg EE and wide range of progestins for 28 days
- **Biphasic:** 20 to 35 µg EE and 0.5 to 1.0 mg norethindrone that is increased about halfway through the cycle
- **Triphasic:** Steady 25 to 35 µg EE and 0.05 to 1 mg progestins in various doses. The progestin dose increases in three phases through the cycle. There are two OCPs available with triphasic estrogen dose and steady progestin dose.

A No delay in return to fertility. A reduction in the risk of endometrial, ovarian, and colorectal cancers has been exhibited with long-term use of combination oral contraceptives.

D Remembering to take a daily pill. Very slight increased risk of venous thromboembolism. Estrogen-related side effects include nausea, breast tenderness, bloating, and headaches. Irregular menstrual bleeding and amenorrhea are more related to the progestins. Breakthrough bleeding is common in the first 3 months of use. Minimal protection from STIs due to increased viscosity of cervical mucus.

FR One-year failure rate: perfect use <1%; typical use 8% rate of pregnancy.

C $35/month. **See Katz 14, Hacker 26.**

Progesterone-Only Oral Contraceptive Pills

M Prevents ovulation, thickens cervical mucus, reduces the activity of cilia in the fallopian tubes.

A Diminished estrogen-related side effects. No delay in return to fertility. Can be used in women who are smokers older than 35 years of age, patients with migraines, diabetics with vascular disease, systemic lupus erythematosus, and thrombophilias, and in patients with risks for cardiovascular disease. Progesterone-only OCPs are a common choice for some breast-feeding mothers because of the small (but controversial) risk that estrogen-containing OCPs may cause a diminution in milk supply/production.

D Menstrual irregularity, irregular bleeding, prolonged bleeding episodes, and amenorrhea. Patient must take a daily pill at the same time each day for best effectiveness. Minimal protection from STIs.

FR One-year failure rate: perfect use <1%; typical use 8% rate of pregnancy.

C $30/month. **See Katz 14, Hacker 26.**

Intramuscular Injection: Depo-Medroxyprogesterone

M Inhibits secretion of pituitary gonadotropins, which prevents follicular maturation and ovulation. Also causes endometrial thinning. Because of its progestin effect, it causes changes in cervical mucus and tubal motility that are hostile to sperm migration.

A	Injections only every 12 weeks, so less dependence on patient motivation.
D	Intermenstrual bleeding, headache, mood changes, weight gain, and breast tenderness. Delayed return to fertility. As much as 30% of women do not conceive within 1 year. Minimal protection from STIs.
FR	Perfect use <1%, typical use 3% pregnancy rate in 1 year.
C	$50/three months. **See Katz 14, Hacker 26.**

Transdermal Patch

M	The transdermal patch contraceptive delivery system (ethinyl estradiol/norelgestromin transdermal) provides continuous sustained delivery of 20 μg of ethinyl estradiol and 150 μg of norelgestromin daily.
A	Convenience of weekly administration, no oral intake. No delay in return to fertility.
D	Bleeding, breast discomfort, dysmenorrhea, application site reactions, (i.e., contact dermatitis), and possibility of increased venous thromboembolism risk. Some patients also have difficulty with patch adherence to the skin. Minimal, if any, protection from STIs.
FR	Perfect use <1%, typical use 8% rate of pregnancy in 1 year.
C	$45/month. **See Katz 14, Hacker 26.**

Contraceptive Vaginal Ring

| M | Each ring contains 2.7 mg ethinyl estradiol and 11.7 mg etonogestrel. These hormones are absorbed through the vaginal epithelium and act systemically. The overall dose of hormonal contraception is lower because of the mode of administration. First-pass effect in the liver does not occur as it does in oral contraceptive use. The combination of the hormones progesterone and estrogen in the birth control ring prevents ovulation. The hormones in the ring also thicken the cervical mucus, decreasing the chance of fertilization. |

A	Convenience of once-a-month use, effects fertility 1 month at a time, does not interrupt intimacy.
D	Does not protect against STIs, can cause increased vaginal discharge, irritation, and risk of yeast infection. Unanticipated ring expulsion can be a considerable problem. Uncommon spotting or breakthrough bleeding can occur. Headaches, weight gain, nausea, breast tenderness, and mood swings are among the side effects because the mechanism of action is systemic.
FR	Failure rate is calculated at 0.1% with perfect use. A failure rate with typical use has not been established.
C	$45/month. **See Katz 14, Hacker 26.**

Levonorgestrel-Releasing Intrauterine Device

M	The levonorgestrel-releasing IUD (Mirena) is an increasingly popular form of contraception in the United States. The levonorgestrel-releasing IUD consists of a T-shaped polyethylene frame with a 52-mg levonorgestrel slow-release reservoir surrounding the vertical arm. The mechanism of action of the levonorgestrel-releasing IUD is through the local progestin effect brought about by slow release of levonorgestrel into the uterine cavity. These effects occur mainly on the endometrium. However, ovulation is inhibited in some women.
A	Along with increased sexual spontaneity, the levonorgestrel-releasing IUD has been shown to have several noncontraceptive health benefits: • Possible protection from endometrial hyperplasia and neoplasia • Protection from pelvic inflammatory disease • Reduction in menstrual bleeding and dysmenorrhea • Decreased pain from endometriosis
D	IUDs are initially costly. The levonorgestrel-releasing IUD can alter the normal menstrual pattern, including inducing amenorrhea or oligomenorrhea. It can also cause breast tenderness, mood changes, and acne. Insertion and removal require an office visit. There is a small risk of uterine perforation.
FR	Calculated at 0.6% to 1.5% with perfect use and 0.8% to 2.0% with typical use.
C	$700/5 years (approximate cost). **See Katz 14, Hacker 26.**

Contraceptive Implants

M The etonogestrel subdermal implant (Implanon) is the only subdermal contraceptive implant currently marketed in the United States. The etonogestrel implant is a single, sterile 4-cm rod implant containing etonogestrel that is inserted subcutaneously into the upper arm. The contraceptive effect is brought about by slow release of etonogestrel into the circulation over 3 years. Several mechanisms play a role in the contraceptive effect, including alterations in the endometrium, suppression of ovulation, and increased viscosity of the cervical mucus, similar to other progesterone-only contraceptive options.

A The advantages of contraceptive implants are as follows:

- Long acting (up to 3 years)
- More than 99% effective
- Does not require daily attention
- Depression and premenstrual symptoms may improve
- Less bleeding, cramping, headaches, and breast tenderness during menstruation

D The disadvantages of contraceptive implants are as follows:

- Requires insertion/removal by clinician
- Complications of insertion and removal
- Bleeding irregularities (most common reason for discontinuation)
- No consistencies in bleeding pattern
- Body weight increase
- Depression and premenstrual symptoms may become worse
- Acne
- No protection against STIs
- If pregnancy occurs, the rate of ectopic pregnancy is higher than in a patient using no contraception
- Implant may be visible or palpable in the upper arm

FR To date, the failure rate reported for contraceptive implants is <1%.

C $500/3 years (approximate cost). **See Katz 14, Hacker 26.**

Nonhormonal

Intrauterine Device: Copper Nonhormonal

M The TCu380A (ParaGard) IUD consists of a T-shaped polyethylene frame wound with copper wire. The mechanism of action of the copper IUD is thought to be related to continuous release of copper ions into the uterine cavity. This interferes with sperm transport, fertilization, and implantation through a local inflammatory reaction.

A The copper IUD is one of the only methods of highly reliable birth control available for women who cannot use hormonal methods of contraception, or who elect against permanent sterilization. IUDs do not require daily attention and allow for sexual spontaneity, unlike the diaphragm or other barrier methods. Copper IUDs are immediately effective and can remain in place for 10 years. Women using the TCu380A specifically have a lower risk of ectopic pregnancy compared with women not using contraception.

D Copper IUDs can sometimes cause heavier menses and dysmenorrhea, both of which are usually well controlled with nonsteroidal anti-inflammatory medications. IUDs do not protect against STIs. Insertion and removal require clinic visits. Although uncommon, IUDs carry a small risk of uterine perforation. IUDs can also be spontaneously expelled.

FR Calculated at 0.6% to 1.5% with perfect use and 0.08% to 2.0% with typical use.

C $725/10 years (approximate cost). **See Katz 14, Hacker 26.**

Barrier Methods: Condoms and Diaphragms
M Condoms prevent direct contact with semen, genital lesions, and subclinical viral shedding on the glans and shaft of the penis. Diaphragms are soft, dome-shaped cups with a flexible rim and should be used with spermicide and placed over the cervix. The female condom is a variant of the more commonly used version.
A Condoms are readily accessible, inexpensive, carried discretely, and may offer some protective effects against certain STIs. Diaphragms also are inexpensive and reversible, but require placement before sexual activity. Barrier methods have no hormonal side effects and may decrease the risk of cervical cancer.
D Condoms fail with inconsistent or incorrect use, or non-use. They may cause decreased sensitivity, negatively effecting erection or enjoyment, require interruption of foreplay to place; require

knowledge and cooperation by the male partner; and should not be used with latex allergies. Diaphragms, under the best circumstances, should be used together with spermicide. Diaphragms must be cleaned after use and must be fitted, particularly after each vaginal delivery.

Diaphragms are associated with an increased risk of urinary tract infection. Effectiveness depends on motivation, skill, and experience.

FR Condoms with perfect use (consistent and correct) have a 2% pregnancy rate in the first year. Typical use results in a 15% pregnancy rate. Diaphragms with perfect use have a 6% rate, whereas typical use has a 16% rate.

C $15/10 condoms; $60/diaphragm. **See Katz 14, Hacker 26.**

Permanent

Laparoscopic Sterilization

M Most common surgical method for interval sterilization. Most common methods of laparoscopic tubal occlusion are bipolar electrodessication, Falope ring, and Hulka clip.

A Opportunity to explore the abdomen for occult disease, small incision, and rapid recovery.

D Unexpected intra-operative findings or complications (i.e. bleeding, organ perforation) may necessitate conversion to laparotomy. Regret after sterilization occurs in 3-25%, associated with change in marital status, etc.

FR The CDC conducted the CREST study and found failure rates higher than previously thought. Overall cumulative failure rate for all sterilization procedures to be 1.9%—more than double what had been accepted as standard failure rate.

C $800. **See Katz 14, Hacker 26.**

Hysteroscopic Sterilization

M A minimally invasive technique, Essure hysteroscopic sterilization is used for nonreversible tubal occlusion. A narrow, 4-cm-long coil is inserted into the proximal fallopian tube hysteroscopically. The device induces growth of surrounding tissue into the coil, leading to tubal occlusion.

A	No incision, lower cost, less time spent in hospital, better procedure tolerance, and decreased postoperative pain compared with laparoscopic tubal ligation.
D	Some women still require neuraxial or general anesthesia. Requires sterile procedure room at a minimum for placement. Requires preprocedure and postprocedure hysterosalpingogram to assess tubal patency. Must use alternative contraception until tubal occlusion is documented 3 months after procedure. Possibility of procedure failure due to inability to visualize tubal ostia, expulsion, perforation, and incorrect placement.
FR	Effectiveness at 5 years is 99.74%.
C	$600. **See Katz 14, Hacker 26.**

Practice-Based Learning and Improvement: Evidence-Based Medicine

Title
Antibiotic prophylaxis for intrauterine contraceptive device insertion (Cochrane Review)

Authors
Grimes DA, Schulz KF

Institution
Multiple institutions

Reference
Cochrane Database of Systematic Reviews 2007(7):CD001327

Problem
Examine the risk of pelvic inflammatory disease (PID) with IUD insertion.

Intervention
IUD insertion

Comparison/control (quality of evidence)
Meta-analysis

Outcome/effect
The review concluded that the risk of PID after the first month after IUD insertion is small. The increased risk of upper genital tract infection seen in the first month after IUD insertion is related to contamination of the uterus with vaginal bacteria, despite sterile technique. In 22,908 IUD insertions, investigators found a risk of PID after 20 days of 1.4 cases per 1000 woman-years of use, compared with 9.7 cases per 1000 woman-years in the first 20 days after IUD insertion. In addition, rates of PID remained low and stable for up to 8 years of follow-up monitoring, which demonstrates that PID is an uncommon event in IUD users after the first 20 days after insertion.

Historical significance/comments
Many patients have scientifically unfounded ideas and fears about IUDs. Many patients need effective, long-term methods of contraception that separate contraceptive efficacy from patient-dependent use. Patients desiring contraception would benefit from counseling on the safety and effectiveness of IUDs. IUDs require one act of motivation and are cost-effective in the long term.

Interpersonal and Communication Skills

Use the "Contraception" Discussion as a Conduit to Discussion of Health Maintenance, Disease Prevention, and Sexuality
A well visit for a patient, which includes consultation regarding contraceptive options, can be an excellent opportunity to review the patient's general state of health and well-being. As physicians, we should strive to establish strong rapport with our patients and encourage them to discuss their health "in general." The doctor–patient relationship is a two-way dialogue that can help satisfy the patient's needs and wants with the best therapeutic modalities and advice we have to offer. Regarding contraception, there are numerous options to help a patient meet her needs. Keep in mind, however, that it is only through open dialogue that these needs are properly recognized and we know which method to recommend. A patient who may want to avoid "hormones," for example, could be offered the copper IUD or a reliable barrier method. A teen with a chaotic lifestyle might be an appropriate candidate for depo-medroxyprogesterone injections four times a year, which you can help her manage.

For the most part, patients are healthy when they present for a discussion of contraceptive options, which offers a great opportunity to review safe practices and the maintenance of a healthy lifestyle. This is often a time when a patient may wish to discuss sexuality or even sexual orientation. Be sensitive to clues that the patient wishes to discuss these matters and do not hesitate to prompt such discussion.

Other issues to be considered at a routine visit for contraceptive counseling might include:

- Reviewing immunizations
- Routine screening mammography
- Exercise
- Smoking cessation
- Calcium supplementation
- Folic acid supplementation
- Future childbearing

Professionalism

Principle: Patient Autonomy

A patient seeking birth control has many options from which to choose. A variety of personal, social, medical, and financial issues may figure into your patient's choice. As a primary care physician, you will be in the unique position of helping her to make this decision. Whenever a patient presents to you asking for medical advice and guidance, you must keep in mind the principle of patient autonomy. At times, you may consciously need to keep your personal, social, or religious views separate from your medical opinions. If you are ever reluctant, for nonmedical reasons, to prescribe birth control (or carry out any other of your patient's wishes), you should refer her to someone else who would be able to help.

Systems-Based Practice

Hospital Ownership and Categorization

You are completing your Ob/Gyn rotation at Saint Anthony's Hospital, a Catholic hospital affiliated with your medical school. Shortly after delivering her third child, a patient informs you that she and her husband have decided not to have any more children, and asks you if she can arrange to have a tubal ligation before discharge. You tell her that because this is a Catholic hospital, tubal ligations cannot be performed, and she will need to make arrangements to have this procedure completed somewhere else. This issue provides us with the opportunity to discuss an important issue: who owns hospitals, and how are they governed?

There are roughly 5000 hospitals in the United States. The vast majority—more than 80%—are nonprofit or government run. About a quarter of these (20% of all hospitals) are government owned, and run by city or state government. Of the remaining nonprofits, most of these are smaller nonprofit facilities owned by the community they serve. The community is represented through a board of trustees, which has ultimate accountability for the management of the hospital. Accordingly, when one of these facilities is purchased by an outside entity (such as a larger health system or a for-profit hospital corporation), the proceeds of the sale are typically spun off into a nonprofit foundation to benefit the community. In essence, the community is being paid for the hospital. Of nonprofit community hospitals, about 625 (or 13%) are Catholic, meaning that they are owned by a Catholic organization, often an order of nuns.

Roughly 1100 hospitals (22%) are teaching hospitals, meaning that they train residents and receive graduate medical education (GME) funding from Medicare. Only 375 of these hospitals (less than 10%), however, are considered academic medical centers (AMCs), also known as major teaching hospitals. These institutions are most often owned by the university or medical school with which they are affiliated, but they can also be stand-alone nonprofits.

Of the 20% of hospitals that are for-profit, many of these are part of large national health system chains, some of which own more than 100 hospitals. Many of the for-profit hospitals are specialty hospitals, often surgical in nature, and are often either partly or completely owned by physicians in the specialty.

Chapter 34
Abnormal Uterine Bleeding (Case 20)

Khaled Sakhel MD and Linda Bradley MD

Case: A 31-year-old woman presents to the clinic with a 10-month history of irregular and heavy menstrual periods.

Differential Diagnosis

Endocrinologic and Hematologic Causes of Abnormal Uterine Bleeding		
Anovulation (hypothalamic/ovarian/pituitary axis)	Von Willebrand disease	Thyroid disfunction

Anatomic and Oncologic Causes of Abnormal Uterine Bleeding		
Endometrial polyp or submucous leiomyoma	Endometrial/uterine cancer	Cervicitis
Atrophic endometritis/vaginitis	Adenomyosis	

Speaking Intelligently

When we discuss menstrual bleeding with our patients, it is important to distinguish between what is normal and what is abnormal. We also need to understand the specific complexities of the medical language that will allow us to communicate about the patient and her concerns in an accurate way in the medical record, and with colleagues. Abnormal uterine bleeding (AUB) is the occurrence of bleeding outside the normal and anticipated menstrual cycle. Normal menses occurs every 24 to 35 days and lasts from 4 to 6 days (see Chapter 31, The Menstrual Cycle). Any bleeding occurring at a frequency of less than 24 days is termed *polymenorrhea.* Bleeding at a frequency longer than every 35 days is known as *oligomenorrhea.* Heavy menstrual bleeding is called *menorrhagia* and intermenstrual bleeding is called *metrorrhagia.* Irregular and heavy bleeding is called *menometrorrhagia.* Historically, any amount of bleeding in excess of 80 mL has also been called menorrhagia, but this is extraordinarily difficult to quantify. As with many gynecologic complaints, the first thing I need to rule out is a pregnancy-associated problem. The next step is to consider the age of the patient and to divide the patients into adolescent, reproductive age, and postmenopausal "categories." I then further subdivide the premenopausal patients into those experiencing ovulatory or anovulatory types of bleeding. This categorization helps me to prioritize my differential diagnosis and the appropriate work-up for the problem.

PATIENT CARE

Clinical Thinking

- Once pregnancy is ruled out, the most serious condition to consider is a gynecologic malignancy. Cancers of the uterus and cervix are the most common malignancies that can present with abnormal bleeding. Each patient needs to be assessed for risk factors for these cancers and should be evaluated accordingly.
- Remember that most AUB occurring in adolescents is due to anovulation. However, coagulation disorders are not uncommon. An expensive and often "low-yield" work-up may not be necessary if the history is suggestive of anovulation in an adolescent.

History

- The most important piece of the history relates to the type (spotting, bleeding, clots), duration, and frequency of the bleeding and other associated symptoms.
- Inquire about recent change in bowel or urinary function.
- Obtain the obstetric, gynecologic, contraceptive, surgical, and past medical history as well as a list of current medications. Be sure to include any over-the-counter herbal medications.

- Obtain a detailed sexual history, specifically with reference to associated bleeding.
- Inquire about any recent pelvic or abdominal ultrasonography or CT that may have been performed.
- Ask about any bleeding disorders in the patient or her family.

Physical Examination
- Perform a complete physical examination and check the skin for signs of a bleeding disorder, especially ecchymoses.
- A pelvic examination is mandatory in all patients with AUB: perform a comprehensive examination with adequate inspection of the vulva, vagina, and cervix.
- Be sure to do a Pap test and sample any lesions for biopsy, especially on the cervix.
- Perform a bimanual examination and assess the size and position of the uterus. A homogeneously enlarged uterus is suggestive of adenomyosis; an irregularly enlarged uterus suggests uterine leiomyomas.
- Try to assess the uterosacral ligaments for tenderness suggestive of endometriosis, and then feel for any adnexal masses.
- If the patient is an adolescent or not sexually active, a rectal examination may be performed instead of a vaginal examination.
- Abdominal and pelvic ultrasonography can be a helpful adjunct to the physical examination.

Tests for Consideration
- **Pregnancy test** (serum or urine): This must be performed for all patients of reproductive age with AUB. — $60
- **Pap test:** This will help rule out any cervical pathology. — $250
- **Endometrial biopsy:** When evaluating a patient for AUB, always consider this test; it can be extremely valuable and is relatively easy to perform. — $250
- **CBC:** Assesses possibility of anemia. — $35
- **Prolactin:** Hyperprolactinemia is a relatively common cause of anovulation. — $100
- **TSH:** AUB can be seen in cases of hyperthyroidism or hypothyroidism. — $60
- **Coagulation profile, including prothrombin time/activated partial thromboplastin time, and platelet count:** Especially relevant if the patient has had long-standing menorrhagia since adolescence. These values should also be evaluated if the patient has had severe anemia or has been hospitalized secondary to menorrhagia. — $160
- **FSH and LH:** Can sometimes be helpful in evaluating the patient for menopause, or premature menopause. — $260

IMAGING CONSIDERATIONS

→**Transvaginal ultrasonography:** Will help in ruling out endometrial pathology such as an endometrial polyp or a submucous leiomyoma. Transvaginal ultrasonography can sometimes be far superior to abdominal ultrasonography and should be requested where available, and used in conjunction with transabdominal ultrasonography. $250

→**Transabdominal ultrasonography:** May be requested if transvaginal ultrasonography is not available. $250

→**Saline infusion ultrasonography** (saline is infused into the uterine cavity while ultrasonography is performed): Can sometimes be useful in the identification of submucous polyps or uterine leiomyomas. $600

Clinical Entities	Medical Knowledge

Endocrinologic and Hematologic Causes of Abnormal Uterine Bleeding

Anovulation (Hypothalamic-Pituitary-Ovarian Axis)

Pφ Anovulatory bleeding is a diagnosis of exclusion secondary to immaturity or dysfunction in the hypothalamic-pituitary-ovarian axis. Usually caused by breakthrough bleeding secondary to unopposed estrogens, with little progesterone production to stabilize the endometrium. Anovulatory bleeding is common in patients with polycystic ovarian syndrome, obesity, and low body mass index.

TP Anovulatory bleeding is noncyclic, with irregular patterns and duration of bleeding. Variants range from spotting to heavy bleeding. Usually associated with *oligomenorrhea.*

Dx This is a diagnosis of exclusion. The history and physical examination are usually suggestive. Hormonal evaluation can be helpful (See Chapter 50, Teaching Visual: Secondary Amenorrhea).

Tx Hormonal manipulation is the mainstay of treatment. Any form of combination hormonal contraception is ideal, especially in patients who require contraception. Cyclic progestins may also be used. If the patient is attempting conception, then ovulation induction using clomiphene citrate may be considered. **See Katz 37, Hacker 32.**

Von Willebrand Disease

Pφ A disease caused by a genetic deficiency in the production of von Willebrand factor, which is required for platelet aggregation and binding to endothelial cells for hemostasis.

TP Heavy menstrual bleeding that begins in the postpubertal years. This may cause severe anemia, requiring hospitalization and even transfusion. In addition, it may be associated with bruising, nose and gum bleeding, and ecchymosis.

Dx Normal platelet count with platelet deficiency–type bleeding is suggestive. A prolonged bleeding time, reduced von Willebrand factor and ristocetin cofactor levels, and an abnormal platelet aggregation test result confirm the diagnosis.

Tx **Desmopressin acetate (**DDAVP**)** can raise the von Willebrand factor level. Antihemolytic factor (factor VII) may be used in preoperative patients. **See Gabbe 40.**

Thyroid Dysfunction

Pφ Both hypothyroidism and hyperthyroidism are associated with AUB. Hypothyroidism may also result in hyperprolactinemia, which is also a cause of amenorrhea or dysfunctional bleeding.

TP Hypothyroidism is also associated with weight gain, cold intolerance, constipation, fatigue, thyroid enlargement, and edema. Hyperthyroidism is associated with weight loss, velvety skin, sweating, thyroid tenderness, and tachycardia.

Dx A high thyroid-stimulating hormone (TSH) and low free thyroxine (T_4) level is diagnostic of hypothyroidism. A low TSH and high free T_4 is diagnostic of hyperthyroidism.

Tx Hyperthyroidism may be treated with beta blockers, radioactive iodine, methimazole, propylthiouracil, or surgery. Hypothyroidism is treated with levothyroxine. **See Katz 37.**

Anatomic Causes of Abnormal Uterine Bleeding

Endometrial Polyp or Submucous Leiomyoma

Pφ Endometrial polyps are pedunculated outgrowths of the endometrial lining that may be a few millimeters to a few centimeters in size. Submucous leiomyomas are tumors of the uterine smooth muscle that arise from or impinge significantly on the endometrial cavity. Both can interfere with the expected regularity of uterine bleeding.

TP Both endometrial polyps and submucous leiomyomas usually cause ovulatory-type menorrhagia. In many cases they may cause irregular bleeding. On occasion, polyps may be associated with tamoxifen use in patients with breast cancer.

Dx A saline infusion sonogram is a highly sensitive and noninvasive technique for diagnosis of endometrial pathology. Other tests that may be performed included a transvaginal ultrasound, MRI, and hysteroscopy.

Tx Hysteroscopy is usually both diagnostic and therapeutic, if the polyps are removed. **See Katz 18, Hacker 33.**

Endometrial/Uterine Cancer

Pφ Uterine cancer most commonly develops in the endometrial cavity. Endometrioid adenocarcinoma is the most common histologic type, but sarcomas can also cause abnormal bleeding. Uterine cancer usually develops in postmenopausal women. Risk factors include age, early menarche and late menopause, nulliparity, obesity, unopposed estrogen, hypertension, and diabetes mellitus.

TP These patients usually have had many years of amenorrhea followed by some form of postmenopausal bleeding. Rarely they may present with an abnormal Pap test result, which is sometimes read by the cytologist as AGUS—atypical glandular cells of undetermined significance.

Dx As with all cancers, the only way to reach the diagnosis is to obtain a histologic sample. Nevertheless, a transvaginal sonogram may be useful. If the endometrial lining is less than 5 mm in thickness, cancer is much less likely. The simplest method of obtaining a histologic sample is an office endometrial biopsy. A hysteroscopy and D&C may also be performed.

Tx The treatment of uterine cancer is surgical staging with hysterectomy, bilateral salpingo-oophorectomy, and sampling the pelvic lymph nodes (see Chapter 52, Endometrial Cancer). **See Katz 32, Hacker 41.**

Cervicitis

Pφ Cervicitis is an inflammatory condition involving the cervix. It is most commonly associated with sexually transmitted infections such as those caused by *Neisseria gonorrhoeae*, *Chlamydia trachomatis*, *Trichomonas vaginalis*, or herpes simplex virus.

TP These patients usually present with intermenstrual or postcoital bleeding, cervical discharge, or dyspareunia. Patients with trichomonal cervicitis sometimes have the classical "strawberry cervix" and those with herpetic cervicitis will have ulcerations on the cervix and other areas.

Dx Cervical cultures and DNA probes are diagnostic.

Tx Treatment is directed at the infectious agent. Gonorrhea is treated with ceftriaxone 125 mg intramuscularly and chlamydial infection is treated with doxycycline 100 mg twice daily for 7 days, or azithromycin 1 g once. Whenever gonorrhea or chlamydial infection is diagnosed, the patient is generally treated for both because they commonly are coinfections. The partner is also treated. Trichomoniasis is treated with metronidazole or tinidazole 2 g orally once, and the partner should also be treated. Herpes simplex infection is treated with acyclovir, famciclovir, or valacyclovir. The dose depends on the history of the infection. Condom use, as well as safe sexual practices, should be encouraged. **See Katz 22, Hacker 22.**

Atrophic Endometritis/Vaginitis

Pφ The decline in estrogen in postmenopausal patients can lead to an inflammatory condition associated with dryness and atrophy of the endometrium and vagina.

TP These patients present with postmenopausal spotting to light bleeding. They may also complain of dyspareunia and urinary incontinence. On examination, the lack of vaginal rugae, mucosal dryness, lack of distinct labia, and other hypoestrogenic effects are suggestive.

Dx This is a diagnosis of exclusion. It is imperative to first rule out other, more serious conditions such as uterine or cervical cancer and endometrial hyperplasia.

Tx Estrogen replacement is usually successful in treating this condition. The estrogen may be administered orally, transcutaneously, or vaginally. **See Katz 42, Hacker 22.**

Adenomyosis

Pφ The presence of endometrial glands and stroma in the myometrium of the uterus is called *adenomyosis*. Adenomyosis causes a homogeneous enlargement of the uterus and interferes with the uterine contractions that aid in hemostasis.

TP The typical patient with a diagnosis of adenomyosis is a multiparous woman in her third or fourth decade of life with menorrhagia and dysmenorrhea.

Dx Definitive diagnosis is obtained by post-hysterectomy histology. However, a homogeneously enlarged uterus in a multiparous patient with menorrhagia or dysmenorrhea is strongly suggestive. MRI can sometimes be helpful.

Tx Definitive treatment is hysterectomy. Other, more conservative and less invasive treatments that may be considered include oral contraceptive pills or endometrial ablation. **See Katz 18, Hacker 25.**

ZEBRA ZONE

a. **Vulvar or vaginal trauma:** Usually suggested by history.

b. **Foreign body:** Uncommon, but should be considered in younger premenarchal girls, the mentally challenged, or elderly women with dementia or Alzheimer's disease.

c. **Cushing syndrome:** Patients with Cushing syndrome usually have other characteristic signs such as moon facies, dorsal hump, central obesity with peripheral wasting, and easy bruisability.

d. **Liver disease:** Should be considered in alcoholics and intravenous drug users. Severe liver disease can cause abnormal production of endogenous clotting factors.

Practice-Based Improvement and Learning: Evidence-Based Medicine

Title
Radiographic imaging techniques for the diagnosis of abnormal uterine bleeding

Authors
Bradley LD, Falcone T, Magen AB

Institution
Department of Gynecology and Obstetrics, Cleveland Clinic
Foundation, Cleveland, Ohio

Reference
Obstetrics and Gynecology Clinics of North America 2000;27:245–276

Problem
Best choices for radiologic evaluation of AUB.

Intervention
Assesses different modalities of imaging.

Quality of evidence
Level III

Outcome/effect
Describes in detail the best studies to evaluate the genital tract and
endometrium in the presence of AUB.

Historical significance/comments
Describes the advantages and disadvantages of the various radiologic
studies available to assess AUB.

Interpersonal and Communication Skills

Overcoming Health Literacy, Language, and Cultural Barriers
Because any significant change in a patient's menstrual cycle may
result in distress to the patient, it is important for the clinician to
ask specific questions regarding the menstrual cycle history, including
duration of cycle, duration of bleeding, time and intensity of
cramping, and any associated menstrual discomfort both at baseline
and at present. The clinician must be able to use language that the
patient can understand, and must also be able to interpret the
patient's descriptions and terms. Make an effort to learn the slang
and colloquial terms for period, cycle, menstrual flow, and intercourse
in the different cultures of the population you serve. Listen to and
communicate with the appropriate cultural, ethnic, racial, age, and
religious sensitivity. You do not have to respond to the patient with
the same words. It is appropriate to respond, "OK, that is what I call
intercourse." At times patients use slang because they are not
familiar with the more commonly accepted terms. It is important to
offer the more appropriate language without making the patient feel
judged. Medical terms are often less emotive than slang, which may
offer comfort for both patient and clinician.

Professionalism

Principle: Commitment to Patient Confidentiality/Commitment to Professional Responsibilities

Your patient is a 32-year-old G2P2 who presents with a missed period and a positive pregnancy test that she administered to herself at home.

She describes her marriage as "stable," but she believes that her husband (with whom she has not had sexual relations in 2 months) is not the father of this pregnancy. The patient requests that you perform an abortion, but asks you to describe it on the medical record as a D&C and attribute it to "abnormal uterine bleeding."

Is this a permissible legal fiction under the circumstances? How do you respond?

Never falsify the medical record. You can reassure your patient that, as with all medical issues, you will keep this matter completely confidential unless she specifically directs you to discuss it with someone else.

Systems-Based Practice

Reimbursement: Medicare

You are evaluating a 67-year-old woman for AUB, and you decide to order some tests. Your office staff asks her what kind of insurance she has. She replies "I have Medicare, of course. But I've been thinking that I should change to a Medicare-HMO program. Should I do that?"

Medicare is the federal insurance program designed to care for the elderly and disabled. Enacted in 1965 as part of President Johnson's Great Society, Medicare was developed in recognition of the fact that the elderly and disabled could not typically participate in the employer-sponsored coverage that had become the cornerstone of U.S. health care coverage. The program, which is administered by the Centers for Medicare and Medicaid Services (more commonly known as CMS), consists of four parts, and in 2006 cost a total of $400 billion.

Medicare Part A covers hospitalizations, and is centered on the DRG system. DRGs (diagnosis-related groups) were developed in 1983, and represent the original "case rate" method of payment. A DRG is a code that represents the diagnosis of a patient; the hospital gets paid a certain amount for each admission depending on the patient's

DRG: for example, the hospital would receive—more for a coronary artery bypass graft, less for a cholecystectomy.

Medicare Part B pays for physician office visits, outpatient care, and durable medical equipment. Physicians are paid based on CPT codes; among these codes are a subset of evaluation and management (E&M) codes that provide for five different levels of patient visits.

Medicare Part C, also known as Medicare Advantage, and formerly known as "Medicare + Choice," was developed as part of the Balanced Budget Act of 1997. It allows Medicare recipients to choose to have their Medicare coverage provided by a private payer. These plans are typically HMO-type plans that save money by limiting their coverage to networks of providers, and then using some of these savings to offer greater coverage of preventive care and drug benefits. To qualify, the person must be enrolled in both Medicare Parts A and B.

Medicare Part D, enacted through legislation in 2003, is the prescription drug benefit component of Medicare. Until then, Medicare did not provide for prescription drugs given outside of the hospital or physician office. Similar to Medicare Part C, Part D is being administered by private insurance plans that are reimbursed by CMS. Medicare recipients have to elect to participate in Part D, unless they are dual-eligible (meaning eligible for Medicare and Medicaid), in which case they are automatically enrolled. There has been significant controversy over Medicare Part D, primarily for two reasons: first, the legislation prevents the government from using its massive purchasing power to negotiate discounts on drugs from drug companies; (many people felt that this was done to appease the drug industry, which has considerable sway over legislators) second, the program has a so-called "doughnut hole" in its coverage. There is no coverage up to the first $295.00; from $296.00 to $2700.00 there is a 25% out-of-pocket expense; from $2702.00 to $6154.00 there is no coverage, all costs being out-of-pocket. Over $6154.00 there is a 5% out-of-pocket cost. In 2006 there were somewhere between 14 and 27 million people enrolled in Medicare Part D.

Adapted from Mann BD: *Surgery: A Competency-Based Companion.* Elsevier, Philadelphia, 2009.

Chapter 35
Vaginitis (Case 21)

Kimberly M. Lenhardt MD

Case: A 34-year-old-woman presents to your office complaining of 3 days of vaginal discharge and irritation.

Differential Diagnosis

Yeast infection (i.e., *Candida* vaginitis)	Bacterial vaginosis	Trichomoniasis
Mucopurulent cervicitis	Foreign body	Hypersensitivity or allergic reaction

Speaking Intelligently

When a patient presents complaining of vaginal discharge, it is important to make sure to take an entire history of the present illness before performing the physical examination. Although a good history is often suggestive of the diagnosis, the physical exam is equally important to help rule out a concomitant or more extensive infection. You need to resist the urge to jump to conclusions based on the history and exam alone. A vaginal pH and wet prep are critical to making the definitive diagnosis. Although patient encounters for vaginitis are generally shorter and more straightforward than others, taking the time to ask the proper questions will not only help you to make the diagnosis, but will key you into behaviors or undiagnosed medical conditions that may predispose the patient to recurrent infections. If you discover that the patient has had recurrent yeast infections (four or more in a year), for example, you need to rule out diabetes and HIV infection. So, a seemingly simple case of vaginitis may actually help you diagnose more serious problems that would otherwise not have become evident until later.

PATIENT CARE

Clinical Thinking

- A patient with vaginal discharge and irritation usually has some sort of vaginitis. The most common types are *Candida* vaginitis, bacterial vaginosis, and trichomoniasis. An examination and wet prep will make the diagnosis.
- The patient may also have cervicitis from a sexually transmitted infection (STI). She needs to be screened for gonorrhea and chlamydial infection. Bacterial vaginosis and trichomoniasis are commonly associated with cervicitis.
- Is she or could she be pregnant? This may affect the type of treatment recommended.
- If the patient reports recurrent yeast infection, is it really recurrent or is it a relapse from incomplete or improper treatment? Patients frequently self-treat *Candida* vulvovaginitis with over-the-counter antifungal vaginal cream. Because the external vulva is not necessarily treated, the symptoms will persist or worsen and the *Candida* vaginitis may redevelop. Many women also mistake bacterial vaginosis (BV) for candidal infections and treat themselves with over-the-counter medications that are ineffective against BV.
- If the patient has a truly separate, recurrent infection, does she have diabetes or is she otherwise immunocompromised? If she has diabetes, how well is it controlled? She needs to be tested for HIV.
- If all routine test results are negative or normal, the possibility of an allergic reaction needs to be considered. However, if you have a high index of suspicion for candidal vaginitis, the patient needs to have a vaginal culture for *Candida* as well.

History

- Menstrual history and the use of contraceptives are important issues to address. This information helps determine the possibility of pregnancy. Many patients develop symptoms of yeast infection immediately before menses. Oral contraceptive pills can increase the risk of yeast infection. Use of condoms in a patient with an unknown latex sensitivity will cause an allergic reaction. Some spermicides have been known to cause symptoms of vaginitis as well. Antibiotics can alter the vaginal flora.
- Inquire about the consistency and appearance of the discharge. Is it malodorous or is it causing pruritus?
  - A white discharge that is described as "cottage cheese–like" with significant pruritus is suggestive of candidal vaginitis.
  - A gray or white vaginal discharge that causes a postcoital fishy odor is suggestive of bacterial vaginosis.
  - A yellow vaginal discharge that causes a postcoital fishy odor may be suggestive of trichomoniasis.
  - A foul, nonspecific vaginal discharge can be associated with a foreign body.

- Mild lower abdominal pain that is crampy in nature is often associated with bacterial vaginosis. Cervicitis with early pelvic inflammatory disease (PID) is possible as well. A urinary tract infection (UTI) should also be considered.
- A patient with trichomoniasis occasionally will complain of dysuria.
- The genital hygiene practices of patients are an important consideration. The use of vaginal douches significantly increases the risk of vaginitis, as well as cervicitis. The use of other feminine hygiene products (e.g., sprays or washes) may also increase the risk of vaginitis. Tub baths can also contribute to the development of both yeast infections and bacterial vaginosis. A patient may also have an allergic reaction after taking a bubble bath. Likewise, the type of material the patient's underwear is composed of is also important. All-cotton underwear is best, but cotton panels are a minimum requirement.
- The social history of the patient may also be relevant. Patients who spend a lot of time in wet or moist undergarments, such as swimmers or those who exercise frequently, have an increased risk of candidal vaginitis.
- The recent use of antibiotics increases the possibility of a candidal vaginitis.
- A history of poorly controlled diabetes, HIV infection, or other reason for immunocompromise increases the possibility of candidal infection.
- Determine if the patient has already tried over-the-counter or homeopathic treatments because this may affect the examination and the results of the tests you may want to order.

Physical Examination
- **Vital signs:** Obese patients are predisposed to yeast infections.
- **Abdomen:** Abdominal tenderness is absent in vaginitis, although may be present with cervicitis and early PID.
- **External genitalia:** Vulvar erythema with satellite lesions or edema is diagnostic of a *Candida* infection.
- **Vaginal speculum:** A thick, white, clumpy, adherent vaginal discharge is pathognomonic of candidal vaginitis. A thin, gray vaginal discharge is consistent with bacterial vaginosis. A yellow, frothy discharge suggests trichomoniasis. Cervical petechiae, described as a "strawberry cervix," is pathognomonic of trichomoniasis. Mucopurulent cervical discharge and "cervical friability" (bleeding with gentle palpation of endocervix) are suspect for cervicitis. A foreign body can be discovered and removed during the examination. Generalized vaginal erythema without discharge is suggestive of an allergic reaction.
- **Bimanual examination:** Cervical motion tenderness suggests cervicitis with PID.

Tests for Consideration

- **Wet prep:** This is the gold standard for diagnosing vaginitis and will almost always make the diagnosis of candidal vaginitis, bacterial vaginosis, and trichomoniasis. The application of potassium hydroxide (KOH) produces an immediate, pungent amine (fishy) odor, known as the "whiff test," in the presence of bacterial vaginosis and, often, trichomoniasis as well. — $60
- **Vaginal pH:** Absolutely necessary. A pH >5.0 suggests bacterial vaginosis or trichomoniasis. A pH <4.5 suggests *Candida* vaginitis. A normal pH is also consistent with hypersensitivity or allergic reaction. The pH of a mixed vaginitis (both bacterial vaginosis and *Candida* vaginitis) can vary and may not be helpful. — $10
- **Gonorrhea and *Chlamydia* culture or DNA probe:** Essential to rule out cervicitis. — $100
- **Herpes simplex virus (HSV) culture:** Possible cause of cervicitis. — $100
- **Urine pregnancy test:** Useful before treating bacterial vaginosis and trichomoniasis because the usual treatments are contraindicated during the first trimester of pregnancy. — $30
- **Urinalysis:** Useful to rule out UTI if suprapubic tenderness is elicited on examination. Also, urine microscopy may reveal yeast buds or trichomonads. — $30
- **Vaginal culture:** Essential if wet mount is negative and index of suspicion is high for *Candida* vaginitis or trichomoniasis. Also useful to isolate specific *Candida* species to better treat recurrent infections. — $250
- **Fasting glucose:** Important to rule out diabetes if patient has recurrent *Candida* vaginitis. — $30
- **HIV screen:** Important to rule out HIV/acquired immunodeficiency syndrome (AIDS) if patient has recurrent *Candida* vaginitis. — $150
- **Radioallergosorbent test (RAST) for latex:** Will determine if a patient is allergic to latex. — $250

Clinical Entities   Medical Knowledge

Candida Vaginitis

Pφ Colonization of the vagina by various *Candida* species, the most common of which is *Candida albicans*.

TP Presentation is characterized by complaints of a "cottage cheese–like" vaginal discharge and pruritus.

Dx Diagnosis is made immediately by examination, wet mount prep, and vaginal pH. Saline microscopy will usually show hyphae with buds, although application of KOH makes them easier to identify. Vaginal pH is <4.5. Vaginal culture for *Candida* species should be performed if the wet mount is negative and there is a high index of suspicion, based on symptoms or vaginal pH. However, the culture results will not be available for a few days. These findings, along with vulvar erythema or edema, are diagnostic of *Candida* vulvovaginitis.

Tx Treatment is with topical antifungal cream or oral fluconazole. **See Katz 22, Hacker 22.**

Bacterial Vaginosis

Pφ Shift from normal vaginal flora of *Lactobacillus* to an abnormal mixed flora of *Gardnerella vaginalis*, anaerobes, and mycoplasmas.

TP Presentation usually consists of vaginal discharge with fishy odor that worsens after intercourse. Patients may also complain of mild, crampy lower abdominal discomfort.

Dx Diagnosis is made immediately by examination, wet prep, and vaginal pH. The speculum exam reveals a thin, gray vaginal discharge, although the appearance can vary. The vaginal pH will be >4.5. Wet prep reveals the presence of clue cells, which are vaginal epithelial cells covered with adherent bacteria. A positive whiff test is evident with the addition of KOH to the slide.

Tx Treatment is with metronidazole or clindamycin, both of which are available in a topical gel form. Metronidazole can also be used orally. Vaginal preparations are not used for treatment of bacterial vaginosis in pregnancy. **See Katz 22, Hacker 22.**

Trichomoniasis

Pφ Presence of *Trichomonas vaginalis*, a flagellated protozoan, in the genitourinary tract. It is transmitted through sexual contact and is considered to be an STI.

TP A patient will usually complain of vaginal discharge with fishy odor that worsens after intercourse. The patient may complain of pruritus or vaginal irritation. Occasionally, dysuria or urinary frequency is present.

Dx Diagnosis is made immediately by examination, wet prep, and vaginal pH. The speculum exam reveals a yellow, frothy vaginal discharge. The cervix may have petechiae, known as a "strawberry cervix." Saline microscopy shows the mobile, flagellated trichomonads. Vaginal pH is >5.0. A positive whiff test may be evident with the addition of KOH to the slide. Vaginal culture is also available, although usually not necessary.

Tx Treatment has traditionally been with oral metronidazole. Tinidazole is also effective and has recently become available for use in the United States. **See Katz 22, Hacker 22.**

Mucopurulent Cervicitis

Pφ Presence of *Neisseria gonorrhoeae* or *Chlamydia trachomatis* in endocervical mucosa. HSV may also cause mucopurulent cervicitis.

TP Presentation may be characterized by complaints of vaginal discharge alone.

Dx Diagnosis is made by history, physical examination, wet mount, and genital cultures. Wet mount will show only white blood cells. Careful inquiry into any new personal hygiene routine (soaps, sprays) or laundry detergent changes may uncover the offending agent.

Tx Treatment is with oral antibiotics based on the result of the gonorrhea and chlamydial culture/DNA probe. If you have a high index of suspicion, you may choose to treat the patient empirically during the visit rather than waiting for the culture results. **See Katz 22, Hacker 22.**

Allergic Reaction/Hypersensitivity

Pφ Immune-mediated hypersensitivity response to an irritant or allergen.

TP Patients complain of vaginal irritation that may be described as burning or itching and is associated with varying amounts of discharge.

Dx History, physical examination, wet mount, vaginal pH, genital culture, and vaginal culture are required because this is a difficult diagnosis to make and is often a diagnosis of exclusion. However, the RAST will identify a latex sensitivity.

Tx Avoidance of the offending agent is the most important form of treatment. **See Katz 18.**

Foreign Bodies

Pφ The intentional insertion of an object or inadvertent failure to remove a temporary hygienic device, such as a tampon.

TP A patient may simply complain of malodorous vaginal discharge with spotting. Alternatively, she may admit to forgetting to remove a tampon. Retained tampons are usually associated with an extremely foul odor.

Dx Diagnosis is made by history and physical examination. A wet mount and vaginal pH should be performed to rule out a secondary infection. A vaginal culture should be considered if a bacterial infection with *Streptococcus* or *Staphylococcus* is suspected.

Tx A foreign body is removed at the time of the exam. Antibiotic treatment for a foreign body, including retained tampons, is not indicated unless the patient is found to have a secondary infection. **See Katz 18, Hacker 22.**

ZEBRA ZONE

a. **Desquamative inflammatory vaginitis:** A rare disorder that causes chronic vaginal discharge and has no known cause.

b. **Fistula:** A vesicovaginal or rectovaginal fistula will cause vaginal leakage of urine or stool, respectively.

c. **Gynecologic lesions:** Vaginal condylomata, a prolapsing leiomyoma, or cervical cancer may cause vaginal discharge.

d. **Erosive lichen planus:** Diffuse ulceration of mucosal surfaces anywhere in the body.

e. **Extensive ulceration:** Ulceration of the vaginal mucosa can cause vaginal discharge.

Practice-Based Learning and Improvement: Evidence-Based Medicine

Title
Nonspecific vaginitis: Diagnostic criteria and microbial and epidemiologic associations

Authors
Amsel R, Totten PA, Spiegel CA, et al.

Institution
University of Washington, Seattle, Washington

Reference
American Journal of Medicine 1983;74:14–22

Problem
Lack of standardization for diagnosis of vaginitis.

Intervention
Examination of 397 female university health center patients to study which criteria (appearance of vaginal discharge, pH, presence of amine odor, presence of clue cells and abnormal amines in vaginal discharge) were associated with vaginitis versus normal vaginal flora.

Quality of evidence
Comparative study, level II-1

Outcome/effect
Development of simple office-based diagnostic criteria to streamline the evaluation of vaginitis.

Historical significance/comments
The criteria created by Amsel and colleagues in this study have become the gold standard for diagnosing vaginitis.

Interpersonal and Communication Skills

Being Direct to Dispel Misconceptions
Although vaginitis is usually a straightforward diagnosis and easily treated, it often results in a patient becoming hypervigilant and worrying excessively that any vaginal discharge is vaginitis. A patient can easily develop the misconception that the problem is due to a lack of cleanliness or poor hygiene. It is helpful to explore the patient's ideas about what she thinks is causing the vaginitis. Take time to educate the patient about normal vaginal discharge, as well as specific symptoms of vaginitis. Explain how recurrent use of over-the-counter medical products may actually increase the risk of recurrent vaginitis. To dispel misconceptions, take time and be direct.

Professionalism

Principles: Commitment to Patient Confidentiality and Primacy of Patient Welfare

When notifying a patient that she has an STI, the information must be delivered in a clear, concise, and nonjudgmental manner. Anticipate that your patient will often react with feelings of anger, doubt, denial, isolation, and betrayal. You will need to help her focus on the need for treatment, both for her own infection and that of her sexual partner. It is very important to emphasize the need for abstinence from sex for both partners until the STI has been successfully treated. This is an ideal time to emphasize further the needs for barrier techniques for the prevention of future STIs.

Although you should always strive to preserve a commitment to patient confidentiality, this commitment should not override a commitment to public health. Think of the community in which you live as your extended patient population. A commitment to public health can easily be seen as an extension of the principle of primacy of patient welfare to include the welfare of the entire community. In certain situations you may be both ethically and legally required to report infections to the Department of Public Health.

Systems-Based Practice

Using Over-the-Counter Treatments

The care and treatment of vaginitis has been estimated to consume millions of health care dollars annually and causes patients considerable inconvenience, discomfort, and time away from work. In some geographic areas vaginitis accounts for as many as one out of four visits to the obstetrician/gynecologist office. Using over-the-counter treatments effectively can be one way of reducing the burden placed on physicians and insurance companies when there is little risk to the patient if she actually attempts to treat herself for the recognized problem.

Although treatment for trichomoniasis and bacterial vaginosis requires a prescription, treatments for candidal vaginitis are widely available over the counter. The availability of medication over the counter for vaginal candidiasis is a relatively recent development, and reflects the confluence of several systems-based forces coming together, widely regarded to be for the benefit of the patient. In this particular instance, the U.S. Food and Drug Administration was able to approve an "over-the-counter" designation for certain anticandidal treatments that are regarded to be extremely safe. Miconazole, found in Monistat and in generic form, is an example. At the same time, drug manufacturers adjusted their pricing of these medications to make them profitable to sell in a nonprescription formulation. Patients often found it inconvenient to make a trip to the office for simple vaginitis, and if the patient has had a yeast infection in the past, she may be well aware of the symptoms and might surmise that she has another yeast infection. To some degree, therefore, patient preference became a driving force in the market-driven concept of making candidal vaginitis treatment easily accessible without a prescription. Physicians and health care providers seem to have come to an understanding that patients now have the opportunity to diagnose and treat themselves. In such an environment, it is important to lower one's threshold to bring a patient in for an examination and evaluation, especially when she states she has failed a course of over-the-counter treatment.

Over-the-counter treatments, however, are not the first choice of all patients and physicians. Many patients often prefer the convenience of prescription oral fluconazole because it is just a single dose and often less cumbersome than the creams and ointment formulations. Both treatments are equally effective. Although the percentage of correct self-diagnoses is unimpressive, it is reasonable for patients to try an over-the-counter yeast regimen or single-dose fluconazole. It will be necessary for the patient to be clinically evaluated, however, if her symptoms persist after the empiric treatment. If her symptoms are not suggestive of *Candida* vaginitis, she should be clinically evaluated immediately. Because trichomoniasis is an STI, it is necessary to make a specific diagnosis so the patient's sexual partner can be treated as well. It is also necessary to rule out chlamydial infection and gonorrhea, which also require the treatment of the partner, because the incidences of chlamydial infection and gonorrhea are increased in the presence of bacterial vaginosis and trichomoniasis. Currently, there are no over-the-counter therapies for bacterial vaginosis or trichomoniasis, but several self-diagnostic kits are now available in most pharmacies that allow patients the opportunity to avoid incorrectly treating bacterial vaginosis or trichomoniasis as a candidal infection.

Chapter 36
Pelvic Pain (Case 22)

Michael Belden MD *and Barry D. Mann* MD

Case: A 22-year-old woman presents to the emergency department with a 12-hour history of right lower quadrant pain.

Differential Diagnosis

Ovarian cyst	Ectopic pregnancy	Intrauterine pregnancy	Threatened miscarriage	Urinary tract infection (UTI)
Ovarian torsion	Pelvic inflammatory disease (PID)/ tubo-ovarian abscess	Appendicitis	Pyelonephritis	Ureterolithiasis/ nephrolithiasis

Speaking Intelligently

When I am asked to see a young woman of reproductive age with pelvic pain, my first question is always: "Is she pregnant?" A quantitative human chorionic gonadotropin (β-hCG) level is mandatory in this population, regardless of birth control use, menstrual history, or, honestly, what sexual history (or lack thereof) is provided to you by the patient. Once I have this information, I prioritize: I separate the gynecologic, gastrointestinal (GI), and genitourinary systems in that order, because missing an ectopic pregnancy could be a very dire mistake. If a urine pregnancy test is *positive*, and the serum quantitative β-hCG is above approximately 1500 mIU, an intrauterine gestational sac should be seen on sonographic evaluation of the pelvis. Cardiac activity should be seen with a β-hCG level of about 11,000. If the urine pregnancy test is *negative*, I reconsider my differential diagnosis. A CBC and urinalysis are helpful. In the face of a fever or increased white blood cell count, pelvic ultrasonography can diagnose the presence of ovarian cysts, ovarian torsion, and other pelvic disease processes. As CT of the pelvis is now really the gold standard for the diagnosis of appendicitis, I usually obtain a CT scan if appendicitis is strongly considered. It is acceptable to perform both ultrasound and CT studies (if warranted), with the ultrasound usually performed first.

PATIENT CARE

Clinical Thinking

- What are the most serious problems you could be faced with? Ectopic pregnancy, ovarian torsion, appendicitis, and miscarriage with hemorrhage can all be surgical emergencies.
- If the clinical picture remains unclear after laboratory and radiologic evaluation and the patient has peritonitis, diagnostic laparoscopy or laparotomy should be considered.

History

- Menstrual history and history of contraceptive use are two critical aspects of the history. But do not rely on these alone regarding assessment of pregnancy: a serum β-hCG value is critical.
- A past history of sexually transmitted infections, human papillomavirus infection, abnormal Pap tests/colposcopy, multiple sexual partners, or ectopic pregnancy in the past raises the strong possibility of pelvic inflammatory disease or tubo-ovarian abscess.
- A history of prior ruptured ovarian cysts, or oral contraceptive pill (OCP) use to control ovarian cysts and suppress ovulation suggests possible recurrence of an ovarian cyst.
- Waxing and waning episodes of excruciating pain suggest torsion, especially in the face of a prior history of known ovarian cyst.
- The onset, quality, quantity, and mitigating or exacerbating aspects of the pain are all relevant. Anorexia may be present with a GI process such as appendicitis, but may also be present in PID or ruptured ectopic pregnancy.
- In your review of GI symptoms, ask about associated bowel symptoms, such as diarrhea, constipation, bloody stools, and family or community illness or food exposures.
- Appendicitis often has a typical prodrome of vague mid-abdominal or periumbilical pain with subsequent migration of the pain to the right lower quadrant (RLQ).
- Dysuria, urinary frequency, hematuria, or pyuria all suggest a urinary tract etiology.
- Renal colic associated with hematuria suggests ureterolithiasis.

Physical Examination

- **Vital signs:** Fever suggests an inflammatory response or infection. Tachycardia or hypotension is of concern for hemorrhage or sepsis.
- **General appearance:** Truly ill patients look ill. They do not smile or laugh. Peritonitis will cause a patient to lie as still as possible. Patients with peritoneal signs (tenderness, guarding, rebound tenderness) often object to being examined. "Colicky" pain, often caused by ovarian torsion or renal calculus, will leave a patient struggling to find a comfortable position.

- **Lungs:** Should be clear bilaterally. Very rarely, pneumonia may present with abdominal pain due to diaphragmatic irritation.
- **Abdominal examination:** Peritonitis, regardless of cause, presents as tenderness, guarding, and rebound. Bowel sounds are usually decreased with peritonitis.
- **Pelvic examination:** Foul or purulent vaginal discharge suggests PID. Cervical motion tenderness is a nonspecific finding suggestive of PID or pelvic peritoneal irritation of any etiology. An appreciable pelvic mass may suggest ectopic pregnancy, torsion, ovarian cyst, or degenerating leiomyoma. In the correct circumstances, genital cultures should be performed as part of the exam. In the absence of obvious cervical pathology, cervical cytology is unnecessary.

Tests for Consideration

- **Quantitative β-hCG:** Essential. $135
- **CBC:** High white blood cell count suggests infection or inflammation. A low hemoglobin may suggest a bleeding ectopic pregnancy or uterine hemorrhage. However, remember that hemoglobin and hematocrit may not drop until late in hemorrhage when equilibration occurs. $35
- **Urinalysis:** Evaluates for pyelonephritis, UTI, and urinary calculi. $38
- **Pelvic ultrasonography:** Essential for evaluation of ovaries, uterus, ectopic, or intrauterine pregnancy. Doppler flow helps with ectopic pregnancy and torsion. $225
- **CT scan:** The study of choice for appendicitis, diverticulitis, or suspected malignancy. $800

IMAGING CONSIDERATIONS

→**CT scan:** Generally diagnostic of appendicitis. If you suspect appendicitis, and the patient has a positive pregnancy test, you should judge how important the CT will actually be in terms of the patient's evaluation. If essential for diagnosis, a CT should be considered even though there is a small amount of radiation exposure to the fetus. $800

→**Pelvic ultrasonography:** Can follow CT, and gives more detailed information in regard to suspected pelvic pathology, especially in light of a positive β-hCG. $225

Clinical Entities	Medical Knowledge

Ovarian Cyst

Pφ Typically physiologic, often a diagnosis of exclusion if all other diagnoses can be effectively ruled out and the patient remains in pain.

TP Pain is often "mid-cycle," but not always. Rare in patients who reliably use hormonal contraceptives such as OCPs or depo-medroxyprogesterone. Pain is often rapid in onset and rapid in regression. Fever and leukocytosis are rare, but mild peritoneal findings may be expected.

Dx A large cyst, hemorrhagic cyst, or collapsing cyst can often be visualized with pelvic ultrasonography. These subtleties are not effectively visualized with CT scan.

Tx Treatment is almost always expectant, except in those rare patients with peritonitis. **See Katz 18, Hacker 20.**

Ovarian Torsion

Pφ Ovarian torsion usually requires the presence of an ovarian mass such as a cyst or tumor. Typically, only when a mass is present will the ovary be able to "torse" on the utero-ovarian and infundibulopelvic ligaments. An ovary free of disease will almost never be involved in torsion. Likewise, pelvic adhesions such as those caused by prior surgery or PID often prevent torsion.

TP Presentation is characterized by intermittent but severe pain. Peritoneal signs are often present.

Dx Diagnosis is made by high clinical suspicion and/or pelvic ultrasonography with Doppler flow, which suggests impeded blood flow and venous return.

Tx Treatment is surgical and can often be accomplished by laparoscopy. Removal of the pathologic process that caused the torsion, or the entire ovary, is reasonable. Simply untwisting the ovary on its vascular attachments is also acceptable in some circumstances, but may allow for repeat episodes and the need for repeat surgical procedures. **See Katz 18.**

Ectopic Pregnancy

Pφ An ectopic pregnancy is a pregnancy that occurs when a fertilized ova implants outside the endometrial cavity. The fallopian tube is by far the most common location. Ovarian, abdominal, or cervical pregnancies are exceedingly rare. One in 30,000 spontaneous pregnancies result in concurrent intrauterine and ectopic pregnancies, known as *heterotopic pregnancy*.

TP Presentation is characterized by lower abdominal pain and bleeding is common. Pelvic ultrasonography reveals an empty uterine cavity in the face of a positive β-hCG.

Dx Diagnosis is made by using the β-hCG level as well as ultrasonography, along with physical examination findings.

Tx Management can be surgical, medical, or even expectant under the correct circumstances. The gold standard of care was formerly laparoscopy, but medical therapy using methotrexate has become widely accepted. In the face of an unstable patient or suspected hemorrhage, immediate laparoscopy or laparotomy is indicated. **See Katz 17, Hacker 24.**

Pelvic Inflammatory Disease and Tubo-ovarian Abscess

Pφ PID and its more chronic counterpart, tubo-ovarian abscess, are caused by ascending pelvic infections, most commonly gonorrhea and chlamydial infection. The infection is often polymicrobial, so broad-spectrum antibiotics should be used until positive cultures are documented.

TP Presentation is characterized by fever, pain, and confirmatory radiologic findings with either ultrasonography or CT scan. Cultures are helpful, but will sometimes be falsely negative.

Dx Diagnosis is made by history of lower abdominal pain with tenderness, cervical motion tenderness, and adnexal tenderness. Supporting criteria include fever of 101° F or greater, abnormal vaginal discharge, and positive cultures for *Neisseria gonorrhoeae* or *Chlamydia trachomatis*.

Tx Treatment is with antibiotics and observation. Rarely, diagnostic laparoscopy with resection or drainage of infected pelvic viscera is indicated. **See Katz 23, Hacker 22.**

Intrauterine Pregnancy

Pφ Normal intrauterine pregnancy can sometimes present with pain and/or cramping. Likewise, threatened miscarriage or incomplete miscarriage often presents similarly.

TP Typical presentation is characterized by crampy midline pain, with a positive pregnancy test.

Dx Diagnosis is made and confirmed by positive quantitative β-hCG, with or without pelvic ultrasonography. Pelvic ultrasonography is extremely helpful, and must be ordered if the possibility of ectopic pregnancy is entertained.

Tx Therapy is expectant with much reassurance. **See Hacker 7.**

Miscarriage

Pφ/TP Miscarriage is most often characterized by uterine bleeding and pain, and can be subdivided into the following categories: *threatened abortion*—bleeding with a closed cervical os; *inevitable abortion*—bleeding with an open cervical os but with no passed tissue; and *incomplete* or *complete abortion*, which simply addresses whether or not all the tissue is passed. A *missed abortion* reveals a nonviable fetus ultrasonographically, but without pain or bleeding. (These categories of abortion are discussed in greater detail in Chapter 20, Early Pregnancy Loss and Miscarriage.)

Dx Diagnosis of miscarriage involves three components: history and physical examination, quantitative β-hCG, and ultrasonographic findings.

Tx Miscarriage can be followed expectantly, or with a surgical procedure if indicated. **See Katz 16, Hacker 7.**

Appendicitis

Pφ *Appendicitis* is an inflammation of the appendiceal wall usually brought about by occlusion of the appendiceal lumen due to a fecalith.

TP Initially, the distended appendix produces vague abdominal pain perceived as a "stomach ache" in the periumbilical region. Within the next 24 to 36 hours, as the serosa of the appendix becomes inflamed, the typical patient becomes aware that the pain has migrated to the RLQ. Usually associated with a mild leukocytosis.

Dx If the prodromal pattern and the subsequent physical findings of RLQ peritoneal irritation are characteristic, a clinical diagnosis of appendicitis can be made and one can proceed to the operating room for laparoscopic or open appendectomy.

Tx Ultrasonography may be helpful to exclude gynecologic pathology as indicated by the history and physical examination. In recent years, CT has been used much more routinely in the diagnosis of appendicitis. A markedly elevated white blood cell count, fever greater than 101° F, or wider distribution of peritoneal findings may suggest perforated appendicitis. **See Katz 8.**

Urinary Tract Infection

Pφ UTIs are extremely common and generally very uncomfortable for patients who acquire them. UTI is a common source of pelvic pain and discomfort.

TP Typical presentation is characterized by pain with urination, possible bleeding or blood in urine, and urinary hesitancy, frequency, and urgency.

Dx Initial diagnosis is made by bladder or suprapubic tenderness and urinalysis, which reveals white blood cells and bacteria; urinary culture confirms infection, identifies the infectious agent, and defines antibiotic sensitivities.

Tx UTIs are treated with appropriate antibiotics; typically an oral regimen is sufficient. Antibiotics may sometimes be started before cultures return. If culture and sensitivities reveal inadequate antimicrobial coverage, a more appropriate antibiotic should be selected. **See Hacker 23.**

Pyelonephritis

Pφ Pyelonephritis is an upper urinary tract infection involving the kidney.

TP Characterized by high fever, painful urination, flank and abdominal pain, and nausea, vomiting, and anorexia. Tenderness at the costovertebral angle is usually present.

Dx Diagnosis is made by physical examination, urine culture, and sometimes-positive blood cultures.

Tx Treatment is either with oral antibiotics or an intravenous regimen. Patients suspected of being poor compliance risks are best treated with intravenous antibiotics as inpatients. **See Hacker 23.**

Urolithiasis/Nephrolithiasis

Pφ Kidney stones, or urolithiasis, is a common condition characterized by the presence of stones in the kidney (nephrolithiasis) or in any position in the system from the bladder to the urethra.

TP Presentation is often rapid in onset, and the pain is severe and generally "colicky" in nature. Many describe pain intensity as near or worse than childbirth.

Dx Diagnosis is made by physical examination findings (which often include tenderness in the costovertebral angle), urinalysis, and often a diagnostic study such as intravenous pyelography, renal ultrasonography, or CT scan with renal protocol.

Tx Treatment usually involves fluid support and generous analgesia. Occasionally stones will need to be retrieved by cystoscopy and ureteroscopy. Extracorporeal shock-wave lithotripsy has been widely proven to be beneficial and is used in some centers.

ZEBRA ZONE

a. Leiomyomata: Relatively uncommon in this age group, but could be a consideration.

b. Bowel obstruction: Should be considered in anyone who has had prior abdominal or pelvic surgery.

c. Gynecologic malignancy: Epithelial ovarian or fallopian tube cancers and germ cell tumors are rare, but may present in this age group.

Practice-Based Learning and Improvement: Evidence-Based Medicine

Title
Nonsurgical treatment of ectopic pregnancy [review]

Authors
Lipscomb GH, Stovall TG, Ling FW

Reference
New England Journal of Medicine 2000;343:1325–1329

Problem
Treatment of ectopic pregnancy with medical therapy instead of surgery.

Intervention
Methotrexate, given intramuscularly, for the treatment of unruptured ectopic pregnancies that meet certain criteria.

Quality of evidence
Review article

Outcome/effect
Resolution of ectopic pregnancy without the morbidity of surgery.

Historical significance/comments
The definitive review article that describes in detail the ground-breaking ability to treat certain ectopic pregnancies with medical management. Previously, ectopic pregnancy was invariably a surgical problem.

Interpersonal and Communication Skills

Communicate Effectively with Patients: Acknowledging Fertility Issues

A young patient about to undergo an operation for a gynecologic problem, either by laparoscopy or laparotomy, is likely to have great concerns, even if unspoken, about future fertility. Certainly, if the suspected diagnosis is pelvic inflammatory disease, ectopic pregnancy, tubo-ovarian abscess, or endometriosis, the issue of future fertility must be addressed as part of the operative consent process. Even if the most likely diagnosis happens to be appendicitis, the issue should still be addressed to reassure the anxious patient that, in most cases, future chances at spontaneous conception will not be significantly diminished. However, if you have a strong suspicion that the patient has a severely diseased pelvis, you should begin the discussion of possible diminished fertility before surgery; if confirmed at the time of surgery, a realistic assessment of the chances of future fertility should be discussed honestly with the patient. It is possible that some patients will not have seriously considered fertility before surgery even when you raise the issue. It is generally wise to monitor your patient after surgery for anxiety about the possibility of diminished fertility, even if the concerns may be unspoken.

Professionalism

Principle: Commitments to Patient Confidentiality and to Patient Welfare

You are called to the emergency department to complete a consult on a 15-year-old girl complaining of pelvic pain. When you arrive, you find the patient in the room with her parents. You know that you will need to ask questions about sexual activity and pregnancy and you decide that to respect the confidentiality of the patient it will be best to ask the parents to step out of the room. Before the parents leave the room, it is important to explain to the patient and her parents that all aspects of the conversation you have with the patient will be confidential unless you are concerned that she is putting her life or someone else's life in imminent danger. When the parents are out of the room, your patient tells you that she has been using intravenous drugs and having unprotected sex. Although this is not grounds to break confidentiality, you, as the physician, need to follow the principle of the primacy of patient welfare. It is your obligation to attempt to convince your patient to involve her parents in her care so that she can receive maximum support in addressing these important issues.

Systems-Based Practice

Hospitals today are busy and complicated places. Although every hospital is unique in some ways, a few general principles usually hold true regarding hospital hierarchical organization. The different branches of a hospital typically meet together primarily in two places: at the bedside and in the executive suite, but in between they are often quite separate. For instance, although nurses, physicians, and case managers typically work closely together on the floor, they each report up through separate hierarchies that meet together through the Chief Nursing Officer (often the vice president for patient care) and the Chief Medical Officer (often the vice president for medical affairs). Ancillary departments—such as laboratory, phlebotomy, physical therapy, and social work—typically report up through entirely separate hierarchies as well. Thus, the social worker taking care of your patient does not typically report to the nurse manager on your floor. Contrary to what many believe, at most hospitals the vast majority of physicians do not work for the hospital but rather for themselves, and have privileges in the hospital. The exceptions to this are often anesthesiologists, radiologists, pathologists, and sometimes emergency medicine physicians, whom the hospital often either employs directly or employs indirectly through contracts with specialty group practices.

Understanding the hierarchical reporting structures becomes important when one wishes to address and remedy a perceived problem in the system.

Chapter 37
Pelvic Inflammatory Disease (Case 23)

Sutthichai Sae-Tia MD

Case: A 20-year-old woman was admitted to hospital with a 2-week history of left lower quadrant pelvic pain, bloody vaginal discharge, and low-grade fever. During the past 2 days, the pain was severe and was associated with shaking chills. She also reported having unprotected intercourse 3 weeks ago. Her pregnancy test is negative, and her urinalysis shows no signs of urinary tract infection or pyelonephritis.

Differential Diagnosis

Pelvic inflammatory disease/ tubo-ovarian abscess	Cervicitis	Endometriosis

Speaking Intelligently

The first and most important step in the evaluation of a clinical problem in a reproductive-age woman is to rule out a pregnancy and its complications. The next step is to approach the patient from the standpoint of her chief complaints, which in this case are pelvic pain, vaginal discharge, and fever. We can either consider a differential diagnosis according to organ systems, including gynecologic, gastrointestinal (GI), and genitourinary; or formulate our differential based on the location of pain, in this case left lower quadrant. Based on the small amount of information we know in the case described, pelvic inflammatory disease (PID) is a likely diagnosis. A good history and physical examination will guide which laboratory studies should be obtained.

PATIENT CARE

Clinical Thinking

- There are three questions we should always ask ourselves when we see a patient with suspected PID. First, is she pregnant? This might change our differential diagnosis. In addition, the selection of laboratory studies, interventions, or medications can be affected by a patient's pregnancy status.
- Second, does she have an acute abdomen that requires emergent surgery? If a patient has signs of peritonitis, including tenderness, rebound tenderness, or guarding, it is important to confirm a diagnosis and initiate a necessary intervention.
- Finally, is she clinically or hemodynamically unstable? If a patient has high fever, tachycardia, and hypotension suggesting septic shock, volume resuscitation will be the most important step to be initiated as the history and physical examination are performed.

History

- A thorough history and physical examination will help us to rule in and rule out our differential diagnoses. It is important to go through the chief complaints of the patient in detail.
- A detailed pain history and the symptoms associated with the pain should be obtained. The onset, characteristics, intensity, location, radiation, and aggravating and relieving factors are important.
- Symptoms such as dysuria and urinary hesitancy or frequency suggest urinary tract infection. Vaginal discharge or abnormal vaginal

bleeding will point toward gynecologic causes. Associated GI symptoms such as diarrhea or bloody stool may suggest possible GI causes.

- In suspected cases of PID, detailed characteristics of vaginal discharge are important. Purulent vaginal discharge will point toward an infectious etiology such as PID or tubo-ovarian abscess.
- A detailed history of menstruation, contraception, and sexual history can help rule in or rule out pregnancy or its complications.
- Look for risk factors associated with PID. Ask about the presence or previous history of sexually transmitted infection (STI), especially chlamydial infection and gonorrhea. A history of PID in the past, sexual intercourse at a young age, multiple sexual partners, and alcohol or illicit drug use are additional risk factors for PID. Recent intrauterine device (IUD) insertion (within 1 month) can increase the risk of PID as well.
- For any patient clinically suspected of having an STI, it is vital to explore the possibility of risk factors for human immunodeficiency virus (HIV) infection, such as unsafe sexual practices, multiple sexual partners, and intravenous drug abuse.
- Recent history of cervical or intrauterine instrumentation should also be considered. Cervical conization, loop electrosurgical excision procedure, D&C, and elective termination of pregnancy are all risk factors for PID in an "at-risk" population.

Physical Examination
- **Vital signs:** These will help us to determine whether a patient is clinically stable. Fever might point to infection such as PID. However, some patients with PID may not have a fever.
- **General appearance:** Patients with septic shock will look extremely ill; we sometimes use the word *toxic*. Such patients may be diaphoretic and confused.
- **Abdominal examination:** Patients with severe intra-abdominal infection might have lower abdominal tenderness, but this finding could be nonspecific. In severe cases, signs of peritonitis, including rebound tenderness, guarding, and rigidity may be present. Bowel sounds may be decreased or absent.
- **Pelvic examination:** The presence of cervical or vaginal mucopurulent discharge will suggest PID. Patients may have either cervical motion, uterine, or adnexal tenderness, but these findings are not specific for PID. In cases of tubo-ovarian abscess, an adnexal mass can sometimes be palpated.
- **Rectal examination:** It is important to test for blood in the stool.

Tests for Consideration

- **Quantitative human chorionic gonadotropin (β-hCG):** Essential for excluding pregnancy. $35
- **CBC:** Elevated white blood cell count suggests infection. $30
- **Urinalysis and urine cultures:** Positive nitrite or leukocyte esterase and the presence of pyuria are suggestive of urinary tract infection or pyelonephritis. $28
- **Vaginal or urine/cervical swab for *Chlamydia trachomatis* polymerase chain reaction (PCR):** Helpful for confirming chlamydial infection. $98
- **Cervical cultures for *Neisseria gonorrhoeae*, *C. trachomatis*, and other bacteria:** Helpful for confirming the cause of infection. Can also identify bacterial causes of PID that might help to dictate antibiotic therapy in situations when the patient is not responding to initial empiric antibiotics. $150
- **HIV test:** Essential to screen a patient with PID for HIV. $100
- **Blood cultures:** Essential in severe cases and in patients with clinical sepsis. Patients with positive blood cultures may require intravenous antibiotics until clinically improved. $250

IMAGING CONSIDERATIONS

→**Pelvic ultrasonography:** Usually the first step in the evaluation of pelvic pathology, and essential for evaluation of pelvic organ structures. Ultrasonography helps in confirming tubo-ovarian abscess, intrauterine or ectopic pregnancy, ovarian cysts or torsion, and endometriosis. Abdominal ultrasonography is often performed in conjunction with transvaginal ultrasonography. Large pelvic masses can sometimes not be fully visualized with an endovaginal approach alone. $250

→**CT scan:** Also useful if the sonogram is unrevealing. CT can be particularly helpful if you suspect a large pelvic abscess. Helpful to rule in or rule out other GI or genitourinary causes such as appendicitis, diverticulitis, or ureteral/kidney calculi. $800

Pelvic Inflammatory Disease and Tubo-ovarian Abscess

Pφ PID is an infection of the upper female genital tract, including the endometrium, adnexal structures, and sometimes the peritoneum. It usually results from ascending infection from the cervix or vagina. Most commonly, it is caused by *C. trachomatis*, *N. gonorrhoeae*, or vaginal bacterial flora, including anaerobic, gram-negative facultative bacteria and *Streptococcus* species. Women at greatest risk are sexually active and younger than 25 years of age. PID can cause significant long-term morbidities including ectopic pregnancy, infertility, and chronic pelvic pain.

TP Presentation is characterized by lower abdominal pain, dyspareunia, fever, back pain, and vaginal discharge or bleeding. Some women have only mild symptoms. Pelvic examination shows cervical or vaginal discharge, cervical motion tenderness, and uterine or adnexal tenderness. A palpable adnexal mass suggests tubo-ovarian abscess.

Dx Diagnosis is made by suggestive clinical symptoms and signs as described, and supported by elevated erythrocyte sedimentation rate or C-reactive protein and laboratory documentation of cervical infection with *N. gonorrhoeae* or *C. trachomatis*. In some cases, pelvic ultrasonography, MRI, or laparoscopic examination might be necessary to confirm the diagnosis.

Tx Treatment should be initiated empirically without delay in any woman at risk for PID with clinical symptoms and signs consistent with PID. Antibiotics must cover *N. gonorrhoeae* and *C. trachomatis*. Even when cultures return only one of these organisms, patients are treated for both because of a 50% coinfection rate. The Centers for Disease Control and Prevention (CDC) website maintains the current antibiotic regimen recommendations. Commonly recommended outpatient regimens usually include a third-generation cephalosporin plus doxycycline. Metronidazole can be added to this regimen. Importantly, the patient's sexual partners need to be treated even though they may be asymptomatic. **See Katz 23, Hacker 22.**

Systems-Based Practice

Creating a System for Accessing Updated Treatment Recommendations

Creating a systems-based practice implies that the practitioner has a system for keeping current in the fields of medicine that evolve continually. Finding the best antibiotic regimen for the treatment of PID is an excellent example of a treatment recommendation guaranteed to evolve during your years of practice. A systems-based method for keeping current on the best antibiotic regiments for PID would be to familiarize oneself with the website of the CDC, the Centers for Disease Control and Prevention. Below are the CDC Recommended Treatments for Pelvic Inflammatory Disease and the URL of the CDC—a site with which you should become acquainted.

Table 37-1 Centers for Disease Control and Prevention Recommended Treatments for Pelvic Inflammatory Disease, 2006*

Regimen A	Regimen B
Inpatient Treatment	
Cefoxitin 2 g IV q6h *or* Cefotetan 2 g IV q12h *plus* Doxycycline 100 mg IV q12h until improved, followed by doxycycline 100 mg orally bid, to complete 14 days	Clindamycin 900 mg IV q8h *plus* Gentamicin 2 mg/kg IV once, followed by 1.5 mg/kg IV q8h
Outpatient Treatment	
Ceftriaxone 250 mg IM in a single dose *plus* Doxycycline 100 mg bid, to complete 14 days *with or without* Metronidazole 500 mg orally bid for 14 days	Cefoxitin 2 g IM single dose and Probenecid 1 g orally concurrently in a single dose *plus* Doxycycline 100 mg bid, to complete 14 days *with or without* Metronidazole 500 mg orally bid for 14 days

*For a more complete list of recommended and alternative treatments from the CDC, see www2a.cdc.gov/stdtraining/ready-to-use/Manuals/PID/pid-notes-2009.pdf.
From Hacker N, Gambone J, Hobel C: Hacker & Moore's Essentials of Obstetrics and Gynecology, 5th ed. Philadelphia, Elsevier Saunders, 2009.

Cervicitis

Pφ Cervicitis is a common lower genital tract infection or inflammatory reaction. It can be caused by *N. gonorrhoeae*, *C. trachomatis*, *Trichomonas vaginalis*, herpes simplex virus (HSV) 1 or 2, or human papillomavirus infection. Cervicitis may also arise as a result of an injury from a foreign object inserted in the vagina, such as a diaphragm.

TP Presentation is characterized by acute vaginal discharge or bleeding, dyspareunia, pruritus, or abdominal pain. Presence of genital ulcers suggests HSV infection. Pelvic examination shows vaginal or cervical discharge, inflamed cervix, and cervical motion tenderness.

Dx Diagnosis is made by history and pelvic exam. Vaginal discharge should be tested using a wet prep and whiff test. Cervical discharge is collected for Gram stain and culture. A Pap test should be done to rule out the possibility of cervical dysplasia or cancer.

Tx Treatment is primarily medical with appropriate antibiotics. The patient's sexual partners must also be treated to prevent reinfection (see the earlier Systems-Based Practice: Recommended Therapy Regimens box). **See Katz 22, Hacker 22.**

Endometriosis

Pφ Endometriosis is the presence of endometrial tissue outside the uterine cavity. Endometriosis can sometimes present with the same sort of nagging, ongoing pain that is seen with PID. Common locations of endometriosis implants include the uterosacral ligaments or rectovaginal space. Endometrial implants may cause irritation and inflammation of localized areas in the pelvis. (See Chapter 48, Endometriosis, for a more comprehensive discussion.)

TP Presentation is classically characterized by dysmenorrhea. Patients might also present with dyspareunia or vaginal bleeding. A low-grade fever or leukocytosis may be present as well.

Dx The presence of tender nodular masses along the uterosacral ligaments, the posterior uterus, or cul-de-sac suggests endometriosis. For definitive diagnosis, laparoscopy with biopsies is required.

Tx Initial management includes control of pain symptoms with counseling, nonsteroidal pain medication, and hormonal therapy—usually oral contraceptive pills. In severe or refractory cases, surgery might be indicated. **See Katz 19, Hacker 25.**

ZEBRA ZONE

a. **Degenerating uterine fibroid:** Not common in young patients, but could present as acute pelvic pain and fever.

b. **Tubo-ovarian abscess due to non-STI causes:** Actinomycosis or tuberculosis are other unusual causes of tubo-ovarian abscess. Actinomycosis is associated with IUD use. If a patient is from a developing country where tuberculosis is prevalent, a tubercular tubo-ovarian abscess should be considered.

Practice-Based Learning and Improvement: Evidence-Based Medicine

Title
Effectiveness of inpatient and outpatient treatment strategies for women with pelvic inflammatory disease: Results from the Pelvic Inflammatory Disease Evaluation and Clinical Health (PEACH) randomized trial

Authors
Ness RB, Soper DE, Holley RL, et al.

Institution
University of Pittsburgh, Pittsburgh, Pennsylvania

Reference
American Journal of Obstetrics and Gynecology 2002;186:929–937

Problem
Evaluate treatment strategies for PID.

Intervention
Inpatient treatment with intravenous cefoxitin and doxycycline and outpatient treatment were compared against a single intramuscular injection of cefoxitin and oral doxycycline.

Comparison/control (quality of evidence)
Multicenter, randomized, controlled trial, level I.

Outcome/effect
Comparison of inpatient and outpatient treatment of PID in preventing long-term adverse outcomes, including decreased pregnancy rate, increased time to conception, recurrence of PID, chronic pelvic pain, and ectopic pregnancy.

Historical significance/comments
This is a randomized, controlled trial demonstrating that inpatient treatment is not superior to outpatient treatment. Therefore, patients with mild to moderate PID can be safely treated in an outpatient setting, as long as compliance with the medication regimen can be ensured.

Interpersonal and Communication Skills

Focusing on the Adolescent Patient

Pelvic inflammatory disease and STIs are always sensitive topics, especially when we encounter them in young patients. As much as it may be difficult, these topics merit adequate discussion. Anticipate two common patient responses: (1) embarrassment and fear; and (2) concern that the physicians will be judgmental when treating for an STI. Your effective interpersonal and communication skills will be tested by this discussion.

It is essential to assure your patient that all the information you exchange is confidential. If the patient is accompanied by others, it is prudent to ask the patient (privately) if she wishes to discuss her case with you alone, or in the presence of those who have accompanied her. You can then request, for example, "I'd like to speak with [the patient] for a few minutes on our own."

All questions regarding sexuality and sexual practices should be asked in a nonjudgmental way: "Are you sexually active?" "Do you have sex with men, women, or both?"

Think carefully about the words you choose and avoid leading questions. Be clear that your patient understands the diagnosis, its significance, the risk of transmitting disease to others, and the plan of management. Certainly the issues of safe sexual practice and HIV testing may be appropriate to incorporate in this discussion—for example, "This is probably a good time to discuss safe sexual practice. Is this okay?"

Be sure to allow your patient to ask questions about what has been discussed, and schedule a follow-up visit, emphasizing the need to return for further discussion.

Professionalism

Principle: Commitment to Professional Responsibilities

A student presents a patient with PID to his attending in the emergency department. Within earshot of the patient's room, the attending physician makes a derogatory comment about the "type of behavior that gets you into this kind of trouble." Even though the attending physician's remarks make the student feel uncomfortable, the student feels unable to report the incident to anyone for fear of receiving a poor evaluation. Medical education is based largely on an apprenticeship model in which students learn by working in close contact with experienced physicians and emulating their practice and behavior. This is an effective way to learn how to manage patients and it is also the way by which a cultural set of behaviors and mores is propagated. Whereas the actual curriculum probably calls for remaining nonjudgmental in situations such as this, the "hidden" curriculum is the body of tenets that gets transmitted by the instructor's actual behavior. As such, the hidden curriculum is often cited as a reason for the perpetuation of unprofessional behavior from one generation of physicians to the next. If the medical profession is to break free of the hidden curriculum, it is incumbent on us to have appropriate mechanisms in place for self-regulation and remediation of unprofessional behavior.

Systems-Based Practice

HIPAA and Compliance with State Regulations

Pelvic inflammatory disease is often caused by STIs, and STIs raise some important issues about government regulations and patient privacy. For one thing, some STIs, specifically syphilis and gonorrhea, are reportable conditions: depending on the state or county in which you practice, the department of health may require notification. Compliance with state regulations is the provider's responsibility. Patients should be made aware that their diseases are reportable and will be recorded in state records, and always be sure to compel your patient to have her partner tested if you highly suspect or diagnose a reportable STI.

Another key issue particularly relevant to STIs is that of patient privacy. The medical profession has always valued the confidentiality of the physician–patient relationship, but before 1996 this was only professional ethic, not the law. The Health Insurance Portability and Accountability Act of 1996 (HIPAA) now requires policies and procedures to protect the privacy of medical information. This has resulted in a significant effort by health professionals and hospitals to be more diligent in protecting information from being obtained by those uninvolved in the care of the specific patient. The use of electronic medical records has raised increased concerns about how patient information is transmitted and made available. This will continue to be an issue throughout your medical practice. For now, as a student or resident, regarding the importance of confidentiality, remember not to discuss cases in elevators or public areas, never to leave documents (including "to-do" lists) with patient information unattended, and to make sure that all documents with patient information are shredded when they are discarded (most hospitals provide special bins for disposal of patient documents).

Chapter 38
Uterine Leiomyomas (Case 24)

Benjamin Montgomery MD

Case: A 42-year-old woman presents to your office in consultation from her primary care physician for an enlarging pelvic mass. She has a negative pregnancy test, and in the course of being evaluated a pelvic sonogram revealed what appear to be normal ovaries.

Differential Diagnosis

Uterine leiomyomas (fibroids)	Uterine malignancy

Interpersonal and Communications Skills

I introduce this chapter with an important matter of terminology and communication: understand that in the field of obstetrics and gynecology, the terms *leiomyoma* (on occasion you will see the plural: *leiomyomata*) and *fibroid* are used interchangeably. This can be confusing at first, but both words mean exactly the same thing. Also, be careful when using the term *tumor*. Although it is true that leiomyomata are benign smooth cell muscle "tumors" of the uterus, many patients equate "tumor" with "cancer."

Speaking Intelligently

Typically, when a patient with a pelvic mass presents to me in consultation, a basic work-up has already been initiated. This work-up usually includes pelvic ultrasonography and pregnancy test, if applicable (never hesitate to order a pregnancy test—you will never be faulted for it). If an ultrasonographic study has not been done, I request one. Ultrasonography is probably the gynecologist's most useful imaging modality because it usually helps to delineate both the origin and likely etiology of many pelvic masses. When considering the differential diagnosis for a pelvic mass, my key concerns are to rule out pregnancy and malignancy: ovarian cancer often presents as a complex ovarian mass(es) with free fluid (ascites) in the pelvis. Endometrial cancer usually presents with abnormal uterine bleeding, sometimes with the accompanying finding of an enlarging uterus. Uterine leiomyomas may present as an enlarged and often irregular uterus with discrete, nodular masses within it; once leiomyomas outgrow their blood supply, however, they degenerate and may appear as complex masses with heterogeneous features within the uterus. This ultrasonographic appearance can complicate the clinical picture.

PATIENT CARE

Clinical Thinking

- Leiomyomas seldom present as a surgical emergency. However, if the patient is hemodynamically unstable from significant menstrual bleeding (menorrhagia), then hysterectomy or uterine artery embolization should be considered in conjunction with a blood transfusion if necessary. Pedunculated fibroids (leiomyomas that have

pedicle-type attachments to the uterine body) may undergo torsion and cause significant abdominal pain. In these situations, diagnostic laparoscopy or exploratory laparotomy may be necessary.
- Once I have determined that the clinical scenario does not require immediate action, I can more thoroughly assess the patient. If heavy vaginal bleeding is a symptom, endometrial biopsy should be performed to rule out any precancerous (endometrial hyperplasia) or cancerous process. If painful cramping (dysmenorrhea) is a symptom, then nonsteroidal anti-inflammatory drugs (NSAIDs) are my first mode of treatment.
- In patients with uterine fibroids who are desirous of future childbearing, a thorough infertility work-up should be initiated to ensure that there are not other causes that could explain lack of conception or early pregnancy loss (e.g., semen analysis, documentation of ovulation, and sonohysterography). For infertility patients who suffer with uterine myomas, sometimes a myomectomy (surgical resection of the leiomyomas from the uterine body, leaving the uterus intact) is the preferred operation if surgery is required.

History
- Common presenting symptoms of uterine fibroids include heavy or irregular vaginal bleeding, painful uterine cramping, and increasing abdominal fullness. However, uterine fibroids can be quite large and still be asymptomatic, so it is important to rule out other etiologies for a patient's complaints.
- A thorough menstrual history is important in isolating uterine fibroids as the source of the patient's complaints. Bleeding secondary to leiomyomas typically presents as regular in interval but significantly heavier at the time of menses. Any intermenstrual bleeding should be evaluated by endometrial biopsy (after confirmation of a negative pregnancy test).
- Painful uterine cramping attributable to uterine fibroids is typically worse at the time of menses secondary to the estrogen dependence of fibroids. However, cramping can be present during the entire course of the menstrual cycle.
- Abdominal fullness is a common but vague symptom of uterine fibroids. Inquiring about a patient's gastrointestinal history may help distinguish between fullness caused by fibroids or a gastrointestinal problem such as irritable bowel syndrome.

Physical Examination
- **Abdominal examination:** A uterus that is enlarged because of fibroids can often be palpated abdominally. However, it can be difficult to distinguish between a fibroid uterus and a large adnexal mass.
- **Pelvic examination:** The pelvic examination permits the examiner to better evaluate and differentiate the etiology of an enlarging pelvic

mass. Freely mobile anatomy is a better predictor of benign disease then a "fixed" pelvis on exam. Also, if hysterectomy is a future consideration, the pelvic examination provides additional information regarding the potential mode of hysterectomy (vaginal vs. abdominal).

Tests for Consideration

- **Quantitative human chorionic gonadotropin (β-hCG):** In a reproductive-age woman with irregular bleeding and an enlarged uterus, this test is necessary. — $135
- **CBC:** In a patient with heavy vaginal bleeding, this test assesses the degree of anemia, if any. The white blood cell count may be elevated in a patient with pain and a degenerating fibroid. — $35
- **CA-125:** This blood test should be obtained any time ovarian malignancy is in the differential diagnosis. — $60
- **Pap test:** Assesses for possible cervical malignancy. — $320

IMAGING CONSIDERATIONS

→**Pelvic ultrasonography:** Best means to image pelvic anatomy. — $225

→**CT scan:** If pelvic ultrasonography is inconclusive, CT may help further differentiate pelvic anatomy. If malignancy is suspected, CT provides important information regarding the possible presence of metastases. — $800

→**MRI:** This is the most common progression for ordering radiologic studies to best distinguish uterine leiomyomas from other pelvic masses. Useful when considering uterine artery embolization. — $1200

Clinical Entities	Medical Knowledge

Uterine Leiomyomas (Fibroids)

Pφ Uterine fibroids are benign, smooth muscle tumors originating from the myometrium. Their exact cause is unknown, but development of these tumors may be estrogen dependent. By the age of 50 years, 67% of white women and 82% of African American women have sonographic findings consistent with uterine fibroids.

TP Uterine fibroids typically present with dysmenorrhea or menorrhagia, or both. Enlarging fibroids can result in increased abdominal girth and a sense of abdominal fullness. Less often, fibroids can result in polyuria if they are anteriorly located and impinge on the bladder. Likewise, back pain and dyschezia can be present if the fibroids are posterior. Dyspareunia can also be an issue because of the mass effect of the enlarged uterus.

Dx Uterine fibroids are diagnosed by physical examination and confirmed by ultrasonography.

Tx For the patient interested in future childbearing, NSAIDs or hormonal management using oral contraceptives could be considered if she is symptomatic. For women interested in preserving their uterus, myomectomy (removal of fibroids) or uterine artery embolization should be considered. Hysterectomy is the definitive means of treating uterine fibroids; however, it should be reserved for women who fail conservative management and do not plan on future childbearing. Gonadotropin analogs (e.g., leuprolide) have a limited use in treating uterine fibroids—this drug can diminish bleeding and reduce uterine volume in preparation for myomectomy or hysterectomy. **See Katz 18, Hacker 19.**

Uterine Malignancy

Pφ Uterine cancers typically arise in the endometrial lining and then progress locally through the myometrium, and then to surrounding pelvic structures in the case of more advanced disease. The most common type of endometrial cancer is endometrioid adenocarcinoma, but there are many other, less common cell types as well.

TP Uterine cancers most commonly present with new-onset postmenopausal bleeding, but can occasionally present as an enlarging pelvic mass in the case of advanced disease.

Dx The diagnosis of uterine malignancy is typically made by tissue biopsy, most commonly an office endometrial biopsy, or by performing a D&C.

Tx Therapy is with surgical resection and staging, and then adjuvant radiation or chemotherapy if indicated. Precancerous lesions can be treated with progestins. The decision for adjuvant therapy is based on the surgical stage and grade of the tumor (see Chapter 52, Endometrial Cancer). **See Hacker 41.**

ZEBRA ZONE

a. **Leiomyosarcoma:** Very rare tumor of the uterus. Leiomyosarcomas are believed to originate from uterine fibroids, but it is estimated that only 1 in 2000 fibroids develops into a leiomyosarcoma.

b. **Adnexal masses/ovarian cysts, benign and malignant:** Adnexal masses, ovarian cysts, or ovarian cancers may present at all ages during a woman's lifetime. In the process of evaluating a patient for a pelvic mass it is crucial that the ovaries and adnexa be evaluated, either with radiologic studies or surgery, if this is indicated (see Chapter 36, Pelvic Pain, and Chapter 54, Ovarian Cancer).

Practice-Based Learning and Improvement: Evidence-Based Medicine

Title
Uterine-artery embolization versus surgery for symptomatic uterine fibroids

Authors
Edwards RD, Moss JG, Lumsden MA, et al., the REST Investigators

Institution
University of Glasgow, Glasgow, Scotland

Reference
New England Journal of Medicine 2007;356:360–370

Problem
Treatment of symptomatic uterine leiomyomas.

Intervention
Randomized trial comparing uterine artery embolization and surgery in women with symptomatic uterine fibroids.

Quality of evidence
Level I

Outcome/effect
Women undergoing embolization for the treatment of uterine leiomyomas had faster recoveries, but were more likely to need further treatment (9%).

Historical significance/comments
Further studies are needed to determine the specific patient who would most benefit from embolization, but this study proved that uterine artery embolization is a safe and effective treatment for many women with uterine leiomyomas.

Interpersonal and Communication Skills

Cultural Awareness
As the country grows more ethnically diverse, physicians need to remain mindful of cultural differences.

Barriers posed by language and ethnic traditions can result in negative health consequences, including:

- Failure to recognize and respond to health problems.
- Inadequate informed consent.
- Misinterpretation of physician's instructions.
- Poor compliance with treatment plans.
- Missed appointments.
- Inaccuracies in medical histories.

Research indicates that language barriers alone are responsible for:

- Fewer clinical visits.
- Longer clinical visits.
- More laboratory tests.
- More emergency department visits.
- Limited follow-up.
- Dissatisfaction with health care services.

Professionalism

Principle: Commitment to Scientific Knowledge
Clinical Research Protocols
Historically, the treatment of uterine fibroids has been either by conservative management with medications such as NSAIDs and hormonal therapy or surgical management by hysterectomy or myomectomy. For a premenopausal woman who wants definitive treatment and wants to preserve fertility, the only option has been myomectomy, which has a risk of being converted intraoperatively to hysterectomy. In the past decade, uterine artery embolization, magnetic resonance–guided focused ultrasound therapy, and laparoscopic uterine artery occlusion have all received considerable attention as uterus-sparing procedures to treat leiomyomata. The research required to ascertain the effects of these therapies on fertility is possible only when clinicians are dedicated to advancing medical and scientific knowledge through clinical research protocols. Participation in such protocols should be part of our commitment as physicians to the advancement of scientific knowledge.

Systems-Based Practice

The Cost of Inpatient Care

Mrs. Jones is a 72-year-old patient in her third postoperative day after hysterectomy for uterine fibroids. She is eating, manifesting normal bowel function, and walking with some assistance. You feel she is ready for discharge. Her daughter is adamant that her mother needs "at least 2 more days" before she is able to return home.

Commensurate with the rise of managed care and increased concern over health care costs, the issue of length of stay (LOS) has become central to discussions of both cost control and quality in health care. Controlling LOS today is also one of the main ways in which a hospital can maintain profitability.

Why does LOS matter? If the hospital is charging patients for each day they are hospitalized, why wouldn't the hospital want patients to stay as long as possible, as would a hotel? The answer is that although hospitals aggregate charges on a daily basis, they are paid—for the most part—on a case rate basis. The majority of hospitalizations in the United States are reimbursed either by the diagnosis-related group (DRG) system through Medicare, or through another comparable case-based system, in which the hospital receives a set payment for the entire hospitalization, regardless of LOS or specific inpatient charges. The hospital, therefore, has an incentive to keep its total costs for hospitalization down because hospital profit (or loss) is equal to the fixed payment less these costs. This is like an all-you-can-eat buffet: once you've paid, the restaurant would prefer you to eat as little as possible and leave as soon as it can get you out. Hospitals can reduce costs in one of two ways: one method is to reduce the cost of supplies and services used in the hospital (e.g., using generic drugs or drugs on the hospital's formulary, avoiding unnecessary laboratory tests and imaging studies); a second means of cost reduction is to reduce LOS (often measured by the hospital's average LOS, or ALOS). Given a fixed payment for a hospitalization, a lower LOS translates to increased revenue per patient day. By discharging a patient sooner, a bed is vacated to admit another patient, increasing the total number of fixed payments the hospital can receive during the year.

Looking at "system" in its largest context, one must keep in mind that even if hospitals were getting paid per day (as some do for some patients) and therefore not losing money for longer LOSs, the overall cost must still be paid. **Someone**, be it the patient, their insurance company (indirectly their employer), or the U.S. government (all taxpayers), must pay for all health care.

Beyond cost, there are other important patient safety reasons to keep ALOS down. Consider the risks of prolonged immobility, nosocomial infection, and the potential for falls and accidents.

Furthermore, patients experience isolation from friends and family, difficulty sleeping, and a propensity for depression. Accordingly, it benefits both the hospital and the patient when hospital stay is only as long as is absolutely required.

Chapter 39
Imaging Tools for Common Pelvic Disorders

Michael Ferrell MD, Ronit K. Devon MD, and Harry Zegel MD

There are three major imaging tools for evaluation of the female patient with abdominal pain. It is often difficult to differentiate between the "abdomen" or "pelvis" as the source of the patient's symptoms, yet this is how most studies are compartmentalized. Pelvic ultrasonography (US), abdominal and pelvic computed tomography (CT), and magnetic resonance imaging (MRI) are the current tools of choice. US and CT are available at any time of day in virtually any emergency department.

Ultrasonography

Gynecologic US is a powerful diagnostic tool. Two types of US probes are routinely used in gynecologic imaging. For the transabdominal/transvesical examination, a curved frequency transducer is placed just above the symphysis pubis, and images are obtained through a filled bladder. This helps get an overall view of the pelvis and assess for large pelvic masses. The quality of the images of the uterus and ovaries depends on the patient's ability to fill her bladder completely, and her body habitus. A patient's body shape and size can have a tremendous impact on the quality of the US images that are attainable. After the abdominal images are obtained, the pelvis is examined transvaginally for more detailed images of the cervix, ovaries, uterus, and cul-de-sac.

The transmitted US signal can also be modified, exploiting the Doppler effect to indirectly visualize flowing blood, measure flow velocity, and even listen to fetal heart tones.

Computed Tomography

Computed tomography is a very sensitive technique and is particularly effective at evaluating the acute abdomen. Diseases such as diverticulitis, nephrolithiasis, and appendicitis commonly have symptoms referable to the pelvis. Performing the examination with intravenous (IV) contrast helps visualize solid organs and the bowel wall more accurately. Examinations done for retroperitoneal hemorrhage or kidney stones are more often performed without IV or oral contrast. Examination 2 to 3 hours after ingesting oral contrast helps further characterize bowel pathology. Because of a number of factors, CT is less effective at evaluating the uterus and ovaries, although it can detect pelvic free fluid, inflammatory changes, or masses that can direct the clinician to further evaluation of the pelvis.

Systems-Based Practice

Patient Safety: The Risks of Radiation

Computed tomography uses ionizing radiation, which has some associated risk. The health risks from CT are complex and multifactorial. Simply put, the more exposures and the greater radiation dose with each exposure, the greater the relative risk of developing a future cancer. This notion is based on observed data for a population, and does not predict what will happen to your patient as a result of her CT scan. However, radiation risk to patients should be routinely assessed and balanced against the severity of their individual clinical scenarios.

If there is any concern, or if the patient is young or pregnant, consult your radiologist or radiation physicist. The radiation delivered from a single CT examination is 100 to 200 times the radiation delivered from a frontal chest radiograph. Also, each pass through the gantry means more radiation, so ordering examinations with and without contrast doubles the exposure to the patient.

Magnetic Resonance Imaging

Magnetic resonance imaging is a complex modality that is reserved for problem solving in the diagnosis and evaluation of pelvic diseases. MRI does not use ionizing radiation like CT, and is less operator dependent than US. Noncontrast MRI is used routinely in pregnancy, and no adverse effects have been yet observed (MRI contrast agents are not safe in pregnancy). Although MRI produces exquisite soft tissue resolution, it does have several limitations. MRI is less available than CT and US. Scan times are longer, and images are much more easily degraded by motion and breathing artifacts. Patient size and claustrophobia are also major limitations. Finally, certain implanted devices are not compatible with MRI, particularly intracerebral aneurysm clips and pacemakers.

Table 39-1 presents a comparison of the imaging modalities discussed previously.

Table 39-1	Comparing Imaging Modalities*		
Entity	**US**	**CT**	**MRI**
Uterus			
Fibroid	Better	Good	Best
Endometrial polyp	Good, best (SHG)†	Poor	Best
Uterine carcinoma	Good	Poor	Good
Adenomyosis	Good	Poor	Better
Ovary			
Endometrioma	Better	Good	Best
Cyst/hemorrhagic cyst	Better	Good	Best
Ovarian carcinoma	Good	Better	Best
Benign cystic teratoma (dermoid)	Good	Good	Best
Torsion	Best	Poor	Too time consuming in the acute setting
Ectopic pregnancy	Best	Poor	Too time consuming in the acute setting
Other			
Appendicitis	Poor	Best	Best, especially in pregnancy
Bowel obstruction	Poor	Best	Poor

*This table summarizes the relative strength of each modality in assessing each of the disease processes discussed in this chapter.
†SGH, sonohysterography.

Imaging Findings

The following are a few examples of the wide range of pelvic disease that can be assessed with US, CT, and MRI.

Uterus

With US, the uterine myometrium is isoechoic to muscle and the endometrium varies in echotexture. In premenopausal women, the normal endometrium varies from 2 to 15 mm depending on the phase of the menstrual cycle. The junctional zone, a transitional region deep to the endometrium and superficial to the myometrium, has a normal thickness of 2 to 8 mm. The serosal surface of the uterus usually cannot be seen with US. After menopause, it is normal to see atrophy of the uterus, with the uterus involuting to a size similar to that of a premenstrual uterus after 15 to 20 years.

On CT, the uterus is isodense to muscle and enhances after contrast administration. Sometimes it is possible to see low density areas centrally within the uterus, which correspond to fluid in the endometrial canal or the endometrial lining.

With MRI, T2-weighted images are the most useful for imaging the uterus, and clearly delineate zonal anatomy. Relative to muscle, on T2-weighted images the endometrium normally is hyperintense, the junctional zone, uterine serosa, and cervix are hypointense, and the myometrium is isointense.

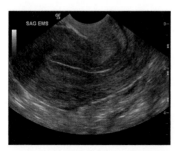

Figure 39-1   Transvaginal US image of the normal uterus.

UTERINE LEIOMYOMATA

Uterine leiomyomata, also called *fibroids*, are the most common tumors of the uterus. Degenerating fibroids can be a source of severe pain when they outgrow their blood supply. This process results in "popcorn"-like calcifications on radiographs. On US, fibroids are usually hypoechoic solid masses. Sometimes fibroids have heterogeneous echogenicity related to calcification and fatty or cystic degeneration. Frequently, they have a typical pattern of shadows with multiple, well-defined, recurring shadows originating from the mass. On MRI, fibroids are often hypointense, but then enhance brightly after contrast administration.

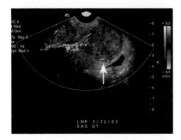

Figure 39-2 Transvaginal US image of a pedunculated leiomyoma, a large intracavitary fibroid. On US, fibroids are typically hypoechoic and can demonstrate degeneration and calcification. The Doppler flow study confirms the blood supply. The *large arrow* points to myoma.

MRI is commonly used in preoperative planning in the evaluation of fibroids. With the advent of uterine fibroid embolization, it is used before and after treatment to assess the degree of bulk reduction and the completeness of embolization. Unfortunately, no imaging characteristics are specific for transformation of a leiomyoma to a leiomyosarcoma, a malignant neoplasm. Postmenopausal enlargement of a fibroid is suggestive of this change, and may lead to hysterectomy.

ENDOMETRIAL POLYP

Polyps in the uterine cavity often present with bleeding shortly before or shortly after the menstrual period. Polyps can also result in infertility. Endometrial polyps are usually diagnosed with US or saline infusion sonohysterography (SHG). In SHG, sterile saline is used to distend the uterine cavity and provide density interfaces to visualize its contents on US.

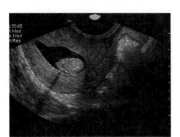

Figure 39-3 Transvaginal US and sonohysterogram showing an endometrial polyp. Sonohysterography confirms the finding of an endometrial polyp.

The differential diagnoses for endometrial polyps must include pedunculated intracavitary fibroids and a polypoid endometrial cancer. MRI is more sensitive for detecting these, but often the diagnosis is definitively made only after biopsy. A polyp will typically be surrounded by normal-appearing echogenic endometrium and have a prominent vascular pedicle (detectable by color Doppler). An intracavitary fibroid will generally be more hypoechoic and fed by less prominent vessels. CT is generally not useful in the evaluation of polyps.

The postmenopausal endometrial stripe is usually not identified, or is hypoechoic and thin. Any thickening over 5 mm should be considered for endometrial biopsy, particularly in patients with vaginal bleeding.

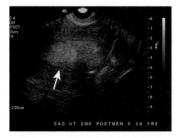

Figure 39-4 Transvaginal US image of endometrial cancer. Note the markedly thickened and heterogeneous endometrium. The *arrow* points to thickened endometrium.

ADENOMYOSIS

Adenomyosis, or the pathologic extension of endometrial implants into the myometrium, can produce pelvic pain and dysmenorrhea. It is best assessed noninvasively with MRI, although US can also be used to suggest the diagnosis. CT is generally not useful.

On US, adenomyosis can be diagnosed by heterogeneity, asymmetric thickening, and replacement of the junctional zone. Multiple foci with posterior shadowing, also called *refractory shadows*, have been described with adenomyosis. MRI is very sensitive for the diagnosis of adenomyosis. Thickening of the junctional zone greater than 12 mm or bright foci within the junctional zone on T2-weighted imaging are characteristic.

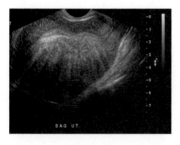

Figure 39-5 Transvaginal US image of adenomyosis. Note the linear shadowing, asymmetric thickening, and loss of definition of the junctional zone.

Ovary

Normal ovarian parenchyma is isoechoic to hyperechoic, and typically has several small follicles scattered throughout. Changes in size, symmetry, echo pattern, or contour can all indicate pathology.

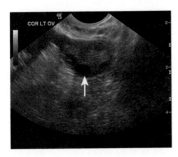

Figure 39-6 Transvaginal US image of normal ovaries. The *arrow* points to normal ovarian tissue.

OVARIAN CYSTS

Ovarian cysts are ubiquitous and are not always a source of pelvic pain. Follicles are physiologic cysts, and a cut-off of 2.5 cm is imposed to differentiate a normal follicle in a menstruating woman from a cyst. For postmenopausal women, this becomes the threshold at which a cyst should be monitored. Cysts greater than 5 cm in size should be considered suspect for neoplasm, and followed carefully with the possibility of need for removal.

On US, a simple cyst has a single, spherical to ovoid wall and absent internal echoes, is well circumscribed, and demonstrates posterior acoustic enhancement (from increased through-transmission of the US waves). The wall thickness in an ovarian cyst can be variable, and blood flow within the cyst wall does not differentiate it from malignant neoplasm. Cysts must be considered as a common cause of pain, especially when they rupture.

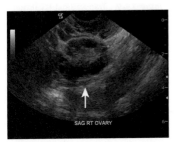

Figure 39-7 Transvaginal US image of polycystic ovary (*arrow*). Multiple, peripherally located cysts in both ovaries are seen in this woman with polycystic ovarian disease. The cysts have a "string of pearls" appearance and there is centrally echogenic stroma on the image, both of which are characteristic.

HEMORRHAGIC OVARIAN CYSTS

Acute hemorrhage in a cyst can distend the capsule and deform adjacent ovarian parenchyma, producing pelvic pain. Hemorrhagic cysts are often difficult to differentiate from endometriomas and can exhibit widely variable patterns, mimicking a number of other adnexal masses. Hemorrhagic cysts can have heterogeneous internal echogenicity—often with "hematocrit" levels and evidence of clot retraction. Like endometriomas, they lack internal Doppler flow. The echogenicity of the blood depends on the state/age of the hemorrhage.

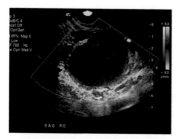

Figure 39-8 Transvaginal US image of hemorrhagic (right-sided) ovarian cyst. This patient presented with right adnexal tenderness. Imaging demonstrates a large cystic structure with layering debris corresponding to hemorrhage. Note the increased color flow in the surrounding tissues from inflammation.

ENDOMETRIOSIS/ENDOMETRIOMA

When normal endometrial epithelium or glands are ectopically located, this process produces the disease spectrum of endometriosis. Symptoms include infertility, dysmenorrhea, and dyspareunia. Large implants can form into the so-called "chocolate cysts" known as *endometriomas*. Classically, endometriomas have homogeneous echogenicity throughout the cyst. Endometriomas, like hemorrhagic cysts, can also have a widely variable appearance. With age, blood products can layer, producing fluid levels that are readily detectable by US. The diagnosis of endometriosis is often confirmed on clinical grounds and the chronicity of imaging findings.

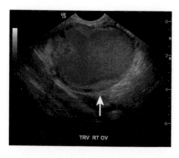

Figure 39-9 Transvaginal US image of endometrioma (*arrow*). Note the homogeneous internal echoes of this classic-appearing chocolate cyst.

OVARIAN NEOPLASM

There are a number of different types of ovarian neoplasms, benign and malignant. Findings in cystic ovarian tumors that suggest malignancy include patient age older than 50 years, size greater than 5 cm, mural nodules or papillary projections, internal septations, increasing size, internal echoes, associated ascites, and evidence of invasion of adjacent structures. No one characteristic by itself is diagnostic of malignancy.

US can suggest the presence of ovarian cancer, and MRI is helpful to determine if there is local invasion. The World Health Organization recommends surgical staging of ovarian cancer, making CT, MRI, and US useful adjuncts for the diagnosis and continued management of a disease process that is challenging to treat effectively.

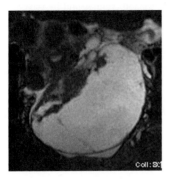

Figure 39-10 T2-weighted MRI of cystic ovarian neoplasm (*arrow*). High intensity signal on the T2-weighted image corresponds to the solid component of the neoplasm. Note the internal soft tissue. Pathology confirmed serous cystadenocarcinoma.

CYSTIC TERATOMA/DERMOIDS

Cystic teratomas, also called *dermoids*, are benign tumors that account for 10% to 15% of all ovarian neoplasms. They are heterogeneous in appearance and can have solid and cystic components composed of mature epithelial elements. This can include a combination of skin, hair, sebum, and even teeth. They are present from birth, are usually soft tumors, and typically grow slowly. Classic findings on US include the "tip of the iceberg" appearance, where most of the mass is obscured by attenuation of the US beam. The absorption of the US beam by multiple interfaces in the mass allows only the nearest portion to be visualized. These density differences are also often evident on CT. Another, more specific, less commonly seen sign is the presence of multiple, interlacing linear echoes that correspond to crossing strands of hair within the mass.

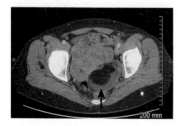

Figure 39-11 CT scan of ovarian dermoid (*arrow*). Note cystic and solid components.

OVARIAN TORSION

Ovarian torsion is a less common cause of pelvic pain, but has an impressive clinical presentation and is a true surgical emergency. Doppler flow studies are crucial to help make this diagnosis. If clinical judgment or US findings suggest ovarian torsion, surgery will be the next step for the patient.

On gray-scale US, a torsed ovary is enlarged and heterogeneously hypoechoic. The presence of multiple small peripheral follicles has also been described. Gray-scale findings can be more important than the absence of arterial and venous flow on pulsed Doppler US, although this does help support the diagnosis of torsion. Clinical correlation is particularly important if the patient is experiencing intermittent torsion. Disease within the ovary that increases its rotational moment of inertia (i.e., increases its diameter) also increases the risk of ovarian torsion, although such masses are often obscured in a torsed ovary because of necrosis and hemorrhage. Ovarian cysts and dermoids in particular can increase the risk of torsion.

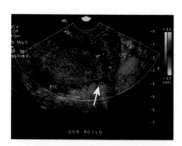

Figure 39-12 Transvaginal US image of ovarian torsion. The ovary is enlarged and has no vascular flow on the color Doppler image. The *arrow* represents the area of torsion where vascular flow ceases.

Pregnancy

Ultrasonography is used extensively in pregnancy, particularly in the second and third trimesters (see Chapter 10, Obstetric Tools: Prenatal Ultrasonography in Each Trimester). First-trimester pelvic US is an extremely important technique that can assess for diseases that are related or unrelated to pregnancy. However, in any woman in her first trimester with severe pelvic pain, ectopic pregnancy should be excluded.

ECTOPIC PREGNANCY

If the serum human chorionic gonadotropin (β-hCG) is at the expected level for the gestational age (calculated either from the LMP or fetal measurements) and there is a pregnancy in the uterus, you have almost entirely excluded the possibility of an ectopic pregnancy.

Patient Care

Caring for a Patient with a Suspected Ectopic Pregnancy
How should you care for a patient with a positive β-hCG but with no obvious pregnancy visualized in the uterus using US? First, it might be too early to detect a gestational sac. Pregnancy dating based on the LMP is often unreliable. Until you see an intrauterine pregnancy, ectopic pregnancy is not entirely excluded, and these patients should be followed clinically or with imaging and serial β-hCG levels.

If you identify ovaries and an adnexal mass in the presence of a positive β-hCG, this is highly suggestive (>90% sensitive) that the adnexal mass is an ectopic pregnancy. Sometimes you can see a fetal pole, or even a heartbeat in the adnexal mass. Both of these findings are highly sensitive and specific for the diagnosis of ectopic pregnancy. Based on the imaging findings and the β-hCG level, you can then triage the patient to medical or surgical therapy.

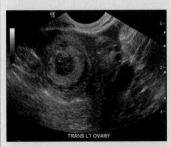

Figure 39-13 Transvaginal US image of ectopic pregnancy. The patient presented with severe left adnexal tenderness and a positive β-hCG. Note the adnexal mass adjacent to the left ovary. Also note the free fluid surrounding the ectopic. A small amount of hemorrhage was present at surgery.

Other Pelvic Diseases
APPENDICITIS

Over the last decade, CT scanning has become the gold standard for diagnosing acute appendicitis. Of course, this helps greatly because it is difficult to differentiate appendicitis from other, less acute causes of abdominal pain. The normal appendix is less than 8 mm in greatest transverse diameter, and fills with contrast or air. In appendicitis, there is obstruction of the lumen, which results in infection and inflammation. This inflammation can extend into the adjacent mesenteric fat, resulting in stranding on CT. If there are inflammatory changes present, the size requirement to diagnose appendicitis is reduced to 6 mm. CT is also extremely useful in determining if an appendix has perforated or if there is an appendiceal abscess.

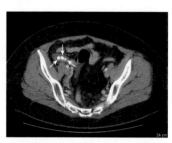

Figure 39-14 CT scan of the pelvis showing acute appendicitis. The appendix is markedly dilated in the right lower quadrant containing multiple calcified appendicoliths. Note the dilated tubular structure and the calcified areas (*arrows*). There is enhancement of the wall of the appendix and surrounding inflammatory stranding in the adjacent peritoneal fat. No perforation or intraperitoneal free air is evident.

SMALL BOWEL OBSTRUCTION

Often, in patients who have been operated on previously, or gynecologic oncology patients who have intraperitoneal malignancy, the CT scan can be enormously helpful in differentiating an obstruction from other causes of abdominal pain. CT shows multiple dilated loops of small bowel and is often helpful in determining the transition point, and what particular bowel pathologic process is resulting in the obstruction (e.g., hernia, adhesions, volvulus, intussusception).

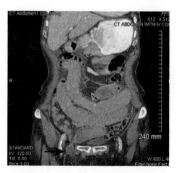

Figure 39-15 Coronal CT scan of a woman with a small bowel obstruction. Note the multiple dilated loops of small bowel, air-fluid levels, and relatively decompressed colon. *Arrow* points to incarcerated right inguinal hernia.

Table 39-2	Imaging Findings*		
Entity	**US**	**CT**	**MRI**
Uterus			
Fibroid	Hypoechoic, multiple recurring shadows	Distorted uterine contour, popcorn calcifications	Size, location, vascularity, embolization/ myomectomy evaluation
Endometrial polyp	Hyperechoic, central feeding vessel, prominent vascular pedicle	Not helpful	Medium signal intensity on T1-weighted imaging, medium to decreased signal intensity on T2-weighted imaging, enhancing postcontrast
Uterine carcinoma	Thickened, heterogeneous endometrium, increased flow	May be helpful prior to staging	Myometrial invasion, spread outside uterus
Adenomyosis	Linear shadowing, asymmetric thickened junctional zone	Not helpful	"Rain in the forest" appearance, multifocal T2 hyperintensities in myometrium
Ovary			
Cyst/ hemorrhagic cyst	Internal echoes, hematocrit levels, clot retraction	Cyst <20 Hounsfield units (HU) Hemorrhagic cyst >20 HU	Variable signal intensity, less complex mass, fewer cystic cavities
Endometrioma	Homogeneous "chocolate cyst," multiseptate walls, past history	>20 HU	Enhancing fibrous tissue surrounding mass, may detect small focal pelvic implants, variable signal intensity
Ovarian carcinoma	Size, internal nodularity, septa, enlargement, invasion	May be helpful prior to staging	Helps assess for local invasion/ extension to lymph nodes

Table 39-2 Imaging Findings*—cont'd

Entity	US	CT	MRI
Benign cystic teratoma (dermoid)	"Tip of the iceberg," interlacing echogenicities from hair	Multiple densities, calcifications	T1/T2 hyperintense fat, fluid-fluid levels
Torsion	Enlarged, heterogeneous echogenicity, no arterial or venous flow	Enlarged ovary	Too time consuming in the acute setting
Ectopic pregnancy	No intrauterine pregnancy, adnexal mass, positive β-hCG	Adnexal mass	Too time consuming in the acute setting
Other			
Appendicitis	Dilated, blind-ending, noncompressible, tubular structure originating from cecum	6-8 mm with inflammation >8 mm no inflammation Nonfilling with contrast	T2 hyperintense, T1 hypointense signal surrounding a dilated appendix; especially useful in pregnancy
Bowel obstruction	Not helpful	Excellent to help determine etiology	Not helpful

*This table summarizes the common imaging findings in the assessment of the disease processes discussed in this chapter.

Systems-Based Practice

Imaging Recommendations

A rule of thumb in imaging the female patient with symptoms referable to the pelvis is to start with US. CT should be used initially in patients with a prior history of abdominal surgery or those for whom you have a high index of suspicion for bowel pathology or kidney stones. MRI is generally used to confirm suspicions raised by findings on CT or US. MRI is also used as an adjunct to help tease out pathologic subtleties. Keep in mind that time constraints, body habitus, and prohibitive cost can all significantly alter utilization. With a good clinical history, US, CT, and MRI are all invaluable tools to help diagnose the pelvic disease processes described in this chapter, as well as many others.

Bibliography

Albayram F, Hamper UM: Ovarian and adnexal torsion: Spectrum of sonographic findings with pathologic correlation. J Ultrasound Med 2001;20:1083–1089.

Ascher SM, Jha RC, Reinhold C: Benign myometrial conditions: Leiomyomas and adenomyosis. Top Magn Reson Imaging 2003;14:281–304.

Baltarowich OH, Kurtz AB, Pasto ME, et al: The spectrum of sonographic findings in hemorrhagic ovarian cysts. AJR Am J Roentgenol 1987;148:901–905.

Baltarowich OH, Kurtz AB, Pennell RG, et al: Pitfalls in the sonographic diagnosis of uterine fibroids. AJR Am J Roentgenol 1988;151:725–728.

Brown DL, Doubilet PM, Miller FH, et al: Benign and malignant ovarian masses: Selection of the most discriminating gray-scale and Doppler sonographic features. Radiology 1988;208:103–110.

Bude RO, Rubin JM: Power Doppler sonography. Radiology 1996;200:21–23.

Carter JR, Lau M, Saltzman AK, et al: Gray scale and color flow Doppler characterization of uterine tumors. J Ultrasound Med 1994;13:835–840.

Chaudhry S, Reinhold C, Guermazi A, et al: Benign and malignant diseases of the endometrium. Top Magn Reson Imaging 2003;14:339–357.

Conway C, Zalud I, Dilena M, et al: Simple cyst in the post-menopausal patient: Detection and management. J Ultrasound Med 1998;17:369–372.

Fleischer AC, Stein SM, Cullinan JA, Warner MA: Color Doppler sonography of adnexal torsion. J Ultrasound Med 1995;14:523–528.

Fried AM, Kenney CM 3rd, Stigers KB, et al: Benign pelvic masses: Sonographic spectrum. Radiographics 1996;16:321–334.

Goldstein A: AAPM tutorials: Overview of the physics of US. Radiographics 1993;13:701–704.

Haynor DR, Mack LA, Soules MR, et al: Changing appearance of the normal uterus during the menstrual cycle: MR studies. Radiology 1986;161:459–462.

Hertzberg BS, Kliewer MA: Sonography of benign cystic teratoma of the ovary: Pitfalls in diagnosis. AJR Am J Roentgenol 1996;167:1127–1133.

Kremkau FW: AAPM tutorial: Multiple-element transducers. Radiographics 1993;13:1163–1176.

Kurtz AB, Tsimikas JV, Tempany CM, et al: Diagnosis and staging of ovarian cancer: Comparative values of Doppler and conventional US, CT and MR imaging correlated with surgery and histopathologic analysis: Report of the Radiology Diagnostic Oncology Group. Radiology 1999;212:19–27.

Lemus JF: Ectopic pregnancy: An update. Curr Opin Obstet Gynecol 2000;12:369–375.

Lin SP, Brown JJ: MR contrast agents: Physical and pharmacologic basics. J Magn Reson Imaging 2007;25:879–880.

Mitchell DG, Schonholz L, Hilpert PL, et al: Zones of the uterus: Discrepancy between US and MR images. Radiology 1990;174:827–831.

Murase E, Siegelman ES, Outwater EK, et al: Uterine leiomyomas: Histopathologic features, MR imaging findings, differential diagnosis, and treatment. Radiographics 1999;19:1179–1197.

Nalaboff KM, Pellerito JS, Ben-Levi E: Imaging the endometrium: Disease and normal variants. Radiographics 2001;21:1409–1424.

Pinto I, Chimeno P, Romo A, et al: Uterine fibroids: Uterine artery embolization versus abdominal hysterectomy for treatment: A prospective, randomized, and controlled clinical trial. Radiology 2003;226:425–431.

Sheth S, Fishman EK, Buck JL, et al: The variable sonographic appearances of ovarian teratomas: Correlation with CT. AJR Am J Roentgenol 1998;151:331–334.

Siedler D, Laing FC, Jeffrey RB Jr, Wing VW: Uterine adenomyosis: A difficult sonographic diagnosis. J Ultrasound Med 1987;6:345–349.

Togashi K, Nishimura K, Itoh K, et al: Adenomyosis: Diagnosis with MR imaging. Radiology 1988;166:111–114.

Zinn HL, Cohen HL, Zinn DL: Ultrasonographic diagnosis of ectopic pregnancy: Importance of transabdominal imaging. J Ultrasound Med 1997;16:603–607.

Ziskin MC: Fundamental physics of ultrasound and its propagation in tissue. Radiographics 1993;13:705–709.

Chapter 40
The Premenstrual Syndrome (Case 25)

Michael Belden MD

Case: A 37-year-old G2P2 with regular menstrual cycles presents with a chief complaint of irritability, fatigue, and anxiety that begins, without fail, 5 days before her menstrual cycle starts and then suddenly abates during the first day of her menstrual bleeding.

Differential Diagnosis

Premenstrual syndrome (PMS)	Premenstrual dysphoric disorder (PMDD)

Speaking Intelligently

When I am asked to evaluate a reproductive-age woman who presents with the constellation of symptoms as described in the case above, PMS is always first on my list of diagnoses. Over the years, I have observed that PMS is more uncommon in patients in their teens and early twenties, and the incidence increases with time, as the patient ages. The average age of onset is thought to be about 26 years, but of course this will vary from patient to patient. PMS and its more severe form, PMDD, can be severely debilitating for many women, and must be taken seriously because although the etiology is not well understood, the methods of treatment are well articulated and are evidence based.

PATIENT CARE

Clinical Thinking

- PMS is a diagnosis of exclusion. Therefore, my first job when evaluating a patient for PMS is to be sure that I have excluded other important diagnoses.
- Rule out depression and thyroid disorders. Less commonly, type 2 diabetes or anemia can present similarly to the previous case.
- As a gynecologist, I am not routinely asked to make the diagnosis of chronic fatigue syndrome. However, this is a plausible diagnosis in a woman presenting with concerns and complaints that can seem very similar to PMS.

History

- The diagnosis of PMS is based on the cyclic nature of the symptoms that characterize the syndrome, and can be validated with a well-organized patient diary or calendar of symptoms.
- A careful history should assess the degree to which these symptoms disrupt the quality of the patient's life.

Common Mood and Somatic Symptoms of Premenstrual Syndrome

Mood-Associated Symptoms
- Hypersensitivity
- Depressive symptoms
- Irritability
- Mood swings
- Tension
- Anxiety
- Fear
- Loss of control
- Anger

Somatic-Associated Symptoms
- Bloating
- Body aches
- Headaches
- Food cravings
- Poor coordination

Physical Examination
- Physical examination for PMS is usually unrevealing.
- Pay careful attention to the thyroid examination, as well as to findings associated with anemia, including lightheadedness, skin pallor, blanching of the nail beds, and so forth.

Tests for Consideration
- **Thyroid-stimulating hormone (TSH):** To rule out hypothyroidism. $60
- **CBC:** To check for anemia. $35
- Interestingly, there are **no measurable differences** in the hormonal profiles of patients with PMS versus asymptomatic patients. Therefore, there is no value in measuring hypothalamic, pituitary, or ovarian hormonal levels.

Clinical Entities   Medical Knowledge

Premenstrual Syndrome

Pφ The pathophysiology of PMS is not well understood, but probably involves an aberration in the metabolism of estrogen and progesterone in the central nervous system that ultimately affects the serotonergic system during the luteal phase. Because patients with PMS are known to typically respond favorably to drugs in the selective serotonin reuptake inhibitor (SSRI) category, the serotonin regulation system is almost certainly involved.

TP The most common presentation involves one or several of the mood and somatic complaints listed in the preceding box.

Dx Diagnosis is reached by history. A symptom diary can be extremely useful, especially in establishing the cyclic nature of the complaints, as well as the degree to which they disrupt the patient's daily life.

Tx Simple reassurance is a mainstay of therapy. In many cases a patient merely needs to hear that she is, in fact, quite normal. Sometimes this is enough to help the patient through the difficulties presented by PMS. There are, in addition, several other therapeutic options that must be tailored to each patient individually: (1) oral contraceptive pills (OCPs) can be helpful and are sometimes used continuously; (2) spironolactone is sometimes helpful, as are OCPs containing drospirenone, a spironolactone analog; (3) SSRIs are sometimes used, especially fluoxetine and sertraline, with either continuous or "luteal phase" dosing; and (4) aerobic exercise is almost universally acknowledged to be helpful. **See Katz 36, Hacker 36.**

Premenstrual Dysphoric Disorder

Pφ PMDD is a more debilitating form of PMS, and is acknowledged by the American Psychiatric Association. The formal criteria from the *Diagnostic and Statistical Manual of Mental Disorders, Fourth Edition, Text Revision* (DSM-IV) are listed in Table 40-1.

TP Symptoms are characteristically much worse than "typical" PMS and result in social impairment that adversely affects the patient's ability to perform her activities of daily living.

Dx Use history and the criteria from DSM-IV.

Tx There is considerable overlap in patients with major depressive disorder (MDD) and patients with PMDD. SSRIs should be used liberally when necessary. There may be a role for gonadotropin-releasing hormone (GnRH) agonists with or without "add-back" therapy to provide relief of symptoms for the most severely affected patients, at least in the short term. Patients who show no real improvement on GnRH agonists are far more likely to have MDD, and *not* PMDD. **See Katz 36, Hacker 36.**

Table 40-1   DSM-IV-TR Criteria for the Diagnosis of Premenstrual Dysphoric Disorder

Five or more of the following symptoms must be present most of the time during the last week of the luteal phase, with at least one of the symptoms being one of the first four. Symptoms should occur for most months within the year, and resolve at or about mid-menses.
- Feeling sad, hopeless, or self-deprecating thoughts
- Anxiety or tension
- Mood lability or crying
- Persistent irritability or anger, and increased interpersonal conflicts
- Decreased interest in usual activities, social withdrawal
- Difficulty concentrating
- Fatigue or lethargy
- Changes in appetite
- Hypersomnia or insomnia
- Subjective feelings of loss of control

Physical symptoms, including "bloating," weight gain, joint or muscle pain

See Katz 36.

Adapted from American Psychiatric Association: Diagnostic and Statistical Manual of Mental Disorders, 4th edition, Text Revision. Washington, DC, American Psychiatric Association, 2000, p 771.

ZEBRA ZONE

a. **Chronic fatigue syndrome:** The pathophysiology of chronic fatigue syndrome is not well understood. It is usually a diagnosis of exclusion. Patients present with multiple symptoms, typically including crushing fatigue, hypersomnolence or hyposomnolence, pain, and difficulty concentrating. Diagnosis is made using a strict definition of symptoms and findings developed by the Centers for Disease Control and Prevention (CDC). Treatment is generally supportive.

b. **Major depressive disorder:** If your history or clinical judgment suggests the patient may be suffering from a more worrisome psychiatric diagnosis, be sure to help the patient set up an appointment with a consultant as soon as possible. Screen for suicidal/homicidal ideation if this seems appropriate.

c. **Hypothyroidism:** A common cause of a generalized sense of non–well-being, and seen more often in women than men. Autoimmune destruction of the thyroid gland is the most common etiology, but hypothyroidism can also be seen after hypothalamic or pituitary damage. Presentation is characterized by fatigue, lethargy, weight gain, depression, constipation, and other somatic conditions that represent a "slowing" of the patient's general metabolic state. Diagnosis is by serum TSH level, which will be elevated. *Subclinical hypothyroidism* is diagnosed when serum TSH is elevated but thyroxine is normal. The treatment is levothyroxine, titrated appropriately.

Practice-Based Learning and Improvement: Evidence-Based Medicine

Title
Effect of a combination of ethinylestradiol 30 micrograms and drospirenone 3 mg on tolerance, cycle control, general well-being and fluid-related symptoms in women with premenstrual disorders requesting contraception

Authors
Borges LE, Andrade RP, Aldrighi JM, et al.

Institution
Laboratorio de Reproducao Humana do Hospital das Clinicas da Universidade Federal de Minas Gerais, Minas Gerais, Brazil

Reference
Contraception 2006;74:446–450

Problem
Addresses usefulness of drospirenone in OCPs for relief of PMS symptoms

Intervention
241 patients with PMS symptoms, requesting OCPs, were offered six cycles of an ethinyl estradiol 30 µg/drospirenone 3 mg, and asked if their symptoms improved.

Comparison/control (quality of evidence)
Nonrandomized cohort study.

Outcome/effect
84.2% reported "great improvement" in PMS symptoms.

Historical significance/comments
A randomized trial is still needed, but this study demonstrated the great promise of drospirenone-containing OCPs for PMS symptoms.

Practice-Based Learning and Improvement

Small Group Learning Program
Residents and students meet to review current information about a specific clinical problem and to reflect on their experiences and challenges with the problem. Group discussion is stimulated by prepared material and led by a trained peer facilitator.

Practical Example: Each week the residents meet with the Program Director or Department Chair to discuss programmatic issues. During the last 15 minutes one of the residents briefly presents one of the American College of Obstetricians and Gynecologists (ACOG) Practice Bulletins. For this particular case, a thorough discussion of Practice Bulletin #15, *Premenstrual Syndrome,* would be germane. Further discussion could include a review of the DSM-IV-TR criteria for PMDD (See Compendium of Selected Publications, American College of Obstetricians and Gynecologists, 2008, 1057–65).

Interpersonal and Communication Skills

Reassurance, But ...
When approaching a patient with PMS, empathy and reassurance are often the most powerful tools available. Patients may feel isolated

and alone during the few days of the menstrual cycle when they are feeling their worst, and they may also have feelings of guilt associated with their emotional lability and its impact on others. It is important to differentiate between what could be considered "normal" PMS symptoms and more worrisome depressive symptoms. This differentiation is one of the most important services you can provide. Acknowledge how difficult this disorder must be for the patient. If the patient's complaints appear to fall within the continuum generally regarded as PMS, then reassurance to the patient and a description of the treatment options available is often all that may be required. Should you decide that the patient's symptoms are beyond your expectations for "standard" PMS, you should offer a psychological/psychiatric referral, explaining that, although exacerbated by the hormonal cycle, her situation may warrant greater clarification and possibly more aggressive treatment.

Professionalism

Principle: Social Justice
"An important AHRQ [Agency for Healthcare Research and Quality] study demonstrated that physician predilection can contribute to differences in access to care for blacks and women. The researchers used well-trained patient actors—two black men, two black women, two white men, and two white women—who described their chest pain using the same scripts, reporting identical clinical symptoms, and reporting the same insurance and professions. Yet even with patients in such identical circumstances, blacks and women had relative odds for being referred to cardiac catheterization, the gold standard for diagnosing coronary artery disease, that were 60 percent of the odds for whites and men. Black women fared the worst, with relative odds that were 40 percent."*

Working actively to fight internal and sometimes subconscious prejudices is only possible if, as a profession, we can acknowledge that these prejudices exist. This is especially important when treating patients for conditions such as PMS who may indeed have many subjective findings.

*http://www.ahrq.gov/news/test52102.htm.

Systems-Based Practice

Selecting Your First Position out of Residency/Fellowship
Probably the most important decision for which most well-trained Ob/Gyn physicians are poorly prepared is finding and selecting that first Ob/Gyn position. Although you are likely to be an expert in

delivering a baby, finding the right position to begin your career is a skill in itself. In fact, it has been estimated that 40% of all physicians leave their first job within 2 years.

The first step in finding the right position is for the candidate to take some time to answer some key questions for himself/herself:

- Is geography important, city versus rural, weather, outside interests, arts, sports, etc., growing community versus an established one?
- Do I want to live near family, in-laws, etc.?
- Are mentorship and further training important?
- How important is money?
- Are there partnership/future opportunities?
- Are teaching and/or research a priority?
- How hard do I want to work in patient care versus balancing other interests?

Once the physician has given these questions some thought, he or she should find out what positions are available. Potential sources for Ob/Gyn positions are journals, conferences, Internet postings (probably the fastest-growing source), and contacting hospitals and practices in a specific region if the physician has chosen a specific area in which to live. Some physicians also use search firms to take on much of this "legwork," which is helpful to avoid this time-consuming task, but the downside is that some hospitals/physician practices are not willing to pay search fees.

When approaching the interview process, it is best to be well rested and well prepared. Develop a list of key questions in advance so you can find out as much about the practice as possible. Also, think through the questions that you are most likely to be asked by the interviewer. If a job appears promising, you may want to ask about conducting rounds with the practice's physicians and talk to the nonphysician employees of the practice, especially the practice manager. It is usually a good sign for a practice if there is minimal employee turnover of staff and young physicians. In selecting a practice in Ob/Gyn, you are selecting a hospital or hospital system, too. Thus, you should probably visit the hospital(s) that the practice uses to ensure that the services that you require are available, such as residency coverage, perinatal backup, and level of neonatal care. In fact, meeting with the chairperson of the Ob/Gyn department, which is a typical step later in the hospital credentialing process, may be worthwhile before you accept a position.

The last major step is the contract process. For any position today, handshakes are nice, but contracts are required. Prepare to retain a lawyer familiar with physician employment agreements, especially with initial contracts. Although these early career contracts should not be extremely complicated, issues for your lawyer and you to address include terms of termination, malpractice coverage partnership, term, salary and bonuses, office, hospital workload and call commitments, and other components of compensation such as paid conferences, time off, pension and profit sharing, and health, life, and disability benefits.

As mentioned, it is estimated that 40% of physicians leave their first job within 2 years, so if your first position does not work out, learn what you can from the experience and find a new position that is a better fit.

Chapter 41
Urogynecology and Urinary Incontinence (Case 26)

Marc Toglia MD

Case: A 45-year-old woman, para 2, presents to the office for an annual gynecologic examination. Just before you leave the room, she admits that she "leaks a little urine" from time to time.

Differential Diagnosis

Stress urinary incontinence	Urge urinary incontinence
Mixed urinary incontinence	Incomplete bladder emptying/urinary retention

Speaking Intelligently

Urinary incontinence is a very common problem in women, although many women are reluctant to discuss it. There are several causes of urinary incontinence (involuntary leakage of urine) and effective therapy differs based upon the etiology. In general, urinary incontinence is either the result of a weakened urethra and pelvic floor (stress incontinence) or a bladder that contracts involuntarily (urge incontinence, also called *overactive bladder syndrome*). It is important to realize that urinary incontinence commonly coexists with pelvic organ prolapse or incomplete bladder emptying (urinary retention). The presence of either condition can dramatically influence treatment.

PATIENT CARE

Clinical Thinking

- Keep in mind that the signs and symptoms of incontinence and urinary leakage can be confusing and clinically challenging—there are only a few bladder symptoms, and the different disorders tend to have overlapping symptoms.
- Obtaining a thorough history is the most helpful strategy that will lead to the correct diagnosis. Given that women are often embarrassed to discuss issues regarding incontinence, be prepared to take the lead to ask very specific questions.
- I prefer to ask a standard list of questions that encompass stress incontinence, urge incontinence, ability to adequately empty one's bladder, and "cystitis-like" symptoms.
- Ask specifically whether these symptoms interfere with sexual activity because many women are too embarrassed to volunteer this information.
- Most important, determine how significant a problem this is for the patient, and exactly what impact it is having on her life.

History

- Many women who complain of urinary incontinence have had prior surgery for prolapse or incontinence. Try to obtain as much detail as possible regarding the exact procedures, surgical approach, and chief complaint for which the initial surgery was performed.
- History can often differentiate between stress and urge incontinence. Leakage of small amounts of urine associated with coughing, sneezing, laughing, and physical activity is more typical of stress urinary incontinence. Irritative bladder symptoms such as urgency (needing to rush to the bathroom), frequent urination, and getting up several times from sleep to void (nocturia) are characteristic of urge urinary incontinence. Leakage of significant amounts of urine in a single episode is also typical of urge incontinence. Some women experience losing large amounts of urine without awareness or warning—this is more typical of urge incontinence.
- Urinary incontinence will often prompt behavioral changes in women—toilet mapping (knowing ahead of time where all the bathrooms are at a destination) and avoiding liquids are two examples of behavioral changes that are typical of patients with urge incontinence.
- Duration and severity of symptoms are perhaps the most important part of the history because they may dictate the level of therapy. Does the leakage occur daily, weekly, or occasionally? More than once a day? Does the woman need to wear protective padding (if so, how often and how many) or change her clothes because of leakage? Has the woman changed her lifestyle to compensate for symptoms?

Patients with more severe symptoms may benefit more from aggressive therapy such as surgery.

- Bladder pain is atypical of urinary incontinence, and should suggest interstitial cystitis as a possible diagnosis.
- A history of recurring urinary tract infections suggests either incomplete bladder emptying or interstitial cystitis. A history of recurring infections without evidence of bacteriuria should raise suspicion of interstitial cystitis.
- Symptoms during sex should be elicited in detail. Leakage of urine associated with orgasm is more typical of urge incontinence, whereas leakage related to thrusting during intercourse can be more typical of stress urinary incontinence. Discomfort either during or after sex is atypical of incontinence but typical of interstitial cystitis.

Physical Examination

- **General appearance:** The treatment of stress urinary incontinence and pelvic organ prolapse is often surgical. Therefore, it is important to get an overall sense of whether the patient is an appropriate surgical candidate. Does the woman appear significantly overweight or undernourished? Significantly younger or older than her stated age?
- **Psychological presentation:** Treatment for incontinence frequently involves a motivated patient and active lifestyle and behavioral modification. Make note of the woman's functional status and affect. Anxiety disorders are extremely commonplace—women suffering from significant anxiety may be very reluctant to consider treatment and may have difficulty deciding between treatment options. Conversely, clearly anxious patients may be overly eager to proceed with surgery "just to get it over with."
- **Abdominal examination:** The presence of an abdominal or pelvic mass is likely to influence treatment options, but unlikely to be the cause of urinary incontinence.
- **Pelvic examination:** The position of the urethra and vaginal walls at rest and with maximal straining effort should be noted. The presence of a fixed urethra (complete lack of any rotational descent with straining) or abnormal elevation of the bladder neck (from previous surgery) are key physical findings. Objective documentation of urinary leakage with coughing is important in the establishment of the diagnosis of stress incontinence. Often, repetitive coughing may be necessary before significant leakage is observed. The amount and force of the urinary stream should also be documented, and correlated with the postvoid residual. The presence of prolapse of the anterior vaginal wall (e.g., cystocele) or apical vaginal compartment (e.g., cervix or vaginal apex) should be documented, as well as the presence or absence of a uterus or cervix. Bimanual examination should first focus on the presence or absence of bladder or urethral tenderness (a sign of interstitial cystitis). Thickening of the bladder

wall, especially in an older woman, is concerning for bladder cancer. The presence of a pelvic mass (e.g., fibroids) should be noted. Tenderness of the pelvic floor muscles either laterally (obturator internus) or deep posteriorly (pyriformis) may suggest the presence of interstitial cystitis or pelvic floor myalgia, and may limit the feasibility of surgical therapy. The ability of the woman to contract her levator muscle should be graded against downward digital pressure of the examiner's index finger.

Tests for Consideration

- **Dipstick analysis:** A clean-catch or sterile urine specimen should be analyzed at each visit, specifically to look for blood or presence of nitrites, because bacterial cystitis is common in women with urinary incontinence. $30

- **Determination of a postvoid residual:** This finding, obtained using bladder catheterization, is critical because treatment options are dramatically altered in the presence of an elevated residual. Ideally, a woman should be catheterized within 15 minutes of voiding. A residual volume of <100 mL can be considered normal, while volumes >200 mL are frequently (but not always) indicative of voiding dysfunction. Values between 100 and 200 mL should prompt (at the least) repeat testing or diagnostic studies (e.g., urodynamic studies). Performed as part of initial evaluation. $10

- **Urodynamic testing:** Frequently helpful in planning therapy, especially for managing stress incontinence and pelvic organ prolapse. Urodynamic testing is standard in several clinical scenarios: consideration of surgical management of stress incontinence; presence of significant pelvic organ prolapse (e.g., leading edge of prolapse beyond the vaginal opening); prior surgical treatment for incontinence or prolapse; failed medical therapy for incontinence; presence of a clinically significant postvoid residual; presence of severe incontinence either by history or demonstration on examination. $1300

- **Uroflowmetry:** Measuring voiding amount, force of stream, and voiding pattern, along with determination of a postvoid residual, is a good screening test for incomplete bladder emptying. Abnormal results should prompt a voiding pressure study. Performed as part of urodynamic testing. $500

- **Cystometry:** Although technically just a plot of bladder pressure related to increases in bladder volume, cystometry is helpful in determining

bladder hypersensitivity and hyposensitivity,
detrusor overactivity, and poor bladder compliance, and in
the objective documentation of stress incontinence.
Performed as part of urodynamic testing. $500

- **Voiding pressure studies:** These combine the
measure of urinary outflow (uroflowmetry) with a
measurement of bladder pressure generated during
voiding. Poor flow of urine associated with elevated
bladder pressure suggests outflow obstruction,
whereas poor flow in the presence of little or no
elevation of bladder pressure is typical of bladder
underactivity. Performed as part of urodynamic testing. $500

- **Cystoscopy:** Examination of the bladder lining
with an endoscope can be helpful, especially with
a prior history of pelvic surgery, or in the presence
of gross or microscopic hematuria. $300

Clinical Entities	Medical Knowledge

Stress Urinary Incontinence

Pφ Reflects an incompetent urethral sphincter, not a dysfunctional bladder. Leakage occurs whenever abdominal/bladder pressure exceeds closing urethral pressure.

TP Leakage typically occurs simultaneously with activity—coughing, sneezing, jumping, running. Leakage tends to be of small dribbles of urine, but with repetitive activity can result in a significant amount of wetness.

Dx Objective observation of leakage with forceful exertion such as coughing is necessary for an accurate diagnosis. Such provocative testing should be performed with both a comfortably full bladder and an empty bladder. Technically speaking, genuine stress incontinence requires leakage of urine during cystometry, in the absence of detrusor overactivity.

Tx Conservative treatment consists of pelvic floor strengthening exercises. Results (typically a reduction in the frequency or amount of leakage) may occur only after several months of daily exercises

Surgical correction, either a pubovaginal sling or urethropexy (to reposition the urethrovesical junction), is often first-line therapy because these procedures are associated with high success rates. **See Katz 21, Hacker 23.**

Urge Urinary Incontinence (Overactive Bladder)

Pφ Urge incontinence reflects a bladder that does not stay voluntarily relaxed. People take for granted that the ability to store urine and defer voiding is simply a socially adaptive behavior learned during childhood. The underlying causes of urge incontinence are multifactorial: poor initial toileting skills and maladaptive behavior (excess drinking of liquids, habit of voiding at either inappropriately short or long intervals) are frequent causes of this problem. In addition, subtle neuromuscular changes in bladder physiology that can accompany pregnancy, childbirth, pelvic surgery, and aging can contribute to urge incontinence. Overt neurologic disease such as stroke, spinal cord injury, or multiple sclerosis can also lead to bladder dysfunction.

TP The triad of urinary frequency, urgency, and nocturia is usually (but not always) the hallmark of urge incontinence, as is leakage of urine followed by a strong urge to void that cannot be deferred for long. The description "when I have to go, I cannot wait" is most indicative of urge incontinence. Some women with overactive bladder syndrome have urgency and frequency without leakage. Others have sudden leakage without warning, and not associated with urgency or frequency. Many women complain of not feeling empty after urinating because they experience a strong urge to urinate shortly thereafter. This is typically associated with normal postvoid residuals and is typical of overactive bladder.

Dx Diagnosis is typically made based on history and in the absence of an elevated postvoid residual urine volume. Urodynamic testing may demonstrate instability of bladder pressures (detrusor overactivity) in less than half of women.

Tx Treatment is typically conservative, and almost never surgical. Behavioral modification, fluid management (drinking fewer liquids, avoiding bladder irritants), toilet retraining (learning how to defer a strong urge to void), and drug therapy are the cornerstones of treatment. Anticholinergic therapy often reduces symptoms, but may not always completely eliminate them.

Urge incontinence commonly coexists with pelvic organ prolapse. It is currently controversial whether surgical correction of prolapse improves bladder symptoms. **See Katz 21, Hacker 23.**

Mixed Urinary Incontinence

Pφ Some women have symptoms of both stress and urge incontinence and are said to have *mixed incontinence*. These women have a combination of both urethral sphincter weakness (stress urinary incontinence) and bladder dysfunction (urge urinary incontinence). Up to a third of all women suffering from incontinence have mixed symptoms.

TP Patients complain of symptoms consistent with both stress and urge incontinence. In these women, it is of paramount importance to understand which symptoms the patient considers the most bothersome.

Dx Diagnosis is based on the same criteria as for stress and urge incontinence.

Tx Therapy is typically sequential. Most experts would suggest treating the urge symptoms first because therapy is conservative and improvements are often seen within a few weeks. Others would suggest that the most bothersome symptoms be treated first.

Incomplete Bladder Emptying (Urinary Retention)

Pφ The pathophysiology of incomplete bladder emptying is poorly understood in most cases. Outlet obstruction occurs uncommonly in women, except in the presence of advanced pelvic organ prolapse or after a surgical procedure that obstructs the bladder neck or urethra. Pharmacologic therapy with anticholinergic agents is an uncommon cause of urinary retention. Denervation of the bladder after pelvic surgery or radiation is also an uncommon cause. Neurologic disease, such as a stroke, spinal cord injury, or multiple sclerosis, can also affect bladder emptying.

TP Clinical presentation varies with the underlying causes. Two patterns are frequently seen. Women with outlet obstruction usually complain of urgency, frequency, difficulty initiating urination (hesitancy), and a poor urinary flow. Other patients have marked reduction in bladder sensation—they void infrequently, have little sense of urgency, and may present only with recurring bouts of cystitis. Some women will present with leakage without awareness, or unexpected loss. Urinary incontinence associated with incomplete bladder emptying has been referred to as "overflow incontinence" in many textbooks. It is likely that this presentation actually reflects either of two conditions: stress incontinence associated with incomplete voiding, or urge incontinence associated with incomplete voiding.

Dx Diagnosis is typically made by the observation of repeatedly elevated postvoid residual urine volumes, typically greater than 200 mL. Urodynamic testing is frequently needed to rule out obstructed voiding, but often only confirms the finding of incomplete bladder emptying and poor bladder sensation.

Tx Current treatment options for incomplete bladder emptying are limited. There are no effective drug therapies that improve bladder emptying. Women with significant pelvic organ prolapse may note improvement in voiding with the use of a pessary, or perhaps reconstructive vaginal surgery. Some women, especially those with neurologic causes for incomplete emptying, may benefit from implantation of a sacral neuromodulator. For most women, however, there is no apparent cause for the incomplete emptying, and diagnostic testing suggests an underactive bladder muscle. For these women, intermittent self-catheterization is the cornerstone of therapy. Women who experience incomplete bladder emptying are also prone to recurrent bladder infections, and may benefit from suppressive daily antibiotic therapy. **See Katz 21.**

ZEBRA ZONE

a. Interstitial cystitis: A poorly understood, chronic condition of the bladder characterized by chronic and sometimes intermittent irritative bladder symptoms such as frequency, urgency, and bladder pain. As such, it typically resembles recurrent urinary tract infections, but urine cultures are typically negative. The symptoms are also similar to those of overactive bladder, except that they are more intermittent, occurring in flares, rather than in a more continuous fashion. Also, pain is an unusual finding with overactive bladder syndrome, and is common with interstitial cystitis.

Practice-Based Learning and Improvement: Evidence-Based Medicine

Title
Stress urinary incontinence

Authors
Nygaard IE, Heit M

Institution
University of Iowa Carver College of Medicine, Iowa City, Iowa

Reference
Obstetrics and Gynecology 2002;104:607–620

Problem
Stress urinary incontinence.

Intervention
Addresses various techniques and procedures that can be helpful with this disease process.

Comparison/control (quality of evidence)
Review article, level III expert opinion.

Outcome/effect
Evaluates treatment strategies for stress incontinence in evidence-based fashion.

Historical significance/comments
This comprehensive and well-written review article sums up state-of-the-art evidence regarding therapy for stress incontinence.

Interpersonal and Communication Skills

Ironically, Specific Questioning Alleviates Embarrassment
Discussing a problem like urinary incontinence is typically very embarrassing for a woman. It is likely that she has suffered in silence with this problem for many years, that her incontinence has affected her sexuality, social activities, and sense of personal image, and that she is unaware that this is a common problem,
Interestingly, I find that probing the problem with personal questions about her "adaptive behaviors" does not embarrass my patient; it helps her to realize that this is a reasonably common problem—and that other women have created the same adaptive behaviors for themselves, which I am able to anticipate.

For example, I specifically ask "Does the urine leakage happen when you laugh, cough, or sneeze? Do you find that you must go to the bathroom as soon as you get home? Do you "map" out where bathrooms are in the course of her daily activities? Do you wear a protective pad, or even an adult diaper?" These inquiries not only allow you to get to the heart of the problem, they make the patient realize that this problem is one she shares with other women and that the aspects of its inconvenience are understood by her physician.

Professionalism

Principle: Patient Autonomy

Even though you may advocate for surgery for a particular patient, competent patients have the right to decline a surgical operation that is advised. During the informed consent process, the physician must decide if a patient has the ability to understand the diagnostic and treatment options and if the patient can generate and defend a rational decision about his or her care. There are times when the patient may appear "incompetent" to make such a decision. *Competence* is a legal term for a patient's ability to make informed decisions about specific medical care. Strictly speaking, all patients are competent to make medical decisions unless they have been determined incompetent by a court of law. When a patient's competence is called into question, it can be a difficult process for the patient, physician, and patient's family. For example, patients on ventilators or those who have a previous psychiatric diagnosis do not necessarily lack decision-making ability, but decisions that appear irrational should be questioned. When patient competence is indeed in question, it is advisable to obtain help from psychiatric consultants and other appropriate hospital resource personnel (e.g., hospital counsel).

From Mann BD: Surgery: A Competency-Based Companion. Copyright 2009, Elsevier.

Systems-Based Practice

Patient Safety: Medical Errors and Quality Improvement Initiatives

After struggling for years with incontinence, your patient elects to undergo a percutaneous suburethral sling procedure, a relatively safe procedure with a low incidence of complications. Unfortunately, during recovery your patient develops a severe infection and ends up requiring a prolonged hospitalization. In reviewing the record, it becomes clear that your patient was not given the standard prophylactic dose of antibiotic that such patients are supposed to be given. Although she eventually recovers from the infection, she rejects her sling and remains incontinent.

Medical errors are the eighth leading cause of death in this country and account for as many as 98,000 deaths per year, and the total cost of preventable adverse events is considered to be between $17 and $29 billion per year.

Quality improvement (QI) initiatives to reduce medical errors and adverse events have gained considerable momentum in the past decade. These initiatives, typically managed by a multidisciplinary team from across hospital departments, are efforts to systematically improve the systems and processes involved in the delivery of care. Some QI initiatives target specific categories of errors across the hospital, such as medication errors. For instance, a QI initiative might attempt to avoid medication errors by having an automatic system for double checking the dose and patient name for certain high-risk medications across the hospital. Other initiatives target the prevention of specific conditions. For instance, many hospitals are putting into place QI initiatives to target ventilator-associated pneumonia (VAP) with a bundle of steps that have been shown to reduce the occurrence of VAP in intensive care unit patients. Finally, other QI initiatives attempt to simplify or standardize a process, such as the use of a standardized preoperative checklist before surgeries, including checking the procedure, site, and patient identification, as well as reviewing potential complications and ensuring the delivery of preoperative antibiotics.

Chapter 42
Menopausal Concerns and Treatment (Case 27)

Asma Ali MD and Beverly Vaughn MD

Case: A 50-year-old woman presents to your office with hot flashes, night sweats, and occasional dyspareunia. She has not had a menstrual period for 18 months.

Differential Diagnosis

Menopause	Hyperthyroidism	Medication side effects: medications that can cause vasomotor symptoms

Speaking Intelligently

Vasomotor symptoms are the most common presenting complaint of women in the perimenopause transition and in menopause itself. Patients may also complain of other signs of diminishing systemic estrogen production such as vaginal atrophy, the main symptoms of which are dyspareunia and vulvar/vaginal itching. In menopausal patients who present with atypical symptoms, other causes should be considered. It is important to obtain a history, paying particular attention to the severity and frequency of the symptoms. We recommend that only severe vasomotor symptoms receive treatment. The traditional definition of "severe" is greater than six hot flashes per day that are troublesome for the patient. Practically, I use the patient's own evaluation of whether or not her symptoms interfere with her quality of life. This is especially true if the flashes are causing sleep disturbance to an extent that the quality of sleep is poor. Many of the other complaints that women have, such as moodiness, difficulty concentrating, and problems with memory can be ascribed to sleep deprivation. The patient's personal and family medical history are essential elements in helping to determine what risks the patient may have, and what course of treatment would be most beneficial.

PATIENT CARE

Clinical Thinking

- Before determining a treatment regimen, evaluate the patient's risk profile for cerebrovascular and cardiovascular disease.
- Does this patient have **documented** cardiovascular disease?
- If the patient has documented thromboembolic disease, she is not an appropriate candidate for hormone therapy.
- Risk factors for osteoporosis? If yes, treatment with hormones will have the likely additional benefit of maintaining her bone mass.
- Family history of breast cancer? Although important, it is not a contraindication for treatment with hormone therapy.
- Focus on improving the patient's symptoms without incurring any unnecessary risk.

History

- Does the patient complain of vasomotor symptoms such as hot flashes?
- Does the patient have a history of any recent postmenopausal vaginal bleeding?
- Review the patient's medication list.
- Inquire about the patient's sexual history and current practices.

- Inquire about current lifestyle considerations, including diet, amount of exercise, and sleep habits.

Physical Examination
- **Vital signs** are important, especially blood pressure.
- **General appearance:** Does this woman seem healthy and happy?
- **Cardiovascular examination:** Pay particular attention to heart rate, and listen for arrhythmias.
- **Thyroid examination:** Is the thyroid normal to palpation?
- **Pelvic examination:** Include Pap test with human papillomavirus (HPV) testing if indicated.
- **Bimanual examination:** Examine the patient with particular attention directed toward uterine leiomyomas, large ovarian cysts, or other causes of dyspareunia.
- **Vaginal inspection:** Look for thinning epithelium, loss of rugae and normal architecture, and pale mucosa. Test for high pH if this seems reasonable.

Tests for Consideration
- **Follicle-stimulating hormone (FSH):** Optional, but can sometimes be helpful in determining true menopausal status if the value is elevated. — $60
- **Thyroid-stimulating hormone (TSH):** Optional, but can sometimes be helpful in the evaluation of patients with sleep disturbances, mood disorders, and other conditions associated with thyroid disorders. — $60

| **Clinical Entities** | **Medical Knowledge** |

Menopause

Pφ Menopause is defined as 12 months of amenorrhea after a final menstrual period. There is ovarian follicular depletion and therefore decreased ovarian estrogen secretion. The primary source of estrogen in menopause is peripheral conversion of systemic androgens to estriol. The mechanisms of vasomotor symptoms of menopause, primarily "hot flashes" or "hot flushes," are poorly understood. There is instability of the central nervous system (believed to occur in the hypothalamus) thermoregulatory set point, and this is the proposed theory of the cause of hot flashes.[1] Hot flashes are **not** necessarily related to a woman's serum estrogen levels.

TP Women older than 45 years of age will frequently present with irregular menstrual cycles, hot flashes, sleep disturbances, vaginal dryness, sexual dysfunction, and breast pain.

Dx Clinical diagnosis of menopause is based on lack of period for 12 months. Measuring serum estrogen is neither helpful nor indicated. FSH levels are not necessary for clinical diagnosis. TSH levels are not recommended unless you suspect thyroid dysfunction. However, thyroid dysfunction is common in this age group and can be part of general health maintenance screening.

Tx Selective serotonin reuptake inhibitors (SSRIs), serotonin-norepinephrine reuptake inhibitors (SNRIs), gabapentin, progestins, or clonidine can sometimes relieve vasomotor symptoms. Alternative therapies such as phytoestrogens have no proven efficacy. Soy food products such as tofu, tempe, and soy milk are said to ameliorate symptoms, but efficacy in studies is variable. Over-the-counter soy capsules have proven to be no better than placebo. Women with new-onset menopause and without contraindications such as breast cancer or known cardiovascular disease are candidates for short-term systemic estrogen therapy if their vasomotor symptoms are debilitating. In women who have not had a hysterectomy (i.e., still have a uterus), estrogen must be combined with synthetic progestin or micronized progesterone because of the increased risk of endometrial hyperplasia or cancer that occurs when estrogen is used in an "unopposed" fashion. Estrogen is not the first line of therapy for prevention of osteoporosis, heart disease, or cognitive function; however, it has been proven to increase bone mass and decrease risk of fractures. Even if using systemic estrogen therapy, patients may need vaginal preparations for atrophic vaginitis. Over-the-counter lubricants are helpful, and some women may require topical vaginal estrogen as well. **See Katz 42, Hacker 35.**

Hyperthyroidism

Pφ Hyperthyroidism is an overactive thyroid gland with excess thyroid hormone production and decreased levels of TSH. Graves disease is the most common cause of hyperthyroidism. Subacute thyroiditis, toxic thyroid adenoma, and pituitary adenoma are less common causes of hyperthyroidism.

TP Hyperthyroidism typically presents with diffuse, nontender, symmetric enlargement of the thyroid gland and symptoms of heat intolerance, diaphoresis, nervousness, palpitations, and menstrual irregularities.

Dx Start by ordering a TSH level. If this value is below the expected range and the diagnosis of hyperthyroidism is considered, an endocrinologist should be consulted as the evaluation moves forward.

Tx Antithyroid medications such as propylthiouracil decrease the oxidation of iodide and iodination of tyrosine, and diminish peripheral conversion of T_4 into T_3. Propranolol is sometimes used to alleviate cardiac symptoms.

Medication Side Effects: Medications That Can Cause Vasomotor Symptoms

- Niacin used in treating lipid disorders
- Direct vasodilators such as nitroglycerin and hydralazine
- Calcium channel blockers
- Cholinergic drugs
- Selective estrogen receptor modulators (SERMs), such as tamoxifen
- Bromocriptine
- Aromatase inhibitors
- Ketoconazole
- Metronidazole
- Chlorpropamide
- Cephalosporins
- Luteinizing hormone–releasing hormone agonists or antagonists

---

ZEBRA ZONE

a. Pheochromocytoma: A neuroendocrine tumor of the adrenal glands that causes increased catecholamine secretion, resulting in diaphoresis, tachycardia, palpitations, and other systemic manifestations.

b. Carcinoid syndrome: A syndrome of findings characterized by flushing and diarrhea. Carcinoid tumors typically arise in the gastrointestinal tract and produce serotonin.

Practice-Based Learning and Improvement: Evidence-Based Medicine

Title
Estrogen and progesterone use in postmenopausal women: July 2008 position statement of the North American Menopause Society

Authors
Utian WH, Archer DF, Bachmann GA, et al; the North American Menopause Society

Institution
North American Menopause Society

Reference
Menopause 2008;15:584–602

Problem
What are the current evidence-based recommendations regarding hormone replacement therapy? Does repleting estrogen or estrogen and progesterone benefit patients?

Intervention
Hormone therapy.

Comparison/control (quality of evidence)
Level 3 (consensus opinion).

Outcome/effect
Addresses strategies to minimize menopausal symptoms without, it is hoped, increasing the untoward risks that can be associated with long-term hormone replacement therapy.

Historical significance/comments
A good review of pertinent evidence to date regarding the benefits and risks of hormone therapy on multiple organ systems.

Interpersonal and Communication Skills

The Menopausal Years and the Role of Health Maintenance
Office visits for the menopausal patient present a unique opportunity for active listening and health education. After sensitively listening to the patient's most acute concerns, I always include a brief description of the cause of hot flashes and their natural history, which most woman find reassuring. I discuss over-the-counter remedies (frequently used by this population) and their potential risks.

In an office visit with a menopausal woman, I find it appropriate to integrate a discussion about healthy lifestyle changes to decrease risks for heart disease, diabetes, and osteoporosis. I also try to help my patients recognize that sexuality does not end with menopause, and I find that my patients often welcome such a discussion, when prompted.

Other issues that deserve being addressed at a routine visit for menopausal treatment include routine screening mammography, screening colonoscopy, exercise, calcium supplementation, and cholesterol screening.

Professionalism

Principle: Commitment to Improving Access to Care

When a perimenopausal woman comes to your office it may be the first time she has seen a primary care physician since she has given birth. In this situation, there are several diseases for which you should consider screening, including osteoporosis, colon cancer, breast cancer, and cervical cancer. It had been well documented that African American women and women from poorer backgrounds were more likely to present with later-stage cancers and to have higher death rates. Programs such as the National Breast Cancer and Cervical Cancer Early Detection Program administered by the Centers for Disease Control and Prevention (CDC) have targeted these communities, among others, for aggressive outreach and access to screening. African American women now have higher-than-average screening rates for cervical cancer and no evidence for overall increased risk of later-stage cervical cancer presentation. This is a heartening example of how efforts to improve access to care can make a positive impact on the health of the underserved.

For more information, see http://www.ahrq.gov.

Systems-Based Practice

Cost Drivers: Drugs

Your patient with hot flashes has just purchased the new, nonhormonal prescription drug you have prescribed that is guaranteed to eliminate hot flashes. The patient telephones your office complaining that the prescription was very expensive.

Indeed, there is much controversy over the cost of drugs, and with good reason: many new drugs on the market are surprisingly expensive, considering that it costs only a fraction of their price to actually manufacture them. The reason for this—the pharmaceutical industry argues—is the enormously high cost of developing new drugs. The typical pharmaceutical company has to start research on 200 novel compounds in order to bring a single drug to market. When that drug reaches market, the company needs to earn back the cost of developing the 199 other drugs that didn't work out. Drug companies feel, therefore, that they have a right to charge high prices for new drugs, especially considering the significant risk they take in the development process.

To help protect these profits, the government enforces a 20-year patent on new drugs: during this time only the drug's developer (or anyone else they allow to) may produce and sell the new drug. (In reality, by the time a drug gets to market usually only 10 to 12 years of the patent are left.) Once this period ends, however, other drug manufacturers can make the same drug and sell it as a generic for significantly less. They can afford to sell it for much less because they do not need to cover the development and marketing cost of the drug. As a physician, it is important to understand this issue. Although many new drugs are worth the high cost, most hospitals have formularies in place that require generics to be used whenever possible.

Reference

1. Speroff L, Glass RH, Kase NG: Clinical Gynecologic Endocrinology and Infertility, 5th ed. Baltimore, Williams & Wilkins, 1994, p 595.

Chapter 43
Osteoporosis (Case 28)

Joseph S. Ferroni MD

Case: A 73-year-old, white G4P4004 presents complaining of nontraumatic middle and lower back pain, which does not radiate. The pain started acutely, has been worsening over the last week, and has been severe enough to wake her from sleep. She has been using analgesics for the pain, with some relief.

Differential Diagnosis

Postmenopausal osteoporosis/osteoporotic vertebral compression fracture(s)	Degenerative disk disease
Osteoarthritis of the lumbosacral spine	Malignancy

Speaking Intelligently

In a postmenopausal woman with back pain unrelated to trauma, you must first consider osteoporotic compression fracture of one or more vertebrae as the likely cause. Up to two thirds of vertebral fractures are asymptomatic; however, a history of having one vertebral fracture is the most common risk factor for subsequent vertebral fracture or even hip fracture. Thus, accurate diagnosis and appropriate management of osteoporosis are essential. The dual-energy x-ray absorptiometry (DEXA) scan is the gold standard for diagnosing osteoporosis, but will not show a vertebral compression fracture unless a lateral vertebral assessment (LVA) is added. If the LVA modality is not available, then spine radiographs can be ordered, which may also help to diagnose or rule out osteoarthritis or degenerative changes in the spinal column. A plain film of the abdomen may be helpful in diagnosing stones in the urinary tract if you suspect nephrolithiasis as a cause of back pain. Above all, and before any testing is begun, a detailed medical history and a thorough physical and pelvic examination are mandatory. Malignancy presentation in this manner, though uncommon, should not be overlooked in this age group.

PATIENT CARE

Clinical Thinking

- Many women experience back pain, although this pain can often arise as a result of chronic conditions such as arthritis or disk disease.
- Back pain arising from a pelvic mass such as a posterior uterine fibroid or a large ovarian mass would be unlikely in this age group, although these causes must be ruled out. Similarly, uterine prolapse with or without pelvic floor relaxation can sometimes cause lower back pain. In cases of pelvic organ prolapse one would expect the patient to be complaining of a bulge at the vaginal introitus.
- If present, kyphosis, or "dowager's hump," would suggest that osteoporotic vertebral fractures are the cause of pain. This forward bending of the upper spine results from the inability of the vertebral column to keep the patient upright. In addition to pain and obvious deformity, this condition causes morbidity by restricting lung volume. Kyphosis is also a cause of ambulatory instability, resulting in falls and additional fractures, often in the bones of the arms or legs.

History

- Ask about age of menopause and the use of hormone replacement therapy.
- Ask about chronic steroid use, or other medicines such as heparin or enoxaparin, which may be associated with bone loss.
- Inquire about sun exposure because of the relationship between vitamin D production and the skin. Vitamin D is vital for healthy bone regeneration.

- Inquire about calcium intake.
- Take a smoking history because smoking is a risk factor for the development of osteoporosis.
- Does the patient perform regular weight-bearing exercise? Is she sedentary?
- Take a good family history looking for relatives who may have had osteoporosis.

Physical Examination

- General appearance is important. Is the patient's spine straight? Do you see evidence of kyphosis or scoliosis? Absence of these signs alone does not rule out vertebral fracture because many patients can have one or more vertebral fractures without showing an obvious deformity.
- Vital signs, including height and weight. Height loss can be caused by osteoporosis, arthritis of the spine, or intervertebral disk shrinkage. A patient with a small frame is generally more at risk for bone loss.
- Palpate the spinous processes. Is this area tender? Unlike a long bone fracture, a compression fracture may not elicit tenderness over the affected vertebra. Patients with arthritis or disk disease may have point tenderness over certain areas, especially over the sacroiliac joint.
- Be sure to do a complete examination of the abdomen. Patients with arthritis often have radicular pain that radiates to the anterior abdominal wall.
- Pelvic examination in the lithotomy position should show a normal cervix and uterus, with no adnexal masses. Examine for cystocele, rectocele, and uterine prolapse.
- Do a thorough extremity examination; straight leg rising can sometimes elicit back pain.
- The neurologic examination is important. Look for evidence of foot drop, which can be a complication of sciatic nerve compression due to a ruptured or bulging intervertebral disk(s).

Tests for Consideration

- **25-OH vitamin D level:** Diagnoses one of the most common causes of osteoporosis: vitamin D deficiency. $60
- **Serum calcium level:** Helps to rule out hyperparathyroidism as cause of bone loss. This should be performed before instituting therapy for osteoporosis. $46
- **Intact parathyroid hormone level:** If calcium is abnormally high, may diagnose primary hyperparathyroidism, a rare cause of osteoporosis. $155
- **Urinalysis:** Microscopic hematuria might suggest renal calculi. $35

IMAGING CONSIDERATIONS

→**Anteroposterior and lateral spine radiographs:**
Diagnostic for vertebral compression fracture due
to osteoporosis and for the diagnosis of
osteoarthritis. $125

→**DEXA scan:** Spinal bone mineral density may be
falsely elevated if osteoarthritis coexists with
osteoporosis. Hip measurements are usually
not affected by osteoarthritis, and can thus
accurately diagnose osteoporosis if the measures
there are abnormal. $800

→**MRI of the spine:** Essential in the diagnosis of disk
disease. MRI is also useful in determining the age
of an osteoporotic fracture and in assessing whether
it can be treated by kyphoplasty. $1500

→**Plain film of the abdomen:** May diagnose renal
calculi or calcified uterine fibroids. $130

Clinical Entities   Medical Knowledge

Postmenopausal Osteoporosis/Osteoporotic Vertebral Fracture(s)

Pφ Between puberty and menopause, bone remodeling is balanced;
that is, the action of bone-resorbing osteoclasts is balanced by
the bone-forming osteoblasts. Estrogen loss after menopause
accelerates bone turnover by increasing osteoclastic resorption.
In addition to menopause, risk factors for bone loss include a
small frame, Asian or white race, smoking, and a family history
of osteoporosis. Bone loss is extremely common in women, with
half of women older than 50 years of age having significant bone
loss and high risk for osteoporotic fracture. Other medical
conditions that can cause bone loss are primary
hyperparathyroidism, chronic eating disorders, celiac disease,
vitamin D deficiency, and long-term treatment with thyroid
hormone or corticosteroids.

TP Osteoporosis is a silent disease, usually causing back pain only
after a vertebral compression fracture has occurred. Height loss
and kyphosis often occur before any painful symptoms. One
vertebral fracture significantly increases the risk of subsequent
fractures, including those of the hip, which may be life-
threatening.

Dx Virtually all postmenopausal women should be screened for osteoporosis at some point because it is such a prevalent disease. The DEXA scan measures bone mineral density at the lumbar spine and at the hip, and is reported as a T-score, which represents the difference (in standard deviations) between the patient's bone mass and the estimated theoretical peak bone mass of a 25–year-old. The World Health Organization defines osteopenia as a T-score between −1 and −2.5, osteoporosis as a T-score below −2.5, and severe osteoporosis as a T-score below −2.5 plus a history of a fragility fracture. Vertebral fractures can be diagnosed by measuring vertebral height on a lateral film. Serum or urine markers of bone formation and bone resorption have limited clinical value.

Tx For the treatment of acute vertebral fractures, kyphoplasty is a procedure in which bone cement is injected directly into the collapsed vertebral body to relieve pain and stabilize the vertebra. For treating osteoporosis, antiresorptive drugs decrease osteoclastic activity and slowly reverse bone loss to reduce the risk of fractures. These drugs include estrogen, calcitonin, the selective estrogen receptor modulator raloxifene, and the class of drugs called bisphosphonates (alendronate, risedronate, ibandronate, and zoledronic acid). Teriparatide, human recombinant parathyroid hormone (1-34), is an anabolic drug that stimulates bone formation when given as a subcutaneous injection. **See Katz 42, Hacker 35.**

Degenerative Disk Disease

Pφ The spinal vertebrae are separated by gelatinous disks that provide cushioning to the spinal column. These disks may herniate from trauma or strain, causing impingement on nerve roots. The lumbar spine area is the most often affected. Disk herniation is often a cause of back pain in women, although the condition is more common in men.

TP Presenting symptom is lower back pain, often radiating to the buttocks and posterior aspect of the leg (sciatica). Tingling, numbness, and muscle weakness in the lower extremity occur in later stages.

Dx A thorough history and physical and neurologic examination will often make the diagnosis. A positive straight leg raising test indicates lumbar disk disease. Spinal CT or MRI will diagnose the level of the disk herniation.

Tx The usual treatment is rest, pain medication, and anti-inflammatory medications, followed by physical therapy. Nonsteroidal anti-inflammatory drugs (NSAIDs) are most often used. Glucocorticoids injected into the epidural space may also be helpful. For some patients, surgical correction is necessary.

Osteoarthritis of the Lumbar Spine

Pφ Spondylosis (spinal arthritis) affects the four facet joints between vertebrae as a patient ages. The cartilage of the affected joint is gradually worn down, eventually causing bone to rub against bone. Bony spurs (osteophytes) develop on the unprotected bones, causing pain and inflammation.

TP Chronic lower back pain, unrelated to trauma, is the presenting symptom. Patients will often complain of stiffness on waking or after sitting for long periods, and then getting relief as they move around. As the joint disease worsens, spinal column deformities such as scoliosis or kyphosis may occur.

Dx Spinal radiographs reveal anatomic deformities and calcifications due to joint deterioration. Patients with spondylosis often exhibit signs of osteoarthritis in other joints, especially the interphalangeal joints of the fingers.

Tx Treatment is symptomatic because this is a chronic, degenerative disease. Mild back exercises may be helpful to strengthen the paravertebral muscles. NSAIDs are often helpful for relief of pain and inflammation. Surgery to remove bone spurs and relieve spinal stenosis is rarely needed.

Malignancy

Pφ A variety of malignancies that may or may not be clinically apparent (including breast and ovarian carcinoma and multiple myeloma) may be initially identified when they present as back pain caused by vertebral metastasis.

TP The typical patient may or may not carry a previous diagnosis of malignancy.

Dx MRI has become the gold standard for anatomic diagnosis of a vertebral metastasis. In a patient with a history or suspicion of breast cancer, a bone scan is an excellent first step and body survey.

Tx Specific therapy (e.g., chemo-, hormonal, radiation therapy and/or intervention for spinal stabilization) depends upon anatomy, tumor histology, and extent of systemic disease.

ZEBRA ZONE

a. **Osteogenesis imperfecta:** This is a type I collagen disorder that causes brittle bones and manifests itself in patients as increased bone fragility with subsequent fractures.

b. **Multiple myeloma:** May initially present as back pain due to vertebral fractures.

c. **Uterine or ovarian mass:** Many women (both premenopausal and postmenopausal) have uterine enlargement due to a posterior wall leiomyoma or adenomyosis. They may also have various types of ovarian cysts or tumors in the cul-de-sac. Any of these conditions may put pressure on the sacrum and cause back pain.

d. **Pelvic floor relaxation with uterine prolapse:** After menopause, relaxation of the pelvic floor can occur, with or without concurrent prolapse of the uterus, especially in (but not exclusive to) women who have had vaginal deliveries. Uterine prolapse can stress the supporting ligaments of the uterus and may cause lower back pain.

e. **Renal or ureteral calculus:** Urinary tract calculi can be a common cause of back pain. Stones may occur in the kidney, ureter, or bladder. Approximately 5% of women and 10% of men will experience a calculus in their lifetime. Calcium stones are most common, followed by uric acid stones. Calculi often recur.

Practice-Based Learning and Improvement: Evidence-Based Medicine

Title
Risks and benefits of estrogen plus progestin in healthy postmenopausal women: Principal results from the Women's Health Initiative randomized controlled trial

Authors
Rossouw JE, Anderson GL, Prentice RL, et al.; Writing Group for the Women's Health Initiative Investigators

Institution
National Heart, Lung and Blood Institute, Bethesda, Maryland

Reference
Journal of the American Medical Association 2002;288:321–333

Problem
To assess the major health benefits and risks of the most commonly used combined hormone preparation in the United States.

Intervention

Participants received conjugated equine estrogens, 0.625 mg/day, plus medroxyprogesterone acetate, 2.5 mg/day, in 1 tablet (n = 8506) or placebo (n = 8102).

Comparison/control (quality of evidence)

Level I. Primary research. Randomized, placebo-controlled, double-blind study.

Outcome/effect

Risks of therapy exceeded benefits, and the study was stopped prematurely after 5.2 years of follow-up. The risks associated with therapy were an increase in invasive breast cancer, stroke, pulmonary embolus, and coronary heart disease. Benefits were a decrease in colorectal cancer, and all fractures, including hip fractures.

Historical significance/comments

After the results of this study were announced, most women who were taking hormone therapy stopped, and most women entering menopause now opt not to begin hormone therapy at all. There has been an approximate 70% reduction in the use of estrogen/progesterone therapy among perimenopausal and postmenopausal women since the Women's Health Initiative study. Consequently, we can certainly expect to see greater numbers of women with bone loss and osteoporotic fractures in the future.

Interpersonal and Communication Skills

Detecting and Discussing Underlying Concerns

A patient whose back pain has been diagnosed as being caused by an osteoporotic fracture will frequently be reminded of one of her relatives who had severe osteoporosis or some related postmenopausal bone issue or fracture. Many women have had a mother or grandmother who had severe spinal deformity related to repeated vertebral fractures, or who may have been confined to a wheelchair or a nursing home after a hip fracture. The past histories of others undoubtedly stimulate fears. In this instance, the patient's fear may be about potential loss of independence. Such "psychological baggage" is common for all us because we all have fears based on memories and previous experiences. Listen carefully and look for cues of such concerns. Encourage your patient to discuss these issues. You will usually be able to allay unfounded fears and this may have a profound impact on your relationship.

Professionalism

Principle: Primacy of Patient Welfare

There is a temptation to become judgmental when one sees a patient in whom lifestyle or lifestyle choices or behaviors have directly contributed to or exacerbated her disease process. An example of this is osteoporosis. This is a disease that has a hereditary basis and is accelerated by the acquired loss of estrogen, but it is also exacerbated by smoking and excessive use of alcohol. As standard treatment for osteoporosis, it is appropriate for the clinician to discuss these matters with the patient and even to state that an integral component to treatment must/should include cessation of smoking and alcohol use only in moderation. It is not appropriate, however, to chastise or belittle patients for behaviors even if we believe them to be counter to their best health interests.

Systems-Based Practice

Capital Investment: DEXA Scanners

In an effort to monitor for signs of osteopenia and osteoporosis, DEXA scanners have become a major part of the care of postmenopausal women. Increasingly, physicians—primary care, obstetricians/gynecologists, and orthopedists—are investing in DEXA scanners in an effort to increase profitability and enhance patient convenience. Because a top-of-the-line central scanner typically costs $75,000 to $80,000, it is important for physicians to determine the financial implications of such an investment before making it.

The central question in any capital investment decision is whether the future revenues generated by the investment will exceed the cost of the investment. One might think that figuring out the cost of an investment like this is easy—it is what the manufacturer is going to charge you. But most large capital investments like this are paid for with loans. In addition to saving the medical group from having to put up a large sum of cash, this allows the group to spread out the cost of the scanner over time, just as the revenues the scanner will generate are spread out over time. This principle of matching costs and revenues in time is a core concept in accounting and finance that allows one to have a better sense of whether something is or is not profitable.

For instance, if the total initial cost of a scanner (including all of the set-up costs) ends up being $100,000, a medical group might take out a 5-year bank loan at 5% interest, with the belief that the scanner should be profitable within 5 years. Such a loan would require 5 years of monthly payments of approximately $5200. In doing this, you have now turned a capital investment into an operating cost that can be matched against the machine's revenues. In addition to the cost of financing the machine itself, you also need to consider other operating costs, such as staffing and supplies. A small practice can typically train an existing staffer to run such a machine, so it would be fair to allocate some part of that staffer's salary—maybe $1400 a month—to the cost of the machine. We also need to allocate the cost of the additional space (say, $500/month), supply costs ($400/month), additional electricity, and maintenance. This brings our operating cost to $2300 a month, plus the $5200 a month for the loan, bringing us to a total operating cost of $7500 a month.

Figuring out revenues involves determining the number of tests you will be able to do, and the expected reimbursements. Let's assume an average Medicare reimbursement for a DEXA scan (CPT Code 76075) of about $138 . Assuming you will schedule scans for weekdays only, and one day off per month for maintenance, one scan per day will generate ($138/scan) × (1 scan/day) × (20 days/month) = $2760 in revenue per month. In order to break even, we will need at least three scans per day:

Scans per Day	Profit
0	($7500)
1	($4740)
2	($1980)
3	$780
4	$3540
5	$6300
6	$9060
7	$11,820

The economics of DEXA scanners has been studied, and the evidence suggests that a referring primary care physician will (on average) generate at most one scan per day. Accordingly, for such an investment to be profitable, one typically needs approximately four or five referring physicians.

The lesson is not to understand the specifics of investing in DEXA scanners, but rather to recognize the basic principles involved in making a capital investment decision—decisions that hospitals and, increasingly, physicians need to make.

Chapter 44
Human Papillomavirus–Related Vulvar Disease (Case 29)

Michelle Vichnin MD

Case: A 27-year-old G2P2 presents for her annual examination with complaints of multiple vulvar "bumps" that have been present for a few months. The lesions are not itchy but have increased in number. Her last gynecologic examination and Pap test were 2 years ago.

Differential Diagnosis

Condylomata acuminata (genital warts)	Skin tags (benign fibroepithelial polyps)	Molluscum contagiosum

Speaking Intelligently

When evaluating a patient who presents with genital lesions, a detailed history (in particular, sexual history) is very important. For example, patients with painful ulcerative lesions are more likely to have genital herpes. Patients with painless lesions are more likely to have genital warts or other viral infections such as molluscum contagiosum. Syphilis and Behçet syndrome can also present as painless vulvar lesions, but these are typically ulcerative. The physical examination should help you confirm what you already suspect from the history.

PATIENT CARE

Clinical Thinking
- Presume the patient has a relatively concerning problem because she is presenting for care and this is not always an easy thing to do.
- Be willing to pursue other problems, especially other sexually transmitted infections (STIs), even if a single STI can be identified.

- Offer human immunodeficiency virus (HIV) testing when appropriate.
- Offer contraception counseling if you know the patient is at risk for pregnancy.
- Encourage safer sexual practices.

History
- Age at first intercourse: The younger the woman is at the age of first intercourse, the higher the likelihood of acquiring human papillomavirus (HPV) infection. Consider asking about time interval between menarche and coitarche: a shortened time frame increases risk owing to increased surface area of the transformation zone on the cervix
- Number of partners: Higher numbers equal higher risk of acquiring an HPV infection.
- Smoking: An independent risk factor for cervical cancer.
- History of prior genital warts: Recurrence is common.
- History of abnormal Pap smear results: Often patients are infected with multiple types of HPV.
- History of any STIs: Having one STI increases the risk of having another.
- History of loop electrosurgical excision procedure (LEEP) or cold knife conization.
- History of immunocompromise (e.g., HIV, transplant): Increases risk of recurrent, difficult-to-treat genital warts as well as cervical dysplasia.

Physical Examination
- **Vital signs:** Check for fever.
- **Full pelvic examination:** Include careful inspection of mons, labia minora and majora, urethra, and perineum and perianal area; note size, number, and shape (papillary, cauliflower-like, or umbilicated appearance) of lesions.
- It is helpful to draw a diagram of your findings in the chart.
- Speculum examination of the vagina with visualization of the cervix and vagina.
- Bimanual examination.

Tests for Consideration
- **Pap test** $340
- **Tests for other STIs:** Gonorrhea/chlamydial infection. $140
- **Biopsy of vulvar lesion:** If unsure of diagnosis. $350
- **Colposcopy:** If Pap test result warrants. Atypical squamous cells of undetermined significance (ASCUS) + high-risk HPV, or a more advanced lesion, would suggest need for a colposcopic examination. $415

Condylomata Acuminata (Genital Warts)

Pφ The human papillomavirus (HPV) causes this condition. HPV types 6 and 11 are known to cause approximately 90% of genital warts. HPV attacks the basal layer of the epithelium, where it multiplies and causes changes in the squamous cells. Typically, lesions occur 3 to 6 months after initial exposure to the virus. However, incubation periods may be underestimated and subclinical infection may be present for months to years before clinical evidence of the disease becomes apparent.

TP Typically, a patient will present with complaints of growths, bumps, or warts on the vagina or vulva. Some women present when they first notice the lesions, whereas others may wait for long periods before seeking treatment. These papillary lesions can be small or large, unifocal or multifocal, and often have the typical "cauliflower" appearance. Warts can also be very small and almost flat in appearance. In immunosuppressed patients, genital warts can be very large and can grow rapidly, often distorting the anatomy. In pregnancy, women often have recurrence of warts; rarely warts grow so large that they obstruct the vaginal canal.

Dx The vast majority of genital warts are diagnosed by visual inspection. However, unifocal lesions can look like skin tags. Smaller, diffuse papular lesions can look like molluscum contagiosum. When the diagnosis is unclear, or if treatment is not working, biopsy is recommended.

Tx There are multiple treatments for genital warts. Treatment can be chosen based on the patient preference and the size, number, and location of the lesions. Response rates to the various therapies range from approximately 5% to 60% and recurrence is common within the first 3 months after treatment. Patients often need several treatments to control the disease.

1. *Trichloroacetic acid (85%):* Desiccant therapy applied to the lesions by the provider in the office setting; can be painful. Clinicians can use petroleum jelly to protect the normal skin around the lesions. May need multiple treatments every week until the lesion is completely gone.
2. *Podofilox (Condylox):* Mechanism of action is unknown. Applied twice a day for 3 days in a row, and may be repeated for 1 to 4 weeks.

3. *Imiquimod (Aldara):* Patient-applied immune modulator medication; applied in the evening for 3 days/week (M/W/F or T/Th/Sat) and patient washes off in the morning. Can be applied weekly for a total of 4 months.
4. *Excision:* When lesions are large and pedunculated, excision works well. Excision is not recommended for multiple lesions spread over the entire vulva because of the pain and disfigurement that surgery can cause.
5. *Laser therapy:* Good choice for lesions recalcitrant to medications or spread over the entire vulva or up into the vagina. This therapy is most often performed as an outpatient procedure. In severe cases, when warts involve the entire vulva, laser treatment can be very painful. Patients sometimes need to be managed postoperatively with pain medication and Foley catheter placement in the inpatient setting.
6. *Cryotherapy:* Uses liquid nitrogen; can be used for smaller, more unifocal lesions.
   See Katz 22, Hacker 22.

Skin Tags (Benign Fibroepithelial Polyps)

Pφ A fibroepithelial polyp is a benign polypoid mass of tissue found on hair-bearing skin of the vulva.

TP Often patients present with the complaint of a lump or bump of the vulva that can be irritated by underwear. Can be confused with genital warts.

Dx Usually diagnosed by inspection; if there is any doubt about the diagnosis, the lesion should be excised or sampled for biopsy.

Tx These lesions do not need to be removed unless they bother the patient.

Molluscum Contagiosum

Pφ The molluscum contagiosum virus, a pox virus, causes these papular, centrally umbilicated lesions that can be present on the vulva as well as other parts of the body. This infection is most common in children 2 to 10 years of age, and lesions are spread by direct skin-to-skin contact as well as by fomites (such as shared towels). In teens and adults, molluscum contagiosum is most commonly an STI. The lesions are often self-limiting, resolving in 6 to 12 months, but sometimes it can take as long a 4 years for complete resolution.

TP Patients may be asymptomatic with this disease. Most often they present to their physicians complaining of small bumps on the vulva and are concerned that they have an STI such as genital warts.

Dx The diagnosis is made on visual inspection if the classic, centrally umbilicated papular lesions are noted. Sometimes the lesions mimic the smaller condylomata, and biopsy is necessary to establish the diagnosis.

Tx There are multiple treatments for molluscum contagiosum. Patients need to be aware that scarring and skin discoloration can occur after treatment.

1. Curettage with a scalpel or tip of an 18-gauge needle.
2. Cryotherapy with liquid nitrogen and a very fine-tipped applicator.
3. Trichloroacetic acid application (as described previously).
4. Large lesions may be excised.
   See Katz 22.

ZEBRA ZONE

a. **Vulvar cancer:** This is a relatively uncommon gynecologic malignancy, representing less than 5% of all gynecologic malignancies. Most vulvar carcinomas are squamous cell in origin, but a small number of vulvar melanomas and basal cell carcinomas can also be seen. HPV-related vulvar cancer occurs most commonly in younger women. The variant of squamous cell vulvar cancer that occurs in older women is not usually HPV related, and is associated with vulvar intraepithelial neoplasia (VIN) III.

   Vulvar cancer usually presents with obvious vulvar lesions that are associated with pruritus. Lesions can appear pink, red, pale, tan, or any combination of these colors. Some have a verrucous appearance. Any suspect lesion of the vulva should be sampled for biopsy. The primary method of treatment for VIN III, which is considered a precursor lesion to vulvar cancer, is wide local excision. After a diagnosis of vulvar cancer is reached with histologic findings, the patient should be staged. The International Federation of Gynecology and Obstetrics (FIGO) introduced surgical staging for vulvar cancer in 1989, and this was further revised in 1994 (Table 44-1).

Table 44-1 International Federation of Gynecology and Obstetrics (FIGO) Staging of Vulvar Carcinoma (1994)

Stage 0	Carcinoma in situ, intraepithelial carcinoma
Stage I	Tumor confined to the vulva or perineum, or both, and 2 cm or less in greatest dimension; no nodal metastasis
Stage Ia	As above with stromal invasion ≤1 mm
Stage Ib	As above with stromal invasion >1 mm
Stage II	Tumor confined to the vulva or perineum, or both, and more than 2 cm in greatest dimension; no nodal metastasis
Stage III	Tumor of any size with: 1. Adjacent spread to the urethra and/or vagina, and/or the anus. 2. Unilateral regional lymph node metastasis, or a combination
Stage IV	
Stage IVa	Tumor invades any of the following: upper urethra, bladder mucosa, rectal mucosa, pelvic bone or bilateral regional node metastasis, or a combination
Stage IVb	Any distant metastasis, including pelvic lymph nodes

From Hacker N, Gambone J, Hobel C: Hacker & Moore's Essentials of Obstetrics and Gynecology, 5th ed. Philadelphia, Elsevier Saunders, 2009.

Much emphasis has been placed recently on vulvar-sparing surgery. In the past, more extensive vulvar resection with bilateral groin and pelvic node lymphadenectomy was the standard of treatment, but this strategy had a very high rate of associated morbidity. Today, wide local excision is commonly performed, with an ipsilateral groin lymphadenectomy performed through a separate incision. Only midline lesions require bilateral lymphadenectomy. Patients with stage Ia disease do not require a lymphadenectomy because the likelihood of lymphatic spread is low.

b. Folliculitis: Superficial inflammation of hair follicles usually caused by bacteria, especially *Staphylococcus aureus*.

c. Epidermal inclusion cysts: Small cysts caused by epidermal cells that have become invaginated into the dermis.

d. Lipoma: Benign soft tissue tumor composed of adipose tissue.

Practice-Based Learning and Improvement: Evidence-Based Medicine

Title
The diagnosis and treatment of human papillomavirus-mediated genital lesions

Authors
Brodell LA, Mercurio MG, Brodell RT

Institution
University of Rochester School of Medicine and Dentistry, Rochester, New York

Reference
Cutis 2007;79(4 Suppl):5–10

Problem
Therapeutic management of genital warts.

Intervention
Assesses diagnosis and treatment options (office-based and home) of genital warts.

Comparison/control (quality of evidence)
Review article.

Outcome/effect
Suggests that newer, home-based treatments can be effective in the treatment of genital warts.

Historical significance/comments
This comprehensive review article articulates several options for home-based care and treatment of condylomata acuminata.

Interpersonal and Communication Skills

Helping Patients Deal with Personal Guilt
When a woman finds out that she has an STI such as genital warts, she may feel "dirty" or "unclean." Anticipate guilt turned inward and anger turned outward. It is helpful to emphasize that HPV infection is common and that nearly 80% of women may be infected with HPV at some point in their lives. While helping your patient to dispel guilt for acquiring the HPV virus, any unsafe sexual practices should certainly be identified and discouraged. Emphasize that this condition is treatable, and in most cases resolves on its own or with minimal intervention.

Professionalism

Principle: Social Justice

A 28-year-old woman presents to the gynecology clinic for a routine health maintenance visit. You finish taking her history and tell her that she should have a pelvic examination and Pap test as part of her visit.

A: The patient says that she would be more comfortable having a *female* doctor perform this part of the exam and asks if there is someone else in the clinic that day.

B: The patient says that she would be more comfortable having a *male* doctor perform this part of the exam and asks if there is someone else in the clinic that day.

The principle of social justice is a very complex concept; a full discussion is beyond the scope of this text. The essence of this principle is that all individuals should be treated justly, in all aspects of life and society, not just in the realm of the law. Physicians should be committed to providing equal and just care to patients of all backgrounds. Patients bring with them all sorts of preconceived notions and beliefs regarding how they can be best taken care of, and who is best equipped to provide the care they need. When it is possible, it is always best to honor a patient's request for a specific physician. When this is not possible, simply explain to the patient that the individual she requests is not available. The patients will then be able to make an autonomous decision whether to be seen or to reschedule. In cases of emergency, explain to the patient that she will be taken care of by the team present.

Systems-Based Practice

Reimbursement: Copayments and Deductibles

You have just examined a woman who has a vulvar lesion requiring biopsy. You escort her to the reception desk to set up a follow-up appointment and your secretary asks her for her copay.

Contrary to what many people believe, the primary reason for these payments is not to reduce the cost of the procedure or office visit to the insurance company. In fact, copays are often only a very small fraction of the cost of the procedure. The real reason is that a small fee deters people from seeking care that they do not need. Health economists have studied this issue—which they call the *elasticity of demand*—extensively, and realized that when health care is entirely free, people seek out unnecessary care above what they need. However, when a small piece of the cost is handed over to the patient, they seek only the care that they need. If the amount is too high (such as with the uninsured) they don't seek out care that they do need. So the trick is to get the amount right—enough that people won't waste health care dollars, but small enough that people will get the care that they need.

Chapter 45
Pap Testing and Cervical Cytologic Surveillance (Case 30)

Janine M. Barsoum DO

Case: A 25-year-old, sexually active woman presents to your office to discuss management of her first abnormal Pap smear. This Pap test was performed about 6 weeks ago at a nearby clinic and she is unsure about the actual wording of the report and the clinical implications.

Differential Diagnosis

Atypical squamous cells of undetermined significance (**ASCUS**)	Low grade squamous intraepithelial lesion (**LSIL**)
Atypical glandular cells of undetermined significance (**AGUS**)	High grade squamous intraepithelial lesion (**HSIL**)

Editor's note to students: Please note that the following terms are commonly used interchangeably in the field of obstetrics and gynecology:
LSIL = LGSIL
HSIL = HGSIL
AGUS = AGS

Speaking Intelligently

A ***Pap test*** is a screening test for precancerous or cancerous changes in cervical cells. The test was first described by Giorgios Papanicolaou, and carries his name. Although an abnormal Pap result does not diagnose cancer, it is used to identify women who require further testing (e.g., colposcopy, biopsy, human papillomavirus [HPV]). In general, I recommend that my patients have an annual Pap test unless there are circumstances that dictate a different surveillance routine. Infection with certain types of HPV is the most common risk factor for an abnormal Pap smear. Women who are positive for high-risk HPV strains (16, 18, and others) are at risk for cervical changes known as ***dysplasia.*** Other important risk factors for abnormal cervical cellular changes include a history of multiple sexual partners or partners with multiple sexual contacts, a history of sexually transmitted infection (STI), human immunodeficiency virus (HIV) infection, chronic immunosuppression, cigarette smoking, and first sexual intercourse before age 17 years. There are several types of abnormal Pap smear results, and each result requires a specific type of evaluation. *Colposcopy* is an office procedure used to magnify the cervix, allowing the clinician to better visualize changes and perform diagnostic biopsies of abnormal areas.

PATIENT CARE

Clinical Thinking
- When managing a patient with an abnormal Pap test, the clinician must consider the patient's age, risk factors, and Pap test history. Diagnostic and therapeutic modalities are affected by these factors.
- It is important to differentiate those cervical lesions that are at risk for progressing to invasive cervical cancer from those that will likely resolve spontaneously over time.

History
- Inquire about past sexual history of STIs and prior HPV status.
- Ask about number of sexual partners and about the sexual behavior of these partners.
- Ask about cigarette, alcohol, and drug use. Include the possibility of prescription drug abuse.
- Note previous Pap test history.
- Obtain a complete medical history, including chronic asthma (requiring steroids), immunosuppressive disorders, organ transplantation, and HIV infection.

Physical Examination
- Use a speculum to visually inspect the cervix and vagina; when indicated, perform a colposcopic examination:
  - The cervix should be prepared with acetic acid and then inspected, using a colposcope, for areas of acetowhite changes. Look for abnormal vascular patterns, and islands of "mosaicism" or punctuations, which generally indicate neovascularization.
  - Lugol's iodine can also be used to define cervical changes; normal epithelium will stain brown and dysplastic areas will not take up the dye and appear pale in comparison.
  - Any visible lesion that is raised, ulcerated, or friable should be sampled for biopsy regardless of prior cytologic findings.

Tests for Consideration

- **Cervical cytology:** Cervical screening Pap test; either conventional smear or newer thin-layer liquid preparation. $250
- **HPV testing:** The main indication for HPV testing in women younger than 30 years of age is to triage women with cytology interpreted as ASCUS. $100
- **Colposcopy:** Diagnostic test; may include cervical biopsies and endocervical curettage. Colposcopy should generally be performed as described previously to evaluate Pap test abnormalities of ASCUS level or greater, per the American Society for Colposcopy and Cervical Pathology Consensus Guidelines (see asccp.org). $300
- **Endocervical curettage** (scraping of the endocervical canal): Performed to identify occult lesions. $50

Clinical Entities	Medical Knowledge

Atypical Squamous Cells of Undetermined Significance (ASCUS)

Pφ Cells display changes not characterized as squamous intraepithelial lesion (SIL), but more marked than reactive changes. Common and often associated with spontaneous resolution. Although there is a low risk of cancer (0.1% to 0.2%), 5% to 17% of ASCUSs may reveal a *pre*cancerous lesion at biopsy.

TP Usually asymptomatic, but can present with postcoital bleeding.

Dx The preferred approach to an ASCUS Pap result is reflex HPV testing; most women with ASCUS and high-risk HPV are triaged to colposcopy for further evaluation. Women with ASCUS who test negative for HPV are followed with repeat cytology in 12 months. The small subset of patients with ASCUS in whom *high-grade SIL cannot be ruled out* are directed to immediate colposcopy because of a higher chance of moderate/severe dysplasia on biopsy.

Tx Treatment of ASCUS depends on colposcopic findings. Biopsies consistent with mild cervical dysplasia are followed with frequent cytology. Biopsies exhibiting moderate or severe dysplasia are treated with either ablative (cryotherapy, electrocautery, or laser) or excisional procedures. **See Katz 28, Hacker 38.**

Low-Grade Squamous Intraepithelial Lesions (LSIL)

Pφ With LSIL changes noted on cytology, the risk of underlying moderate/high-grade dysplasia is 15% to 30%. Up to 80% of women with LSIL are HPV positive, so testing is not used in management. LSIL is common in adolescent women and is conservatively managed because clearance of HPV in this population is high and cancer rates are low.

TP Usually asymptomatic, but can present with postcoital bleeding.

Dx Colposcopy is recommended for most women; adolescents may be followed with repeat cytology if compliance can be ensured.

Tx Treatment of LSIL depends on colposcopic findings. Biopsies consistent with mild cervical dysplasia are followed with frequent cytology. Biopsies exhibiting moderate or severe dysplasia are treated with either ablative (cryotherapy or laser) or excisional procedures. **See Katz 28, Hacker 38.**

High-Grade Squamous Intraepithelial Lesions (HSIL)

Pφ A result of HSIL carries a 70% chance of underlying moderate/severe dysplasia, and a 1% to 2% risk of invasive cancer.

TP Usually asymptomatic, but can present with postcoital bleeding.

Dx Cervical colposcopy should be performed. The entire vagina should be inspected, especially in the absence of an obvious cervical lesion. Endocervical evaluation completes the evaluation.

Tx Treatment of HSIL depends on colposcopic findings. Biopsies consistent with mild cervical dysplasia are followed with caution. Cytology and biopsy histology should be reviewed.

In the absence of biopsy proven high-grade dysplastic lesions noted on colposcopy (reflecting a discrepency between Pap test screening and colposcopic findings), an excisional procedure such as a cold knife cone biopsy or loop electrocautery excision procedure (LEEP) should be performed to ensure no dysplasia has been missed. Biopsies exhibiting moderate or severe dysplasia are treated with excisional procedures. **See Katz 28, Hacker 38.**

Atypical Glandular Cells of Undetermined Significance (AGUS)

Pφ The finding of atypical glandular cells (AGC) includes subcategories based on histologic location (endocervical vs. endometrial), and degree of cellular change ("not otherwise specified" vs. "favor neoplasia"). This category also includes adenocarcinoma in situ and adenocarcinoma. AGC is associated with a 9% to 41% risk of moderate/severe dysplasia. If "favor neoplasia" is the result, the risk is 27% to 96%.

TP Often asymptomatic, but can present with postcoital bleeding, abnormal vaginal bleeding, and postmenopausal bleeding.

Dx All women should undergo complete cervical and vaginal colposcopy as well as endocervical curettage. Any woman with atypical endometrial cells should also have an endometrial biopsy to evaluate the uterine lining. Any woman with an AGC Pap result who is older than 35 years of age should also have endometrial sampling.

Tx The treatment of AGUS Pap findings depends on the findings of the examination described previously. **See Katz 28, Hacker 38.**

Practice-Based Learning and Improvement: Evidence-Based Medicine

Title
A randomized trial on the management of low-grade squamous intraepithelial lesion cytology interpretations

Authors
ASCUS-LSIL Triage Study (ALTS) Group

Institution
Multicenter

Reference
American Journal of Obstetrics and Gynecology 2003;188:1393–1400

Problem
Study undertaken to compare alternative strategies for the initial management of LSIL cytology. More simply put, what is the best way to follow patients who have LSIL Pap test results?

Intervention
A large sampling of patients (1572) with a community-based LSIL interpretation were randomly assigned to immediate colposcopy, triage based on enrollment HPV DNA testing and liquid-based cytology at a colposcopy referral threshold of high-grade squamous intraepithelial lesion (HSIL), or conservative management based on repeat cytology at a referral threshold of HSIL.

Comparison/control (quality of evidence)
Level I: large, randomized study that compared follow-up and triage strategies for ASCUS and LSIL.

Outcome/effect
Advocated use of HPV status as triage tool for ASC; provided treatment algorithms for ASC and LSIL (see 2006 Consensus Guidelines for the Management of Women with Abnormal Cervical Cancer Screening Tests, ASCCP, 2006. Available at http://www.asccp. org/consensus/cytological.shtml.)

Historical significance/comments
Provided information on natural history of cervical intraepithelial neoplasia. Confirmed relationship of abnormal cytology, histology, and HPV results to moderate/severe dysplasia.

Practice-Based Learning and Improvement

Evidence-Based Medicine Curriculum
Residents rotate as leaders of a group session to discuss the application of evidence-based medicine to the care of one of their own patients. In preparation, the presenting resident should develop a focused clinical question, conduct a literature search, critically appraise the evidence, and then demonstrate application of the evidence to the care of his/her patient.

Consider, for example, an issue in the management of cervical cytology, the focus of this chapter: widespread use of HPV testing is not yet commonplace throughout the medical community. Inattention to HPV testing data can lead to the over-treatment of pap test abnormalities, particularly in adolescents and women with low-grade lesions. A careful review of *Algorithms: 2006 Consensus Guidelines for the Management of Women with Cervical Cytology Abnormalities,* an evidence-based guideline published by the American Society for Colposcopy and Cervical Pathology (ASCCP), could potentially be very beneficial in this clinical circumstance.

Interpersonal and Communication Skills

Smoking Cessation
For reasons that are not entirely understood, cigarette smoking has a high correlation with Pap test abnormalities and cervical dysplasia. Although cigarette use is generally diminishing in the general population, cigarette use among teens and women in their twenties (a population at high risk to acquire HPV infection) continues to be prevalent. It is estimated that 13% of pregnant women in the United States smoke during pregnancy. At an office visit in which you address an abnormal Pap result, other health maintenance issues (when appropriate) should be integral parts of your management discussion, including safe sexual practices, drug abuse, and smoking cessation. In the population of your patients who may become

pregnant, you should indicate that smoking while pregnant is a cause for concern. Discuss the availability of smoking cessation support groups, nicotine patches and gum, and sustained-release bupropion as possible options.

Professionalism

Principle: Commitment to Maintaining Appropriate Relations with Patients

Human papillomavirus is a central factor in the development of cervical dysplasia and cervical cancer. It is also an STI. A discussion of risk factors for the development of HPV infection will often raise many sensitive issues, including the number of one's sexual partners and questions about specific sexual practices. The clinician must not be judgmental in asking such questions. Instead of asking, for example, "Have you been sleeping with a lot of people recently?" it would be more appropriate to phrase your question, "How many sexual partners have you had in the past six months?" The former phrasing is judgmental and implies that "you've been sleeping with 'a lot' of partners," whereas the language of the latter phrasing is a neutral question and, therefore, more appropriate.

Systems-Based Practice

Clinical Practice Guidelines

Management of abnormal cervical cytology has changed recently with the advent of HPV testing and ground-breaking studies describing the regression and progression of various cervical lesions. The main focus of management should stress treatment for lesions associated with progression and conservative management of lesions likely to be self-limited.

Part of the movement toward evidence-based medicine has been the development and maintenance of clinical practice guidelines— roadmaps of care—that reflect the best treatment decisions given the current literature. There are multiple guidelines for the management of abnormal cervical cytology.

Which guideline one follows is often a factor of the institutional affiliation or opinion of the clinical leadership in the community. Nevertheless, despite the fact that such guidelines are considered to reflect the best care, and result in the best outcomes, there is significant evidence showing that there is considerable variance in adherence to such guidelines.[1] Some of this variance in adherence is due to differences in opinion, but much is due to the lack of willingness among many physicians to accept that any standardized guideline can provide better care than their own clinical judgment. This sentiment, however, increasingly stands in conflict with the evidence; and, as physicians are increasingly required to practice evidence-based medicine, it is likely that clinical guidelines will play an increasing role in the care of patients.

Reference

1. Singhal R, Rubenstein LV, Wang M, et al: Variations in practice guideline adherence for abnormal cervical cytology in a county healthcare system. J Gen Intern Med 2008;23:575–580.

Chapter 46
Breast Cancer Screening (Case 31)

Robin M. Ciocca DO, Paula H. Termuhlen MD, and Ari D. Brooks MD

Case: A 54-year-old woman presents for her yearly gynecologic examination. She has a benign breast examination and you recommend routine mammographic screening for early detection of breast cancer.

Speaking Intelligently

When I am asked to see a patient, one of my first questions is: "Should this patient be receiving annual screening mammography?" The widespread use of screening and diagnostic mammography has contributed significantly to the decrease in death from breast cancer seen over the past several decades. Patients need to be educated on the importance of yearly mammography and monthly self-breast examination. As physicians who sometimes act as the primary care doctor for women of childbearing age, it is incumbent on the obstetrician/gynecologist to take an active role in recommending and arranging appropriate mammographic screening. As the primary care provider for many women, it is imperative that you are able to guide the care of patients who have palpable masses or suspect radiologic findings. Make sure you know who does the mammography in your area. Get to know their radiology practices and, most important, what system the radiology practice uses to notify patients and referring physicians of abnormal findings. How do they ensure patients return for additional images? Do they track the outcomes of their abnormal mammograms? Establish a system to review all your patients' radiology reports in a timely fashion. Your role in keeping your patients in touch with the radiology center needs to be clear, so that no follow-up study or biopsy is delayed or missed. You need to know the published guidelines for breast cancer screening as well as the language of the Breast Imaging Reporting and Data System (BI-RADS®) lexicon for the categorization of mammographic findings, both of which are included in the following text.

Breast Cancer Screening Recommendations

- **Mammograms:** Should be ordered yearly on all women older than 40 years of age per American Cancer Society guidelines. For women with a significant family history for breast cancer, mammography should begin 10 years before the age of the family member diagnosed at the youngest age (i.e., for a woman whose aunt was diagnosed at age 45 years, she should begin at age 35 years).
- **Clinical breast examination (CBE):** Should be performed as part of routine physical examination at least every 3 years for women 20 to 40 years of age and yearly for women older than 40 years of age.
- **Self-breast examination (SBE):** Women should be encouraged to perform SBE on a monthly basis; information is available from the American Cancer Society as well as multiple other sites to educate patients on proper technique.

The BI-RADS® Lexicon

The American College of Radiology's BI-RADS® lexicon (Table 46-1) is a systems-based approach to reporting the results of mammography that standardizes a common language to facilitate communication between radiologists, referring physicians, and patients.

Table 46-1 Breast Imaging Reporting and Database System (BI-RADS®)

Category	Assessment	Follow-up Recommendations
a. Mammographic Assessment Is Incomplete		
0	Need additional imaging evaluation and/or prior mammograms for comparison	Additional imaging and/or prior images are needed before a final assessment can be assigned
b. Mammographic Assessment Is Complete—Final Categories		
1	Negative	Routine annual screening mammography (for women over age 40)
2	Benign finding(s)	Routine annual screening mammography (for women over age 40)
3	Probably benign finding—initial short-interval follow-up suggested	Initial short-term follow up (usually 6-month) examination

Category	Assessment	Follow-up Recommendations
4	Suspicious abnormality—biopsy should be considered Optional subdivisions:* 4A: Finding needing intervention with a low suspicion of malignancy 4B: Lesions with an intermediate suspicion of malignancy 4C: Finding of moderate concern, but not classic for malignancy	Usually requires biopsy
5	Highly suggestive of malignancy— appropriate action should be taken	Requires biopsy or surgical treatment
6	Known biopsy-proven malignancy— appropriate action should be taken	Category reserved for lesions identified on imaging study with biopsy proof of malignancy prior to definitive therapy

*A subdivision may be used **in addition to** the Category 4 final assessment; MQSA does **not** allow a subdivision to replace a Category 4 final assessment. Use of subdivision is at the discretion of the facility it is not required by the FDA. From the American College of Radiology (ACR). ACR BI-RADS®—4th Edition. ACR Breast Imaging Reporting and Data System, Breast Imaging Atlas; BI-RADS. Reston, VA. American College of Radiology; 2003. *Reprinted with permission of the American College of Radiology. No other representation of this material is authorized without expressed, written permission from the American College of Radiology.*

PATIENT CARE

Scenario 1: The Mammogram of Minimal Concern

Most (95% of the time) your patient's mammogram will be read as a BI-RADS® 1, 2, 3, or 0:

- Negative (BI-RADS® 1): There was no significant mass, calcifications, or architectural distortion seen. There is a less than 1% chance of malignancy.

- Benign findings (BI-RADS® 2): A benign-appearing mass is seen, benign-shaped calcifications are seen, or a finding is re-demonstrated as unchanged. There is about a 1% chance of malignancy.
- Probably benign (BI-RADS® 3): A new finding of a benign-appearing mass, change in a benign calcification pattern, or other change from previous images. There is a 3% to 6% chance of malignancy.
- Assessment incomplete; need prior films or additional studies (BI-RADS® 0).

If the findings of the patient's mammogram are either negative or benign, it is recommended that you continue with routine annual screening. A BI-RADS® 3 finding usually requires reimaging (with mammography or ultrasonography) after some interval. Order the follow-up test, schedule it with the patient, and note the date it is due. If the assessment is incomplete, urge the patient to obtain old films or schedule the recommended additional films in a timely fashion. Make sure to look for the new report.

Scenario 2: The Mammogram of Significant Concern

Unfortunately, your patient's study may be concerning to the radiologist (<5%). Typical BI-RADS® 4 or 5 interpretations will read as follows:
- Suspicious (BI-RADS® 4): A finding of calcifications with morphology that could be malignant (pleomorphic, clustered, branching pattern, or associated with a mass), or a finding of a mass that has indistinct borders or significant density. About 15% to 30% of these will turn out to be malignant.
- Highly suspicious (BI-RADS® 5): A finding of a mass with spiculation and associated parenchymal or skin changes or calcification patterns that are most likely malignant. About 80% to 95% of these will turn out to be malignant.

Clinical Thinking

- Patients in Scenario 2 above need a biopsy, usually accomplished in consultation with a surgeon.
- The surgeon will determine if the patient satisfies the criteria of the *Triple Test:* **clinical examination, imaging,** and **pathology** are three important tools to determine the diagnosis of a breast mass. If all are not concordant with the clinical diagnosis, further work-up is needed.
- The differential diagnosis of a breast mass stays consistent, but the likelihood of malignancy changes with the patient's age and risk factors. The older the patient, the more likely the mass is malignant.
- The goal is to obtain a tissue diagnosis by fine-needle aspiration (FNA) biopsy, avoiding open surgical biopsy when possible. This enables the surgeon to plan a single definitive operation for cancer in many instances.

- In patients with a palpable or ultrasonographically visible suspect mass, an FNA or ultrasonography-guided needle biopsy is the preferred method of diagnosis.
- In patients with a mammographic finding that is not palpable or visible by ultrasonography, a stereotactic biopsy is indicated. This is a core needle biopsy done under mammographic (or MRI) guidance.
- If these procedures are not possible because of location or patient factors, a surgical biopsy can be performed. Often these procedures require a localizer needle to be placed preoperatively under mammographic or ultrasonographic guidance.

History
- Inquire about new breast masses, skin changes, nipple retraction, or nipple discharge.
- Ask about breast pain. Is it cyclic or constant, unilateral or bilateral, burning or sharp? Make sure to differentiate tenderness from pain.
- Ask about previous history of breast biopsies.
- Ask about use of oral contraceptives or hormone replacement therapy.
- Ask specific questions about family history of breast and ovarian cancer. Take a full pedigree, if necessary.
- Ask about prior breast cancer history; if positive:
  - What surgical management did the patient undergo? This dictates what to look for on physical examination (postmastectomy, reconstruction, or lymphedema risk) and your subsequent screening plan.
  - Did she have radiation therapy? You may find radiation changes in the breast examination on that side; there is also a slight increased risk for sarcomas in the radiated field.
  - Did she receive chemotherapy? This may produce long-lasting sequelae such as cardiomyopathy (doxorubicin) or neuropathy (taxanes).
  - Is she on an estrogen blocker (e.g., tamoxifen, raloxifene) or an aromatase inhibitor (e.g., anastrozole)? The estrogen blockers may help prevent osteoporosis, and aromatase inhibitors may increase osteoporosis. Estrogen blockers are associated with an increased risk of endometrial cancer, so look for postmenopausal bleeding. All of these agents are associated with an increased risk for deep vein thrombosis.

Physical Examination
- Breast examinations should be performed both in the upright and supine positions with the patient in a gown that is open in the front.

- Examine the neck and supraclavicular lymph nodes. (It is often perceived as less threatening to touch the neck and supraclavicular fossa first, and then the breast.)
- In the upright position, examine the axillae; push the fingertips against the chest wall after having the patient place her *relaxed* arm on your shoulder or across your arm. Pull your hand down tracing your fingers down the chest wall. Palpable nodes will get caught on or bounce by your finger tips.
- While examining in the upright position, have the patient raise her arms over her head. Observe for symmetry, skin changes, or obvious masses. Have the patient place her hands on her hips and press down, looking for skin dimpling or breast distortion. Lift the breasts gently, palpating with a sweeping motion.
- Assist the patient to lie supine or in a reclining position. Examine the breast with the pads of the fingertips in an organized fashion such as in concentric circles or radially. It is important to develop a system by which you examine **all** of the breast tissue. Do not become distracted by an obvious abnormality and forget to examine the remaining tissue. As a rule, it is better to examine the unaffected breast first.
- Remember that breast tissue can extend to the edge of the sternum, the clavicle, below the inframammary fold, and to the mid-axillary line.
- Determine if there are any areas that are tender, and ask the patient to show you any areas about which she may have concern. Ask if the area is best appreciated in the upright or supine position. Reexamine the patient after she identifies areas of concern.
- When you are palpating a breast mass, be thoughtful about the texture: is it rubbery or hard, or smooth or nodular? Note carefully the size and shape of any masses, and whether they are discrete or nondiscrete; note mobility: is the lesion movable? Is it fixed to the skin overlying it or to the muscle beneath it?
- If a patient had prior breast surgery or radiation, take note of the scar location and characteristics on inspection and palpation.
- Document your findings in the chart. This should include a description of the abnormality (size, position on the clock or quadrant, and distance from the nipple) as well as a plan of action.
- Be sure to discuss your findings with the patient.

Treatment Options
- Most women with breast cancer qualify for breast conservation surgery. This involves removal of the cancer and surrounding normal margin with radiation therapy to prevent recurrence in the breast.
- Some women are not eligible for breast conservation; large tumors, multiple tumors, and second cancers in the same breast are the main

disqualifiers. Some women elect to undergo mastectomy to avoid radiation therapy; others elect to undergo bilateral mastectomy so they don't have to worry about new cancers in the future. Most women can undergo some type of plastic surgical reconstruction to look cosmetically "normal" after treatment.

- Management decisions in any cancer rely on complete staging information, including tumor extent, lymph node involvement, and presence or absence of distant metastases. In breast cancer, we use the sentinel lymph node biopsy to find, remove, and evaluate the single lymph node most likely to contain metastatic cancer cells. If that node is negative, there is no need to perform an axillary dissection.

- Adjuvant chemotherapy is offered to most women with stage II and III breast cancers. Ductal carcinoma in situ (DCIS; stage 0 breast cancer) does not require chemotherapy.

- After surgery, chemotherapy, and radiation therapy are completed, patients may be maintained on an antiestrogen drug for 5 years to prevent progression and new cancer development.

IMAGING CONSIDERATIONS

→**Mammography:** Considered the standard of care for breast cancer screening; this consists of two views of the breast: mediolateral oblique (MLO) and craniocaudad (CC). $250

→**Diagnostic mammography:** May include magnification and spot compression views. Diagnostic mammography is indicated if the patient has any area of concern or a specific complaint (i.e., skin changes). $550

→**Breast ultrasonography:** Not a good screening test; used as a focused radiologic evaluation of the breast when there is an area of concern on physical examination or a mammogram. $300

→**Breast MRI:** Not a screening test; sometimes used when a patient has known cancer and there is concern for multifocal disease. Can be used as an adjunct to mammography in patients with equivocal findings. Often used to evaluate postsurgical breasts (augmentation, or significant scarring from prior surgery); the exact guidelines for use of this test remain under scrutiny. $1500

Differential Diagnosis

The most likely underlying causes leading to a report of abnormal mammographic findings as in **Scenario 2** are as follows:

Simple Schema for Categorization of Mammographic Findings			
	Calcifications	**Mammographic masses**	**Architectural distortion**
Benign	• Sclerosing adenosis • Intraductal papilloma • Degenerated fibroadenoma	• Breast cysts and fibrocystic changes • Fibroadenoma (Generally ovoid and smooth borders)	• Scarring from previous biopsy
Malignant	• Breast cancer • DCIS	• Breast cancer (Generally irregular, spiculated)	• Malignancy • Recurrent malignancy

Calcifications

- *Calcifications* are the deposition of calcium in the breast tissue or its elements. Calcifications are divided into three types: *benign, indeterminate,* or *high probability of malignancy.*
- *Benign calcifications* may be coarse, rodlike, associated with blood vessels, round, popcorn shaped, or milk of calcium (concave).
- *Malignant calcifications* are more likely pleomorphic, heterogeneous, clustered, linear, or branching.
- Linear, branching calcifications are commonly associated with DCIS. Calcifications can also be associated with the common premalignant lesion atypical ductal hyperplasia (ADH)

Mammographic Masses

- Masses in the breast are space-occupying lesions seen on at least two views of the mammogram. Well-circumscribed and smooth masses are suggestive of a benign etiology.
- The typical benign mass is either a cyst or a fibroadenoma. Ultrasonography will differentiate.
- Malignant masses typically show an irregular contour, with linear extensions or areas of branching.

Note: *10% to 15% of cancers may present as smooth masses, particularly in the elderly population.*

Architectural Distortion

- **Architectural distortion** may be the earliest sign of breast cancer. (Some distortions are also associated with scars from previous biopsies or surgery.)
- Accordingly, after any breast biopsy, it is recommended that a new follow-up baseline mammogram be obtained 6 months after surgery.
- When a mammogram is obtained after surgery, scars are marked externally to aid in identifying architectural distortions in the breast. Biopsy is indicated only if recurrent cancer is suspected.

Clinical Entities   Medical Knowledge

Breast Cancer

Pφ Approximately 80% of breast carcinomas are infiltrating ductal carcinomas, arising in the epithelium of the ducts of the breast. Other histologic types include medullary, papillary, and inflammatory cancers. On occasion, cell types can be mixed.

TP Typically presents as a new palpable mass; with widespread mammography, most tumors can be diagnosed before masses are palpated. This is particularly true in the case of DCIS, the earliest form of breast cancer. DCIS is usually diagnosed when new calcifications are seen on mammography and presents as a palpable mass only in about 10% of cases.

Dx Invasive breast cancer typically presents as a spiculated, irregular mass on mammography. Some palpable masses do not show up on mammography or ultrasonography, and negative imaging studies do not end the work-up of palpable masses. The patient should be referred to a surgeon for possible image-guided or open biopsy if the clinical presentation warrants it.

Tx Breast-conserving surgery with postoperative radiation has been shown to be equivalent to mastectomy for the treatment of early breast cancer in many prospective, randomized studies. Appropriate patient selection as well as patient preference are the main factors in the type of treatment selected. **See Katz 15, Hacker 29.**

Breast Cysts and Fibrocystic Changes

Pφ Usually, but not always, these entities occur in younger patients. The etiology of these cystic changes is not well understood, but they likely represent the patient's breast tissue response to fluctuations in systemic estrogen and progesterone production. Fibrocystic change almost always represents a benign process, except in cases where cellular atypia is noted. These cysts sometimes progress to invasive disease.

TP Typically presents as a well-circumscribed, mobile mass in premenopausal women. These cysts can oftentimes be painful, which is the driving force for the patient to seek care.

Dx Often does not appear on mammography. However, breast cysts are usually easily seen on ultrasonography as anechoic, well-circumscribed masses with posterior acoustic enhancement.

Tx If a mass meets all sonographic criteria for a cyst, most can be monitored without intervention. If the presence of the cyst creates anxiety or significant pain for the patient, or the lesion does not meet the sonographic criteria for a simple cyst, it can be aspirated directly or with sonographic guidance. If a cyst recurs, persists after aspiration, or contains bloody fluid, surgical excision is warranted. **See Katz 15, Hacker 29.**

Fibroadenoma

Pφ A benign mass of predominantly fibrous tissue, sometimes containing a glandular component as well.

TP The most common breast mass in women younger than 30 years of age; may be multiple, and may sometimes grow to an impressive size.

Dx Usually found on clinical examination, this lesion appears as a round or lobulated mass with well-circumscribed borders. Fibroadenomas will appear as a solid mass on mammography and ultrasonography, with a heterogeneous appearance compared with the surrounding breast tissue.

Tx FNA or core needle biopsy should be done. If pathology confirms the diagnosis of fibroadenoma the mass can be monitored. However, many patients are not comfortable with the presence of the mass, so surgical excision is warranted if the patient is anxious or has significant pain, or if pathology is inconclusive. **See Katz 15, Hacker 29.**

Benign Breast Nodularity

Pφ Normal breast tissue can have a nodular texture and pattern in some women. This is more marked in the upper outer quadrants and is often very tender in response to normal cyclic hormonal variations. This cyclic tenderness is more pronounced as women become perimenopausal and often one breast is affected more than the other.

TP The typical patient is premenopausal and complains of an intermittently tender mass that seems to fluctuate in size. The pain is characteristically worse in the 7 days before her cycle and then begins to abate with the onset of menses.

Dx Mammograms and sonograms typically show normal breast tissue.

Tx If the palpable mass is thought to be suspect or if the patient's anxiety requires it, a biopsy should be performed despite negative imaging studies to exclude malignancy.

ZEBRA ZONE

a. **Paget disease of the breast:** A form of carcinoma in situ; presents as a scaly, flaking lesion of the nipple and areolar skin that may be associated with itching or pain; often initially misdiagnosed as eczema or contact dermatitis; diagnosis can be confirmed with a skin punch biopsy.

b. **Inflammatory breast cancer:** A form of breast cancer that involves the skin of the breast; presents with erythema, edema, and a heaviness of the breast; frequently misdiagnosed as cellulitis or mastitis; patients are often treated with a course of antibiotics and local care without resolution of symptoms, leading to delay in diagnosis; mammography and ultrasonography often fail to show a discrete mass; skin biopsy shows infiltration of the dermal lymphatics with tumor cells; neoadjuvant chemotherapy is the first-line treatment for this aggressive type of breast cancer.

Practice-Based Learning and Improvement: Evidence-Based Medicine

Title
Projecting individualized probabilities of developing breast cancer for white females who are being examined annually

Authors
Gail MH, Brinton LA, Byar DP, et al.

Institution
National Institutes of Health, Bethesda, Maryland

Reference
Journal of the National Cancer Institute 1989;81:1879–1886

Problem
Breast cancer risk assessment.

Intervention
Developed a personal risk assessment tool.

Comparison/control (quality of evidence)
Case-control study of 284,780 women in a prospective cohort study.

Outcome/effect
An easily applied tool for risk evaluation in asymptomatic women.

Historical significance/comments
In 1989, Gail and colleagues set out to evaluate a large cohort of
women who participated in a mammography screening trial 10 years
earlier for epidemiologic factors predictive for the development of
breast cancer within 5 years. They found that risk increases with age,
number of breast biopsies, number of first-degree relatives with
breast cancer, and age at first live birth or nulliparity, and was
inversely proportional to age at menarche. By asking each patient
these questions, it is possible to calculate her risk of developing
cancer in 5 years and over her lifetime (see http://www.cancer.gov/
bcrisktool/). This model is useful to identify "high-risk" women for
interventions such as prevention or close surveillance by a breast
physician.

Interpersonal and Communication Skills

Anticipate and Discuss Sensitive Issues with Patients: Alleviating Fears Regarding Breast Cancer Prognosis

A possible diagnosis of breast cancer is one of the greatest fears of
many women today. Widespread media coverage adds to this anxiety.
It is not unusual for a patient to present with a small mass in her
breast that she has recently discovered on BSE or to be faced with a
report of an abnormality on screening mammography, and then
immediately express her concerns about the possibility of dying from
breast cancer to her gynecologist. In your discussion of breast cancer
screening and abnormal results with the patient, it is important to
stress the positives regarding breast cancer diagnosis, treatment, and

survival. The most important statistic is that the overwhelming majority (>90%) of palpable masses and abnormal mammograms are caused by benign disease. Adherence to a routine screening program has lowered breast cancer mortality each year in the United States. Biopsies are increasingly minimally invasive, without significant scar or anesthetic risks. Early detection leads to treatment options that do not require chemotherapy and are associated with a 92% 10-year survival for women with breast cancers detected in stages 0 and 1. Breast complaints warrant a systematic work-up and referral to a breast specialist for any clinically suspect lesion regardless of patient age or radiologic findings. Many women, however, consider their Ob/Gyn provider as their primary care physician. Therefore, although you may not be the physician in charge of the actual treatment of the breast cancer, you will become the patient's advocate and source of advice and information.

Professionalism

Principle: Commitment to Professional Competence

Delay in diagnosis of breast cancer is one of the most common reasons for medical malpractice claims. As a physician, one must be vigilant in maintaining adherence to appropriate guidelines for screening examinations *and appropriate follow-up of test results.* In particular, in regard to mammographic surveillance, the American Cancer Society has made specific, easy-to-follow guidelines regarding timing of mammography, clinical breast examinations, and BSEs (see www.cancer.org). The clinician must know the latest guidelines for screening and the latest methods to optimally detect this disease.

Systems-Based Practice

Profiling by Family History to Determine Risk Assessment Is Systems-Based Practice

Prevention and early detection strategies for cancer depend on proper patient selection. I use key information from the patient's history to build a risk profile for breast and ovarian cancer. The Gail model is a good way to begin this assessment; as I explore a patient's family history of cancers, I go past first-degree relatives and look at three generations if available, which includes grandparents and their siblings (maternal and paternal aunts/uncles) and offspring (maternal/paternal first cousins) and, finally, the patient's siblings and first and second cousins. In this pedigree, I look for families with more than one or two breast cancers or any cases of ovarian cancer. I also look for early onset of these cancers to gauge genetic risk. We know that about 10% of breast and ovarian cancers are associated with *BRCA1* or *BRCA2* mutations. *BRCA* positivity is more likely in families with ovarian cancer and breast cancer histories, families with two or more first-degree relatives with breast cancer, families with male breast cancer, and families of people with early-onset breast cancer (before 50 years of age).

In these individuals, I offer the option of genetic testing to identify mutations in *BRCA1* or *BRCA2* so that the patient and I can better plan her preventive therapy strategy.

Patients need to be counseled about two main risks from genetic testing:

1. If a patient tests positive, she may suffer from significant stress or depression related to a fear of cancer. She may be qualified as having a "preexisting condition" that would prevent her from obtaining life insurance, and possibly health insurance. She may feel compelled to undergo radical procedures that may or may not be life saving.
2. If she tests negative, she could still develop breast or ovarian cancer.

If the patient does test positive for *BRCA1* or *BRCA2*, she is now officially at "high risk" for breast and ovarian cancer. I usually counsel young women about the benefits of prophylactic oophorectomy as soon as they feel their childbearing is done. Women older than 60 years of age are much less likely to benefit from prophylactic oophorectomy. As far as breast cancer prophylaxis is concerned, we can step up the screening with MRI and frequent follow-up examinations, or we can offer prophylactic bilateral mastectomy.

Professor's Pearls: Cases in Gynecology

Consider the following clinical problems and questions posed. Then refer to the professor's discussion of these issues.

1. A 45-year-old woman with type 1 insulin-dependent diabetes mellitus presents with heavy and irregular menstrual bleeding for the past 2 years. She had her fallopian tubes ligated 10 years ago and has had normal Pap tests. Her most recent normal Pap test was 3 months ago at her family physician's office. She denies any history of cancer.

2. A 25-year-old G0 presents complaining of vaginal discharge, pruritus, and urinary urgency. She occasionally uses condoms for contraception. The speculum examination reveals a copious, frothy, yellow vaginal discharge and cervical petechiae. The cervix begins to bleed when cultured with a cotton swab. The vaginal pH is 5.0 and the wet mount reveals flagellated organisms.

3. A 63-year-old G0P0, menopausal since age 52 years, presents with abdominal pain, bloating, nausea, vomiting, and intermittent diarrhea and constipation. She has persuaded her physician to prescribe unopposed estrogen therapy for the last 11 years to help with her complaints of insomnia, hot flashes, and vaginal dryness. She has been unable to tolerate progesterone.

4. A 53-year-old postmenopausal G2P2 complains of bothersome urinary leakage. She informs you that she "cannot hold her urine" and must find a bathroom immediately when she feels an urge to go. She complains of the need to void frequently, and gets up twice at night to urinate. She sometimes does not make it to the bathroom in time and starts to leak as soon as she sees the toilet and closes the bathroom door. She isn't sure that she empties her bladder completely because she frequently feels the need to urinate a second time, shortly after leaving the bathroom.

5. A 19-year-old G0P0 NCAA Division I long-distance runner, who has not had a menstrual period in the last 2 years, presents to the emergency department. An x-ray shows a fracture in her right third metatarsal. She is 5 feet, 6 inches tall, and weighs 96 lbs.

Discussion by Dr. Mark B. Woodland, Drexel University College of Medicine, Philadelphia, Pennsylvania

Answer 1: Clinical Considerations: Evaluation of Abnormal Uterine Bleeding

Before one gets caught up in the medical illnesses of this patient, keep it simple. You are presented with a 45-year-old woman who has irregular periods. There could be many causes of this problem, but first and foremost, you must evaluate the endometrial lining. The good news is that you already have a normal Pap test that can help you to eliminate cervical abnormalities. Ultrasonography is a good first step and will also provide a glance at the adnexa to help you to either eliminate or guide your diagnostic testing toward the ovaries, uterus, or both. You will not only have to consider uterine polyps or fibroids, but issues of hyperplasia, endometrial abnormalities, and potential cancer. For patients in this age group, blood work may be helpful. A baseline follicle-stimulating hormone and estradiol level will help establish the patient's menopausal status if this is not clear from the history. This not only will become important later in helping to make critical decisions about ongoing care, but also may help in making decisions for ultimate therapy for this patient. Finally, consideration of the patient's medical illness will be important in planning the ultimate therapy. Minimally invasive approaches may give this patient the best possible outcome with the least potential for major complications that may be affected or caused by her underlying disease process. Remember, patients with diabetes have increased risk of renal problems, not to mention infections.

Answer 2: Clinical Considerations: Evaluation and Management of Cervicitis and Vaginitis

Once again we are presented with a complex case that we need to take apart and consider not only the end point, but the process that brought the patient to this point—specifically, unprotected sexual intercourse. Trichomonads have been known to be self-infected through poor hygiene from rectal colonization, but the most commonly accepted manner of transmission is through vaginal sexual intercourse. To treat this, the clinician will have to prescribe appropriate oral or vaginal antibiotics. In general, metronidazole preparations are the best. However, trichomonads may not be her only problem. This patient may also have been exposed to other sexually transmitted infections such as hepatitis, human immunodeficiency virus (HIV), syphilis, chlamydia, gonorrhea, and herpes. Testing for these problems must be done, and should be done at the time of the first diagnostic intervention. Treatments should be guided by positive tests. Finally, the patient needs to remember that she may have also been exposed to the human papillomavirus (HPV). A Pap test must be done, but you may have to postpone this until after the acute inflammatory process is over. The patient should come back to be evaluated within the following week. If the Pap smear is inconclusive or her cervicitis does not clear with antibiotics, a biopsy should be done of the most affected area to rule out a dysplastic or even neoplastic lesion. Although the HPV vaccine has not been proven to help those patients who are already been exposed to HPV, this patient should be offered the vaccine based on the possibility that she may not yet have been infected. Finally, unplanned pregnancy accounts for over 50% of all pregnancies. This patient needs to be counseled about the potential of pregnancy. If she is within 72 hours of intercourse, you may consider offering her emergency contraception of any type. Check a urine pregnancy test, and if she is not pregnant offer her emergency contraception and plan for future contraception. Also emphasize to her the importance of condoms.

Answer 3: Clinical Considerations: Evaluation of Abdominal Pain and Bloating in a Postmenopausal Patient

Let's deal with the most obvious breach in physician–patient relations. This patient should never have been able to persuade her physician to do anything outside the guidelines of practice broadly interpreted as "standard of care." Patients may make requests, but clinicians should not feel obligated to fulfill these requests. Nor should a patient feel entitled to have her requests blindly met. Menopausal symptoms can be overwhelming for women and use of hormone therapy does treat these symptoms in a "natural" way. For women with an intact uterus, progesterone should be added to the hormone therapy regimen to protect the lining of the uterus from potentially developing abnormalities as a result of unopposed estrogen therapy. Progesterone may carry with it undesired side effects (e.g., fluid retention, weight gain, bloating, and moodiness) and the patient may opt not to take combination therapy. The clinician should proceed with caution. The patient's need for hormone therapy and the status of her endometrial lining should be monitored frequently, and her compliance with monitoring should be assessed annually. Vaginal ultrasonography can be very helpful in these circumstances. If the endometrial stripe is thickened or irregular, consider doing an office hysteroscopy followed by endometrial sampling or guided sampling. I am not an advocate of blind endometrial sampling because although it is highly specific for what it samples, it may not be as sensitive for the disease you want most to rule out. Having said all of this, the risk of severe consequences as a result of use of unopposed estrogen in the menopausal woman with an intact uterus is small.

Back to the case at hand, while you are thinking of the hormone therapy use, don't get distracted from other issues that might carry even greater consequences for this patient: specifically, the issue of cancer; more specifically ovarian, pancreatic, and colon cancer. This patient will need to have a colonoscopy, a CT scan of the abdomen and pelvis, and routine blood work. The blood work should not only look at routine laboratory values such as fasting lipids and glucose, but should check liver functions and thyroid levels and include a CBC and coagulation profile. If there is any evidence of intraperitoneal masses, tumor markers can also be ordered such as the CA-125 or carcinoembryonic antigen (CEA). Any abnormalities should be pursued aggressively to catch any problems at the earliest possible time for intervention. Early diagnosis has been linked with more favorable outcomes. Although I did not address it at the beginning of this discussion, a good history and physical will be helpful for you to prioritize testing and intervention.

Answer 4: Clinical Considerations: Evaluation of Incontinence

This is a distressing story that is all too frequent in our offices. Unfortunately, sometimes we as clinicians forget to ask questions regarding continence, or don't pay attention to the answers. Patients feel self-conscious and don't want to ask the questions and are embarrassed by the answers. It can be a vicious cycle that results in very little positive outcome for the patient. Let's go back to basics: we need a better history and a good physical. We need to find out if she ever had this problem before, and if in fact she can start or stop her urinary stream at will. Because of her postvoid retention, you will have to be a little more invasive and perform bladder catheterization after she has voided. This will give you information about her postvoid function and quality of her urine, and also rule out infection. If she can control her urine, you may achieve relief by treating the patient with an anticholinergic medication. This will not only stabilize the bladder, but may improve her emptying. I have found that treating the "neurogenic" bladder for a period of 3 to 6 months is very helpful, and patients may then be able to stop their medications for a time until the problem recurs. Certainly, if the patient gets no relief she deserves a more comprehensive evaluation. More invasive procedures will give you a better idea of the different pressure gradients in the bladder and bladder neck (cystometrics) and guide you to interventions that may have a bigger impact, such as collagen injections, urethral support procedures, and vaginal support procedures. As part of any good work-up, the clinician should include cystoscopy to evaluate for any lesions within the bladder.

Answer 5: Clinical Considerations: Amenorrhea in a Teenager

Given that teen obesity is one of the major developing epidemics in this age group, this 19-year-old should be applauded for her physical activity. Unfortunately, she needs to be educated about the effect that this activity may have on her body. In addition, she should be educated about the efficacy and safety of intervening with oral contraceptive pills to provide her with a more balanced hormone state to help prevent further problems. Finally, the clinician needs to consider whether this young lady is running for the sport and the psychological benefits, or if she is in fact running *from* other issues, including weight management or anorexia. To evaluate this young patient, you will need to develop an appropriate doctor–patient relationship with her. She needs to trust you and understand your concerns. You will need to be patient and reach out to her in ways to help gain her confidence and compliance. A detailed history will be very important. Follow the history with an in-depth examination that should include vaginal probe ultrasonography. You should consider performing blood tests consistent with amenorrhea, such as thyroid screening, pituitary function screening, ovarian function screening, and baseline hemoglobin and electrolytes. Although there was no mention of sexual activity, you should ask about this and check her human chorionic gonadotropin (β-hCG) level. During this time, make sure she has a good podiatrist and consider helping her offset the physical punishment of running with lower-impact exercise such as swimming or bike riding. Finally, you need to seriously consider intervening with low-dose oral contraceptive pills. If she does not like to have menstrual periods, she can use continuous dosing regimens that can reduce the cycle to four times a year or less. Don't forget to ask her about sexual activity, check cultures if indicated, and consider the HPV vaccine.

Section VI
CASES IN REPRODUCTIVE ENDOCRINOLOGY

Section Editor
Keith Issacson MD

Section Contents

Chapter 47
Evaluation of the Infertile Patient (Case 32)

Shahab S. Minassian MD

Case: A 34-year-old G0 has had no success conceiving a pregnancy for 30 months.

Differential Diagnosis

Ovulatory factor infertility	Male factor infertility	Unexplained infertility
Cervical factor infertility	Tubal factor infertility	

Speaking Intelligently

When I see patients for an initial infertility evaluation, I make certain that I consider all possible causes because multiple infertility factors may be present. I perform a thorough screening evaluation for all possible known causes of infertility, including male factor, tubal/pelvic, ovulatory, cervical, and other, unexplained causes of infertility. Keep in mind that, in fact, many cases of infertility are "unexplained" in that there is no obvious diagnosis for the patient's inability to conceive once the evaluation is completed. Because the infertility evaluation is sometimes grueling, my staff and I must include patients in treatment plan decisions and provide emotional support, and sometimes financial counseling as well.

PATIENT CARE

Clinical Thinking

- Consider how you can focus the evaluation to arrive at an efficient and timely diagnosis. Be guided by clues in the history and physical examination, particularly patient age, menstrual history, and sexually transmitted infection (STI) history.
- A great majority of patients will have one of the following factors: ovulatory, male factor (in the cases where the patient has a male partner), or tubal factor. Other important but less common causes of infertility include a uterine factor and a cervical factor. Unexplained

infertility occurs in up to 5% of patients. Multifactor infertility is also common. It is critical to make sure that the patient is evaluated for all these possibilities.

- It is common to see women older than 35 years of age for an infertility evaluation. They should be given a diagnosis of infertility after 6 months of attempting conception without pregnancy. Women younger than 35 years are given the diagnosis after 1 year.
- If there is a male partner it is important to obtain a good history and perform a semen analysis to screen for male factor. Up to 40% of male partners are found to have male factor infertility on initial evaluation.

History

- Patient age is important. Women older than 35 years undergoing infertility evaluations are defined as being of advanced reproductive age. Their fertility rates on average are reduced owing to ovarian aging and resistance, with decreased ovum quality.
- The menstrual history will provide an almost immediate diagnosis in some cases. Menstrual irregularities such as amenorrhea and oligomenorrhea strongly suggest anovulation and therefore an ovulatory factor. A history of significant weight gain or loss may coincide with irregular menses and must be included. A history of hirsutism, acne, and weight gain suggests polycystic ovary syndrome (PCOS). Galactorrhea suggests hyperprolactinemia. Cold intolerance, weight gain, somnolence, and fatigue suggest possible hypothyroidism.
- A past history of pelvic inflammatory disease (PID) places the patient at a high risk for tubal factor. Any STI history (even with ambulatory treatment, such as with *Chlamydia trachomatis* infection) should make you suspicious of a tubal factor.
- A past history of pelvic surgery such as ovarian cystectomy, myomectomy, or ectopic pregnancy increases the risk of postoperative pelvic adhesions. This may lead to peritubal or periovarian adhesions or the loss of a tube or ovary, and result in tubal/pelvic factor.
- A history of dysmenorrhea, dyspareunia, or pelvic pain suggests endometriosis, which can result in pelvic adhesions or ovarian endometrioma formation. Dysmenorrhea may also suggest chronic PID.
- Consider social and family histories: smoking increases the risk for tubal infertility. Significant alcohol and caffeine use can adversely affect fertility. Family histories of endometriosis and thyroid disease predispose patients to these disorders.
- If there is a male partner a thorough history should be taken. Concentrate specifically on past medical and surgical history. Diabetes or prostate disorders may result in impotence. Hypertension and the medications prescribed to treat it may cause male sexual dysfunction.
- Patients should be advised to bring the records of any previous infertility evaluation they have had. This portion of the history can help focus the evaluation and eliminate duplicate testing.

Physical Examination

- **Vital signs:** A body mass index (BMI) is calculated from height and weight. A BMI less than 18 and greater than 30 often correlates with menstrual irregularities.
- Skin changes such as hirsutism and acne in patients with irregular menses suggest PCOS.
- On breast examination, galactorrhea suggests hyperprolactinemia; thyroid enlargement or nodularity may suggest thyroid disease.
- Tenderness, masses, or nodularity on pelvic examination raise suspicion for endometriosis, chronic PID, or ovarian cysts, which can result in tubal/pelvic factors.

Tests for Consideration

- Patients with ovulatory infertility are required to have a serum evaluation for four specific entities: (1) PCOS, (2) hyperprolactinemia, (3) thyroid disease, and (4) hypothalamic dysfunction. Appropriate tests include **thyroid-stimulating hormone (TSH), prolactin, luteinizing hormone (LH),** and **follicle-stimulating hormone (FSH). Dehydroepiandrosterone (DHEA) sulfate, testosterone,** and **free testosterone** are serum androgen tests that are useful to screen for PCOS. PCOS is the most common reason for ovulatory infertility in women.   Total: $760

- Low serum **FSH** and **LH** levels are frequently found in hypothalamic amenorrhea. If the patient is older than 35 years of age she should be screened for the possibility of ovarian resistance. A serum FSH level is drawn on the third day of the menstrual cycle; an elevated (>10 mIU/mL) level is considered diagnostic for ovarian resistance. $200

- A **semen analysis** of a male partner is an essential part of the infertility evaluation. $250

- **Postcoital test (PCT):** Diagnoses cervical factor infertility. It is performed by evaluating the cervical mucus of the patient after having intercourse during or just before ovulation. Ideally, the couple will have intercourse 4 to 18 hours before the test. Cervical mucus is removed using a disposable aspiration pipet, placed on a glass slide with a coverslip, and evaluated with gross and microscopic examination. $250

  - Thin, watery, and stretchable mucus with motile sperm, preferably >10 per high-power field, indicates a normal test.
  - Thin mucus or poor to no sperm survival indicates a possible immunologic factor with rejection of sperm by antisperm antibodies.

- A leukocytic infiltrate with thick mucus indicates possible cervicitis.
- If no sperm are seen in good-quality mucus, a poor sperm count, sexual dysfunction, or immunologic infertility can be suspected.
- If immotile or poorly moving sperm are seen in good-quality mucus, immunologic infertility is highly suspected.
- It is important to note that there is significant controversy over whether the PCT is clinically useful.

IMAGING CONSIDERATIONS

→**Hysterosalpingography** (HSG) is the preferred screening test for tubal factor infertility whether or not the patient has a history of PID. HSG is performed by placing a disposable intrauterine catheter or a cervical cannula into the endocervical canal and injecting radiologic dye into the uterus under fluoroscopy. Tubal patency and endometrial cavity abnormalities can be evaluated. Be mindful that diagnostic laparoscopy is sometimes the preferred method of evaluation if there is a documented history of PID or if there are abnormalities on pelvic examination suggesting PID or endometriosis. $350

→**Sonohysterography** is a useful and highly sensitive and specific test for the evaluation of the endometrial cavity. This test allows screening for intracavitary masses that may suggest endometrial polyps, intrauterine fibroids, or adhesions. $550

Clinical Entities   Medical Knowledge

Ovulatory Factor Infertility

Pφ PCOS is the most common cause of ovulatory factor infertility. Hypothalamic amenorrhea/dysfunction, thyroid disease, and hyperprolactinemia are also frequently encountered and must be considered. All causes result in infrequent or absent ovulation.

TP Irregular menses or complete absence of menses is most commonly encountered. Patients may demonstrate evidence of endocrine dysfunction. In PCOS these may include obesity, hirsutism, and acne; in hyperprolactinemia galactorrhea is usually noted; in thyroid disease, skin, gastrointestinal, central nervous system, and metabolic changes may be noted.

Dx Diagnosis is made by history, physical examination, and serum hormonal screening. Ultrasonographic evaluation is useful in the diagnosis of PCOS.

Tx Medications such as clomiphene are commonly used to induce ovulation. Injectable FSH or FSH/LH is used when ovulation does not occur with clomiphene. Adjunctive medications to treat underlying endocrine disorders are used to increase ovulation rates. Examples of these include metformin for PCOS, bromocriptine for hyperprolactinemia, and thyroid supplements for hypothyroidism. **See Katz 41, Hacker 34.**

Tubal Factor Infertility

Pφ *C. trachomatis* infection is the most common cause, although gonorrheal infection remains significant. Repeated infections will result in damage to the tubal serosa and mucosa. Eventually, proximal (cornual or isthmic) or distal (hydrosalpinx) occlusion of the tubal lumen occurs. Adnexal adhesions are also observed. Capture of the ovulating ovum by the tube will be decreased or eliminated.

TP Most patients with tubal factor infertility present with no history of pelvic infection. The risk for tubal factor infertility greatly increases if a patient does have a history of PID. The pelvic examination is most often unrevealing, but some patients will present with uterine or adnexal tenderness, or with adnexal masses and immobility of the pelvic structures noted on bimanual examination.

Dx HSG is the screening test of choice for tubal factor infertility. Diagnostic laparoscopy is sometimes indicated in patients who have a history of PID or if the HSG is abnormal.

Tx In vitro fertilization (IVF) is the ideal treatment for patients with tubal factor and offers the best treatment outcomes. Laparoscopic correction of tubal factor—including lysis of adhesions and opening of distal tubal occlusion—is also a standard of care and can be offered at the time of laparoscopic diagnosis. **See Katz 41, Hacker 34.**

Male Factor Infertility

Pφ The most common etiologies of male factor infertility include idiopathic causes, infectious causes (prostatitis or urethritis), failure of spermatogenesis, and sexual dysfunction. Failure of spermatogenesis can result from testicular failure due to chromosomal causes (examples include classic or mosaic forms of Klinefelter syndrome or a microdeletion of the Y chromosome), hypothalamic/pituitary failure or dysfunction (examples include Kallmann syndrome or pituitary neoplasms), "Sertoli cell–only" syndrome (lack of spermatogonia), or testicular damage from chemotherapy or radiation therapy.

TP Most men with male factor have no presenting history or signs/ symptoms. Occasionally, the male partner's history may be significant for radiation or chemotherapy treatment, sexual dysfunction, or lack of secondary sexual development. The latter may be noted on examination by a urologist on referral.

Dx Semen analysis may show low sperm counts, sperm motility problems, or abnormal sperm morphology. Microscopic analysis of the semen may reveal leukocyte infiltrates (leukocytospermia). Low semen volumes may indicate ejaculatory dysfunction. In cases of azoospermia, a karyotype and Y-deletion analysis are indicated. Serum gonadotropins, testosterone, and prolactin are indicated to evaluate for endocrine causes. Testicular biopsy may also be indicated in patients with azoospermia and normal gonadotropins to assess testicular sperm production.

Tx A urology referral for a complete examination is indicated once an abnormal semen analysis is encountered. IVF is the ideal treatment choice for severely low sperm counts. Milder cases of male factor can be treated with intrauterine insemination of washed sperm (separated from the seminal fluid) at the time of ovulation. Endocrine causes can be treated by correcting the endocrine abnormality, and antibiotics are used for infectious causes. **See Katz 41, Hacker 34.**

Cervical Factor Infertility

Pφ Immunoglobulin A (IgA) antibodies, found in cervical mucus and directed against sperm, result in sperm immobilization and infertility. Surgical procedures like cone biopsies can cause a loss of cervical mucus glands and lack of cervical mucus to support sperm. Cervicitis, most commonly from *C. trachomatis* infection, is also a known cause of cervical factor infertility.

TP Although the great majority of patients are asymptomatic, patients with cervicitis may note pain or an abnormal discharge.

Dx Postcoital testing is diagnostic. This test will reveal lack of sperm motility, poor-quality cervical mucus, or a leukocytic infiltrate.

Tx Intrauterine insemination (IUI) of sperm, separated from the seminal fluid by centrifugation by a process called sperm washing, is indicated for immunologic and surgical causes. IVF is an ideal alternative. Antibiotic treatment is indicated for cervicitis. **See Hacker 34.**

Unexplained Infertility

Pφ Possible reasons for unexplained infertility may include fertilization, embryo, and implantation abnormalities. Also theorized are defects in ovum pickup by the fallopian tube and embryo/gamete transport in the female reproductive tract.

TP There is no specific presentation for this disorder.

Dx Unexplained infertility is diagnosed when all testing returns negative, including the ovulatory history, PCT, semen analysis, HSG, and diagnostic laparoscopy.

Tx Ovulation induction with clomiphene or injectable FSH or FSH/LH is used in conjunction with IUI as a treatment option. IVF is an ideal alternative. **See Katz 41, Hacker 34.**

Medical Knowledge

Intrauterine Insemination
Intrauterine insemination is a potentially beneficial intervention for cervical factor infertility, mild male factor infertility, and unexplained infertility. Semen is obtained after 2 to 4 days of abstinence, and after being "washed" and concentrated at an appropriate center, this sperm is then placed in a thin pipet and injected directly into the endometrial cavity at about the time of ovulation. The cervix should be appropriately prepared before the procedure. Sometimes ovarian hyperstimulation using clomiphene citrate or FSH analogs (injectable gonadotropins) is also incorporated into this treatment strategy.

Medical Knowledge

In Vitro Fertilization

In vitro fertilization is an incredibly valuable infertility treatment that is useful for virtually all causes of infertility except uterine anatomic causes such as intracavitary leiomyomas or adhesions. An IVF "cycle" is begun with ovarian hyperstimulation, typically using injectable gonadotropins. The stimulated oocytes are then retrieved using a vaginal approach, and then combined with the partner's sperm in a specially equipped laboratory. The resulting embryos are evaluated for quality, and then a small number (typically 2 to 4) are placed in the endometrial cavity using a soft pipet 3 to 5 days after the initial retrieval. IVF is an effective treatment for ovulatory dysfunction, tubal/pelvic infertility, male factor infertility, and unexplained infertility. The usual success rate is about 25% per cycle, but can be much higher in some centers.

Practice-Based Learning and Improvement: Evidence-Based Medicine

Title
Metformin increases the ovulatory rate and pregnancy rate from clomiphene citrate in patients with polycystic ovary syndrome who are resistant to clomiphene citrate alone.

Authors
Vandermolen DT, Ratts VS, Evans WS, et al.

Institution
Medical College of Virginia, Richmond, Virginia

Reference
Fertility and Sterility 2001;75:310–315

Problem
Clomiphene-resistant infertile women.

Intervention
Adjunctive metformin treatment.

Comparison/control (quality of evidence)
Randomized, placebo-controlled study comparing clomiphene alone to clomiphene and metformin.

Outcome/effect
In anovulatory women with PCOS who are resistant to clomiphene, metformin use significantly increased the ovulation rate and pregnancy rate from clomiphene treatment alone.

Historical significance/comments
This study was one of the initial reports supporting the use of metformin treatment for patients with PCOS undergoing clomiphene induction of ovulation.

Interpersonal and Communication Skills

Listening for Cues to Depression

Half of all women destined to suffer with depression will be diagnosed during the reproductive years. The emotional stress, self-doubt, and frustration experienced by many women during an infertility work-up can be contributing and sometimes triggering factors for a depressive episode. When working with patients going through this type of work-up, clinicians should be very attentive to the symptoms and presentations of depression, such as loss of interest in previously enjoyable activities, persistent physical symptoms such as chronic pain or headaches, exaggerated depressive response to miscarriages, stillbirth, or infertility, and dyspareunia or sexual dysfunction. Your patient may not volunteer the information that she is depressed. She may not recognize her symptoms as depression. Through effective listening and observing vocal characteristics (e.g., tone, pace, and volume) and body language, you may be able to recognize a depressive episode. If you suspect depression, it is likely you will need to use heightened sensitivity not only in phrasing questions but in "really" hearing what the patient is conveying through words and actions.

Professionalism

Principle: Commitment to a Just Distribution of Finite Resources

With the field of reproductive endocrinology and infertility rapidly expanding, we are now able to help many couples with infertility problems to have their own biologic children. Although the work-up of an infertile patient starts with simple, cost-effective measures (e.g., effective history taking and behavioral modification), expensive laboratory and radiographic tests become important very quickly. In our current model for medical payment, those without medical insurance are often unable to avail themselves of the more expensive measures used to overcome infertility, and third-party carriers are often responsible for deciding how to best allocate limited resources. It is our responsibility not only to think about judicious use of resources on an individual level, but to advocate for what we believe to be judicious use of resources at the level of hospitals, insurance companies, and even entire health care systems.

Systems-Based Practice

How Hospitals Decide Which Specialists to Hire

How does a hospital or health system (a group of hospitals) decide on which specialists to recruit? One of the primary strategies in the strategic plans of most hospitals/health systems is the recruitment of selected specialists. In most health care organizations, the first step in developing this strategy is conducting a physician community needs assessment to quantitatively measure which specialties are in a surplus or deficit position based on the supply of physicians and the population. The community needs assessment drives the medical staff plan, setting forth the physician recruitment priorities for that year and beyond.

Let's say, or example, that Hospital A's strategic plan includes the expansion of its Ob/Gyn services. In considering specific tactics to act on this strategy, it is discovered that most patients in Hospital A's community had their babies delivered at Hospital A, except for the patients who required infertility services at Hospital B in another nearby community; those infertility patients ended up using Hospital B for delivery because of the infertility group that practices at Hospital B. Not surprisingly, when Hospital A performs its physician community needs assessment, it realizes that the community it serves is not lacking general Ob/Gyn physicians, but is lacking a number of Ob/Gyn subspecialists, including infertility. Based on these facts, Hospital A decides to recruit an infertility specialist to better serve the patients in its community.

When looking for a position in a specific community, contacting the local hospital president/CEO would be a good way to find out if your specialty is a recruitment priority at that hospital. Most well-managed hospitals have a strategic plan and medical staff recruitment plans as described in the foregoing example, and the hospital management leadership is usually willing to share this information for a physician's given specialty. Although you can certainly succeed in locating in a community where your specialty is not a strategic priority, having the support of the hospital increases the likelihood of success.

Chapter 48
Endometriosis (Case 33)

Christian Perez MD *and John Orris* DO, MBA

Case: A 30-year-old nulligravid woman presents to the office complaining of 8 years of dysmenorrhea and dyspareunia. She has been unsuccessful in achieving pregnancy during the last 3 years, and she has a sister who has been diagnosed with endometriosis. Her menstrual periods are characterized by heavy bleeding. She has been treated in the past with anti-inflammatory medications, antibiotics, and progesterone with poor response. She is asking for a better pain control, and inquires regarding the possibility of pregnancy in the near future.

Differential Diagnosis

Endometriosis	Adenomyosis	Pelvic adhesions
Pelvic inflammatory disease (PID)	Pelvic congestion syndrome	

Speaking Intelligently

Endometriosis is a relatively common cause of pelvic pain and infertility, but is not an easy diagnosis to confirm. Endometriosis occurs when endometrial tissue implants are found *outside* of the lining of the uterus. We speculate that there is about a 10% prevalence in the general population. We find endometriosis in up to 32%, 42%, and 50% of women undergoing laparoscopy for pelvic pain, sterilization, or infertility, respectively. The most common affected sites are (in order) ovaries, cul-de-sac, broad ligament, uterosacral ligaments, uterus, and fallopian tubes. Less commonly involved sites are the vagina, cervix, rectovaginal septum, ileum, abdominal wall, peritoneum, and urinary tract. Chronic dysmenorrhea and dyspareunia in the presence of infertility represents the classic triad associated with endometriosis. These are the sorts of general thought processes that go through my mind when I first begin to suspect endometriosis in a possibly affected patient, and I sort this all out using my history and physical, ultrasonographic evaluation of the pelvis, and, in many cases, laparoscopy. As a general rule, after the history and physical examination, transvaginal ultrasonography is the best initial approach to diagnosis because it may detect endometriomas (large, fluid-filled endometriosis implants) and serve to evaluate the pelvis for the presence of other pathology. The diagnosis of endometriosis can be confirmed only through laparoscopy or laparotomy, with tissue biopsies. Surgical or hormonal treatment modalities should be considered based on the severity of the disease and the desire for childbearing.

PATIENT CARE

Clinical Thinking

- When approaching a patient with suspected endometriosis, the clinician must remember that there are no signs or symptoms pathognomonic of endometriosis.
- A detailed history and physical with special attention focusing on quality and character of pain as it relates to menses and intercourse

are of paramount importance. Urinary, bowel, and musculoskeletal symptoms should also be addressed. Initial evaluation should include urinalysis, endocervical cultures, pregnancy test, and transvaginal ultrasonography to rule out other conditions associated with chronic pain (i.e., uterine fibroids and ovarian cysts). Urinary or pelvic infections should be ruled out.

- At this point, the necessity of laparoscopy is dictated by the severity of symptoms, the patient's age, and her desire to achieve pregnancy.
- Patients with mild or moderate pain and no interest in future fertility may receive empiric medical treatment with oral contraceptives, progestins, danazol, or gonadotropin-releasing hormone (GnRH) analogs. Those with more severe symptoms or those whose symptoms do not respond to medical therapy are good candidates for laparoscopic exploration with possible intraoperative intervention according to the findings. Those interested in optimizing reproductive potential should also undergo laparoscopic surgical intervention.
- After the severity of the disease has been adequately classified, an individualized treatment plan can be implemented.

History
- Many women are totally asymptomatic and present with a negative history. Endometriosis is often documented as an incidental finding during gynecologic and general surgical procedures.
- However, most patients with endometriosis have a long-standing history of dysmenorrhea, dyspareunia, low back pain, pelvic pain, or infertility. The aforementioned symptoms may present as a single symptom or in any combination.
- The most frequent chief complaint is pelvic pain that can be persistent during the menstrual cycle. Alternatively, pain may be described as increasing just before menstrual flow. Significant exacerbation of pain is often associated with active bleeding. Pain may present with various grades of severity.
- The presence of bowel or bladder symptoms often makes it very difficult to differentiate endometriosis from irritable bowel syndrome or interstitial cystitis.

Physical Examination
- A wide range of physical findings may be present at once, individually or in combination, or not be present at all.
- The patient's abdomen is typically soft with different degrees of lower abdominal and pelvic tenderness. Tenderness is generally consistent with serial examinations.
- Cervical and vaginal visual examinations are often normal.
- Bimanual examination may demonstrate a retroverted uterus (secondary to posterior cul-de-sac adhesions), cervical motion tenderness, or uterosacral ligaments with nodularity and tenderness.

Pelvic organ fixation (i.e., "frozen pelvis") with or without adnexal masses may be appreciated with more severe cases.
- Blue, brown, or black nodules can be found in previous laparoscopy or laparotomy surgical sites.

Tests for Consideration
- **Laparoscopy:** The gold standard for the diagnosis and initial treatment of endometriosis. $700
- **Depo-leuprolide treatment:** Hormonal or GnRH agonist treatment can be considered as an adjunct to help with diagnosis, but it cannot reliably tell the whole story. $300
- **Pathologic biopsies:** From the laparoscopy. Implants can be described in various ways (e.g., gunshot, powder burn), have different colors (e.g., white, red, black, brown), present in various locations (e.g., peritoneal, ovarian, bowel), and can also be described with different grades of severity (minimal, mild, moderate, and severe). $500

IMAGING CONSIDERATIONS

→ **Ultrasonography** is often the first choice for an imaging study. Ultrasonographic scans are useful to discover and describe endometriomas. Endometriomas appear as intraovarian cystic structures with internal echoes and hazy borders. This noninvasive study also helps to exclude other causes of chronic pelvic pain that may be secondary to adnexal or uterine masses. $250

→ **CT** and **MRI** are occasionally helpful to characterize pelvic pathology (e.g., adenomyosis), but should not be ordered routinely in this context.   CT: $800   MRI: $1500

Clinical Entities   Medical Knowledge

Endometriosis

Pφ Endometriosis is characterized by implants of endometrial tissue at "ectopic" or unexpected locations in the pelvis. There are competing theories as to why endometriosis develops in some patients and not others. The etiology of endometriosis remains elusive and controversial.

TP Typical presentation is as previously described, and can include chronic pelvic pain, dysmenorrhea, infertility, and abdominal or pelvic masses.

Dx Diagnosis is generally reached at the time of laparoscopy or laparotomy, but the physician may have a high index of suspicion based on history, examination findings, and ultrasonographic findings.

Tx Therapy can include surgical removal of the implants, fulguration of the implants, or hormonal suppression of endogenous estrogen production because estrogen is presumed to be the hormonal agent that drives the development and growth of the implants. **See Katz 19, Hacker 25.**

Adenomyosis

Pφ Defined as the presence of endometrial glands and stromal tissue in the myometrium. The endometrial tissue described may be functional, causing cyclic pelvic pain and congestion. Adenomyosis may present with endometriosis or fibroids.

TP A broad spectrum of symptoms are associated with adenomyosis. Various degrees of dysmenorrhea, dyspareunia, and abnormal bleeding are often reported. The uterus can be found to be enlarged, globular, soft, or boggy. Adenomyosis is more often associated with parous women.

Dx The diagnosis can be clinically suspected and histologically confirmed. Ultrasonography may be helpful but MRI is the study of choice if adenomyosis is a part of the differential diagnosis. Endometrial biopsy is used only to rule out any other associated cause of abnormal bleeding.

Tx Conservative management is recommended in young patients, especially those desiring fertility. Treatment strategy should mirror that for endometriosis. Surgical treatment (i.e., total abdominal hysterectomy) can be entertained in patients with severe pain who have completed childbearing. **See Katz 18, Hacker 25.**

Pelvic Adhesions

Pφ The adhesive process results as a consequence of an inflammatory event (appendicitis, pelvic infections, endometriosis) or trauma (surgery) on or around the pelvic organs. During the process of healing, some pelvic organs become unintentionally adherent to one another, leading to anatomic distortion, functional alterations, and pain.

TP Patients present to the office with history of pelvic surgery, infection, or inflammatory process. There is no typical presenting sign or symptom. If present, pain is typically chronic (i.e., not related to the cycle) and may increase with intercourse or activity. Intestinal symptoms or even obstruction might develop if there is bowel involvement. Fallopian tube involvement invariably results in tubal factor infertility.

Dx Laparoscopic visualization of the pelvic and abdominal cavity is the method of choice. No imaging diagnostic techniques are recommended in these cases.

Tx The studies evaluating the efficacy of laparoscopic lysis of adhesions for pain control have shown contradictory and inconsistent results. This approach is currently recommended after the other causes of pain have been excluded. **See Katz 8, 11; Hacker 21.**

Pelvic Inflammatory Disease

Pφ Inflammatory reaction caused by pathogens ascending to the upper genital tract, including the fallopian tubes and pelvic peritoneum. Often caused by infection with *Neisseria gonorrhoeae* and *Chlamydia trachomatis*. Less commonly caused by anaerobes, such as *Hemophilus influenzae*, group A *Streptococcus*, and *Pneumococcus* species.

TP Patients present with the typical triad of fever, pelvic pain, and cervical motion tenderness. A mucopurulent vaginal discharge may also be present.

Dx Swab for Gram stain and culture of endocervix is mandatory. Other nonspecific laboratory findings may include leukocytosis and an elevated C-reactive protein and erythrocyte sedimentation rate. Ultrasonography will help to document the presence of tubo-ovarian abscesses. Laparoscopy will visually confirm the presence of inflammation, purulent secretion, or abscess. Surgery should be avoided if an acceptable response to antibiotics is appreciated.

Tx Different modalities are available according to the degree of severity:

Inpatient therapy:

- Intravenous third-generation cephalosporin plus intravenous doxycycline
- Intravenous clindamycin plus gentamicin

Outpatient therapy:

- Second-generation oral cephalosporin plus oral doxycycline
- Oral fluoroquinolone plus oral metronidazole

See Chapter 37, Pelvic Inflammatory Disease, for a more comprehensive discussion of PID diagnosis and treatment. **See Katz 23, Hacker 22.**

Pelvic Congestion Syndrome

Pφ Pelvic venous congestion (similar to varicosities in the legs) has been described as one of the causes of chronic pelvic pain in women. It has been postulated that the smooth muscle dysfunction of the pelvic veins is the result of autonomic nervous system dysfunction in response to stress and hormonal actions.

TP Women of childbearing age are the most commonly affected, often complaining of bilateral lower abdominal and back pain before and during the menstrual period, occasionally associated with dyspareunia and abnormal bleeding. Pelvic examination reveals diffuse lower abdominal and parametrial tenderness.

Dx Ultrasonography and MRI may reveal dilated pelvic veins and varicosities. This may also be demonstrated during diagnostic laparoscopy. Venography, however, is the gold standard for diagnosis.

Tx Again, after ruling out other causes of chronic pelvic pain, we may initially approach the problem medically (with hormone suppression therapy—progestins, continuous oral contraceptives, etc.); however, if the pain is incapacitating and affects daily living, we may offer other, more invasive treatment modalities such as embolization or salpingo-oophorectomy. A hysterectomy and bilateral salpingo-oophorectomy may be entertained as possibly therapeutic in more severe cases. **See Katz 8, 36; Hacker 21.**

ZEBRA ZONE

a. **Ovarian remnant syndrome:** Results from residual ovarian tissue left in the abdominal cavity after oophorectomy. The pain is the product of ovarian remnant encasement in fibrotic adhesions.

b. **Urethral syndrome:** Suprapubic and vaginal pain, dyspareunia, associated with urinary symptoms (dysuria, frequency, urgency) of unknown etiology, in absence of bladder or urethral abnormalities.

c. **Myofascial pain:** Characterized by diffuse lower abdominal, vaginal, or pelvic pain in association with multiple trigger points distributed mainly in lower abdominal quadrants.

d. **Diverticular disease:** Characterized by the presence of outpouchings of sigmoid colon wall, usually asymptomatic if noninfected. May present as a long history of diarrhea, constipation, bloating, and pain.

e. **Psychogenic pain:** Commonly present in patients with history of depression, psychiatric events, or sexual abuse.

Practice-Based Learning and Improvement: Evidence-Based Medicine

Title
Ovulation suppression for endometriosis

Authors
Hughes E, Fedorkow D, Collins J, Vandekerckhove P

Institution
Department of Obstetrics and Gynaecology, McMaster University, Hamilton, Ontario, Canada

Reference
Cochrane Database of Systematic Reviews 2003;(3):CD000155

Problem
Determination of ovulation suppression effectiveness in the treatment of endometriosis.

Intervention
Patients with diagnosis of endometriosis were subject to ovulation suppression with danazol, medroxyprogesterone, gestrinone, contraceptive pills, or GnRH analogs compared with placebo.

Comparison/control (quality of evidence)
Randomized, controlled trials comparing ovulation suppression agents versus placebo from 1985 to 2002 were systematically analyzed.

Outcome/effect

The results of this study suggest that the use of study medications do not justify the risk of side effects when used as therapy for endometriosis-associated infertility.

Historical significance/comments

Although ovulation suppression appears to be beneficial for endometriosis-related pain, there is evidence that is not useful for endometriosis-associated infertility. In this group of patients the surgical approach is preferred.

Interpersonal and Communication Skills

Endometriosis: Counseling Partners of Patients

Endometriosis can be a distressing diagnosis both for your patient and her partner. Research on patients with endometriosis demonstrates a patient perception that their disease surrounds them with a sense of powerlessness, frustration, and ongoing grieving. Partners of patients with endometriosis can be affected by similar feelings, particularly powerlessness, frustration, and guilt. They will also face many challenges, including unanticipated life changes and natural grief reactions. When counseling your patients, be sure to show empathy and provide emotional support to partners as you sense this is required. Keep in mind that your patient's partner is surely involved with her life and should be, to some degree, involved with her care. Involve them as much as is appropriate in discussions with your patient and empower them to help if possible.[1]

Professionalism

Principle: Commitment to Patient Welfare

Endometriosis as a source of pelvic pain is one of many disease processes in which pain has both physiologic and psychological roots. To provide best care, the clinician must seek out and understand both of these components and be able to discuss them openly with the patient in a shame-free environment. Knowledge of the patient's social situation and emotional well-being obtained through discreet and comfortable dialogue will be helpful. Holding such conversations early while formulating a treatment plan lets the patient know that the physician acknowledges that psychological components of the pain are just as real as the physiologic. The clinician must be able to manage the process in a holistic, comprehensive manner.

Systems-Based Practice

Do We Have a "Right" to Health Care?

One of the challenges of the U.S. health care system surrounds the question of whether people inherently have a right to health care. Many people feel that everyone—regardless of ability to pay—should have a right to basic care. Others argue that like other goods or services, health care needs to be delivered in a free market. The question of treatment for infertility takes this question to another level. Although many agree that everyone should have a right to basic emergency health care (e.g., treatment of acute appendicitis) and even more would agree that it is appropriate for health insurance plans to cover reasonable necessary nonemergency care (e.g., primary care visits or treatment of hypercholesterolemia), there is much less agreement on whether it is appropriate for health care plans to cover treatment of infertility, which is not medically necessary. Although some argue that infertility itself is a medical disorder and deserves treatment on par with any other medical disorder, others maintain that because it does not present any clear danger to a patient, and is in many cases the natural result of advanced maternal age, it falls beyond the appropriate use of health care dollars, and should have to be paid for by patients themselves. In the United States, most insurance companies have come to something of a compromise on the matter, in which they will cover some limited forms of treatment for infertility (such as a diagnostic work-up, drug therapy, and in some cases a single attempt at IVF), whereas more extensive treatment, including repeated attempts at IVF, is left for patients to pay out of pocket.

Reference

1. Fernandez I, Reid C, Dziurawiec S: Living with endometriosis: The perspective of male partners. J Psychosom Res 2006;61:433–438.

Chapter 49
Approaching Secondary Amenorrhea (Case 34)

Jessica M. Mory DO *and*
Cynthia Carrole Sagullo MD, FACOG

Case: A 35-year-old G1P1 presents to your office complaining of amenorrhea for the last 8 months.

Differential Diagnosis

Hypothalamic dysfunction	Pituitary dysfunction	Premature ovarian failure
Uterine scarring: Asherman syndrome	Polycystic ovary syndrome (PCOS)	Hypothyroidism

Speaking Intelligently

There are two types of amenorrhea. Primary amenorrhea can be diagnosed if the patient has no spontaneous menses by the age of 16 years. (The evaluation for **primary amenorrhea** is complex, and is addressed in **Hacker 32, pp 355–358**.) **Secondary amenorrhea,** characterized by absence of menses for 6 months or more, is far more common. The most important tool for evaluating the etiology of secondary amenorrhea is a comprehensive history. A stepwise approach to this involves a thorough knowledge of the physiology that controls the various aspects of the menstrual cycle: the hypothalamus, pituitary, ovaries, and uterus. Of course, first I always rule out the most common cause of secondary amenorrhea— pregnancy.

PATIENT CARE

Clinical Thinking
- First, establish that the problem is indeed *secondary* amenorrhea by careful history taking.
- Mentally work cephalic to caudal, thinking of each system, organ, or anatomic cause that could affect the menstrual cycle. Consider the hypothalamus, pituitary, and thyroid; then ovaries, uterus, and cervix.

- Prioritize the differential diagnosis in order to be efficient and cost effective. Proceed with a focused examination and appropriate testing.

History

- Begin with the patient's menstrual history. Be sure to include age at menarche, then work chronologically to the present. Establish whether there have been prior episodes of amenorrhea and if a cause was discovered in the past.
- Ask the patient if she has ever been diagnosed with a disease process that could be responsible for the amenorrhea: specifically, inquire about thyroid or pituitary dysfunction, PCOS, tumors, or other systemic illnesses.
- Rule out recent stressful events that may lead to hypothalamic amenorrhea, such as change in diet, weight, exercise habits, or severe illness.
- Check the patient's medications for drugs known to cause amenorrhea such as danazol, progestins, or drugs that affect prolactin levels—like metoclopramide and certain antipsychotics such as risperidone.
- Ask about symptoms such as headache, visual changes, fatigue, palpitations, polydipsia, or galactorrhea. These findings can represent hypothalamic or pituitary dysfunction.
- Are there signs of estrogen deficiency that could be caused by premature ovarian failure such as hot flashes or vaginal dryness?
- Ask about events that may have caused uterine scarring (Asherman syndrome), such as previous uterine infection or D&C; or surgical procedures that may have led to cervical stenosis and hematometra, such as cervical conization or cauterization; or spontaneous stenosis secondary to hypoestrogenism.

Physical Examination

- Does the patient have any signs of hyperandrogenism such as acne, hirsutism, or voice changes?
- Examine the skin, looking for acanthosis nigricans, vitiligo, skin thinning or thickening, bruising, or striae.
- Measure and record height and weight. Consider both extremes of the body mass index (BMI). A BMI greater than 30 kg/m^2 is seen in more than 50% of women with PCOS. Keep in mind, however, that there are thin patients with PCOS as well. If the patient's BMI is less than 18.5 kg/m^2, it is important to consider hypoestrogenism as a cause of amenorrhea, and consider cachexia as a possible sign of an eating disorder or other systemic illnesses.
- Perform a thorough breast examination with gentle compression toward the areola looking for the presence of galactorrhea.
- A careful pelvic examination is essential in diagnosis of a cervical, uterine, or adnexal pathology.

Tests for Consideration

- **Human chorionic gonadotropin (β-hCG):** To rule out
  pregnancy. $135
- **Prolactin:** To rule out hyperprolactinemia. $100
- **Thyroid-stimulating hormone (TSH):** To rule out
  thyroid disorders. $60
- **Follicle-stimulating hormone (FSH):** To rule out
  ovarian failure. $100
- **Dehydroepiandrosterone sulfate (DHEAS)** and
  testosterone: To rule out hyperandrogenism. $200

IMAGING CONSIDERATIONS

→**Pelvic ultrasonography:** If adnexal pathology
suspected on physical examination. $250
→**Hysteroscopy:** If indicated based on history of risk
factors for Asherman syndrome. $355
→**Cranial imaging—MRI:** If prolactinemia is diagnosed
on two separate occasions and cannot be attributed
to another cause such as an antipsychotic medication. $2150
→**CT of adrenal glands:** In presence of
hyperandrogenism that does not suppress with
administration of dexamethasone. $800

Clinical Entities   **Medical Knowledge**

Hypothalamic Dysfunction

Pφ Functional hypothalamic amenorrhea arises as a result of
decreased gonadotropin-releasing hormone (GnRH) secretion by
the hypothalamus.

TP The patient may present with a history of anorexia nervosa, high
stress state, or excessive exercise. In some instances there is no
identifiable contributing factor. There may be the presence of the
"female athlete triad": amenorrhea, eating disorder, and
osteoporosis/osteopenia.

Dx May be seen in patients with BMI <18.5, or more than 10%
below ideal body weight. Clinical signs of low estrogen (hot

flashes, vaginal dryness), as well as normal to low FSH (with FSH > luteinizing hormone).

Tx Weight gain by increasing the ratio of caloric intake to energy expenditure, under the supervision of a dietician. Possible psychiatric counseling or cognitive behavioral therapy. Treatment of osteoporosis with bisphosphonates if indicated. **See Katz 38, Hacker 32.**

Pituitary Dysfunction

Pφ Increased prolactin secretion suppresses hypothalamic GnRH secretion, leading to low gonadotropin and estradiol concentrations.

TP Amenorrhea associated with the onset of galactorrhea. This may be associated with the start of a new medication, such as an antipsychotic like risperidone or the antiemetic metoclopramide.

Dx Serum prolactin concentration above 15 to 20 ng/mL (15 to 20 µg/L). Cranial imaging (MRI) is indicated if prolactin is elevated on two occasions and it cannot be attributed to other causes such as medication.

Tx There are several options for the treatment of pituitary dysfunction, ranging from medication to surgery.

- **Dopamine agonists** (cabergoline, bromocriptine, pergolide) are used most commonly, and allow the pituitary-GnRH axis to resume normal function. This is the first-line treatment for hyperprolactinemia as a result of pituitary dysfunction, and this therapeutic approach is often successful, resulting in resumption of normal menses.
- **Trans-sphenoidal surgery:** *Considered* when dopamine agonists fail, or when the adenoma is >3 cm and the patient desires pregnancy.
- **Radiation therapy:** Rarely used except to prevent regrowth after excision of a macroadenoma.
- **Estrogen** (with progestin): An option for patients with hyperprolactinemia secondary to antipsychotic therapy. Sometimes estrogen therapy can be prescribed for patients who fail dopamine agonist therapy and do not wish to become pregnant.
  See Katz 38, 39, Hacker 32.

Hypothyroidism

Pφ Hypothyroidism can occur either at the level of the pituitary gland, with decreased TSH production, or at the level of the thyroid gland itself, with decreased thyroid hormone production.

TP Classic signs and symptoms of hypothyroidism such as depression, weight gain, or somnolence accompanied by secondary amenorrhea.

Dx Abnormal TSH or thyroid hormone levels, usually seen with other physical findings consistent with hypothyroidism as listed above.

Tx Correct the thyroid dysfunction as indicated with medication, therapy, or surgery, and await return of regular menstrual cycles when euthyroid state is achieved. **See Katz 39.**

Polycystic Ovary Syndrome

Pφ PCOS is a complicated and not entirely well understood condition that arises in the face of insulin resistance and hyperandrogenism. Very often, but not always, it is associated with obesity.

TP Throughout her reproductive life the patient may have irregular menstrual cycles punctuated by prolonged periods of amenorrhea. Hirsutism and obesity are very common physical examination findings.

Dx For a diagnosis of PCOS, a patient must have two of the following three:

- Hyperandrogenism
- Oligomenorrhea or amenorrhea
- Polycystic ovaries on ultrasonography

Tx The treatment of PCOS begins with a compassionate discussion with the patient regarding the fact that the etiology of this disorder is poorly understood, and that there may be a familial component as well. Treatment then proceeds with counseling regarding the risks and benefits of combined estrogen and progestin hormone replacement. Birth control pills are a convenient and well-tolerated therapeutic option. The first-line treatment of PCOS is usually oral contraceptives for patients who do not currently desire pregnancy. Oral contraceptives contain estradiol, which prevents androgen excess by inhibiting the hypothalamus-pituitary-ovarian axis, and progestin, which prevents endometrial hyperplasia. Other therapies to consider are progestins, glucocorticoids, GnRH agonists, and oral hypoglycemic agents such as metformin. **See Katz 40, Hacker 32.**

Premature Ovarian Failure

Pφ Occurs when the supply of oocytes is depleted before the age of 40 years, resulting in a premature menopause causing estrogen deficiency, endometrial atrophy, and cessation of menstruation.

TP Increasingly irregular menses throughout the course of reproductive life, often accompanied by other signs of menopause. The patient may have a family history of premature ovarian failure.

Dx Premature ovarian failure can be diagnosed with three measurements of "day 3" (i.e., the third day of a normal menstrual cycle) FSH and serum estradiol. This is done over the course of three consecutive menstrual cycles. The FSH will be elevated and the estradiol will be low.

Tx Premature ovarian failure is usually treated with repletion of estrogen and progesterone, if the patient is symptomatic and so desires. **See Katz 38, 42.**

Uterine Scarring: Asherman Syndrome

Pφ Asherman syndrome is characterized by intrauterine adhesions, called *synechiae* (the sequela of intrauterine trauma and scarring), which result in amenorrhea. Think of this condition as an occlusion of the normal endometrial cavity.

TP Patients complain of prolonged amenorrhea after a uterine procedure. Most typically, Asherman syndrome occurs after a vaginal delivery complicated by a postpartum hemorrhage secondary to a retained placental fragment. Curettage and subsequent endometritis in the immediate postpartum period is the most likely cause in this situation. Endometrial scarring can also occur after routine D&E or D&C procedures.

Dx Diagnostic hysteroscopy is the gold standard for diagnosis. However, radiologic imaging studies, such as a hysterosalpingography (HSG) or sonohysterography, may be helpful.

Tx The primary treatment is lysis of adhesions with operative hysteroscopy. The prevention of adhesion reformation in the immediate postoperative period can be achieved by the administration of high-dose estrogen followed by a progesterone-induced withdrawal bleed, or the intraoperative placement of a cavity-filling device such as a pediatric Foley balloon within the uterus, which can remain for up to 10 days. **See Katz 38, Hacker 19, 32.**

ZEBRA ZONE

a. **Premature ovarian failure:** Caused by fragile X syndrome, Turner syndrome (45X), or 47,XXY and mosaicisms.

b. **Secondary empty sella turcica syndrome:** This occurs after a large pituitary adenoma is surgically removed and can result in amenorrhea.

c. **Infiltrative diseases of the hypothalamus:** Lymphoma, Langerhans cell histiocytosis, sarcoidosis.

d. **Hypothyroidism:** Secondary to Sheehan syndrome (pituitary dysfunction after severe postpartum hemorrhage with hypoperfusion of the pituitary gland, resulting in cell death), radiation, infarction, nonlactotrophic adenomas, and infiltrative lesions of the pituitary gland.

Practice-Based Learning and Improvement: Evidence-Based Medicine

Title
Current evaluation of amenorrhea

Authors
The Practice Committee of the American Society for Reproductive Medicine

Institution
American Society for Reproductive Medicine, Birmingham, Alabama

Reference
Fertility and Sterility 2006;86(5 Suppl):S148–S155

Problem
Amenorrhea.

Intervention
Diagnosis algorithm and management.

Comparison/control (quality of evidence)
Practice bulletin.

Outcome/effect
Advocates and instructs for better, more thoughtful evaluation of amenorrhea.

Historical significance/comments
Current consensus on diagnosis, evaluation, and management of women with amenorrhea presented as a practice bulletin from the American Society for Reproductive Medicine. Describes current expert opinion and evidence-based approaches to the diagnosis and management of amenorrhea.

Interpersonal and Communication Skills

Talking about Adoption

The nature of obstetrics and gynecology presents the need and opportunity for physicians to speak with patients about adoption both in the context of an infertile couple's desire to adopt a child and in the case of a patient wanting to give up a child for adoption. In fact, one of the most important interventions a clinician can provide to such patients is a referral to a well-established, well-respected adoption service. Such agencies provide crucial needs, including counseling, home studies, and legal advice.

Because premature ovarian failure is one of the more common causes of secondary amenorrhea, such conversations will often arise in this context. For patients with premature ovarian failure who have not begun or completed childbearing, the options for reproductive success are significantly diminished. The only real option for many of these patients is "donor-egg" programs, which can be complicated, costly, and in many instances unsuccessful. Rather than pursue donor programs, many patients will instead elect to pursue adoption.

Obviously, a second context when the topic of adoption arises is when one is faced with a patient who has an unwanted pregnancy who is considering giving up the child for adoption. When discussing adoption, it is important to be candid and forthright but gentle in conversation. When you are providing care for adoptive parents or to parents who are giving up their child for adoption, maintain a compassionate approach. From both perspectives, it is likely that there will be very strong emotions. Consider the patient's unique perspectives on these matters and differentiate them from your own perspectives, lest you be judgmental. Counseling about adoption is highly specialized and a clinician's confident referral to reputable agencies is likely to be an enduring support for patients.

Professionalism

Principle: Commitment to Primacy of Patient Welfare

Understanding when a patient is likely to be receptive to your advice is part of the "art" of medicine. Consider, for example, that a patient presents to you with secondary amenorrhea and you diagnose her with an eating disorder. Surely, your responsibility should not end abruptly with a summative formulation and explanation of a treatment plan. Young women with eating disorders will often have very complex underlying psychopathology and even though you may feel unprepared or unqualified to deal with the psychological underpinnings of a patient with an eating disorder, referring this patient to a counselor at the first visit could engender resentment and prove counterproductive. In such a case it is prudent to work through several visits to create an atmosphere of trust and respect. Identify social supports in the patient's life who might be able to work as allies with the health care team. Although your goal should be to eventually get your patient involved with a treatment team that includes a counselor, a nutritionist, and the primary care physician, timing is important. Part of the art of medicine is to decide *when* your patients will be most receptive to the "correct" interventions and when it is advisable to wait before moving forward with your recommendations.

Systems-Based Practice

Use of Practice Guidelines

The American Society for Reproductive Medicine (ASRM), as well as the American College of Obstetrics and Gynecology, publishes evidence-based practice guidelines that can serve as general templates for "best practices" regarding diagnosis and treatment. For example, the work-up of a patient similar to the one cited at the beginning of this chapter is outlined in the ASRM practice bulletin discussed in this chapter's Practice-Based Learning and Improvement box. This practice bulletin recommends that you first:

- Take a history and perform a physical examination.
- Rule out pregnancy with a serum quantitative β-hCG.
- Check FSH and prolactin levels.

Based on these few simple and easy-to-interpret test results, you can then move on to more advanced diagnostic testing should it be required. Practice bulletins are typically drafted by committees of experts, incorporate most of the recent data regarding the clinical problem, and are regularly updated. Evidence-based practice guidelines prevent or discourage unnecessary or unhelpful testing, allow easy access to the most relevant strategies for diagnosis and treatment, and contain bibliographies of the most useful references.

Chapter 50
Teaching Visual: Secondary Amenorrhea
Anthony Lee Yu and Michael Belden MD

Objectives

- Describe the differential diagnosis of secondary amenorrhea.
- List the appropriate laboratory studies to evaluate secondary amenorrhea.

Medical Knowledge

Secondary amenorrhea is one of the most common complaints an obstetrician/gynecologist will be asked to evaluate in the clinical setting. It can be a particularly vexing disorder, especially to the patient who has had essentially regular cycles throughout the majority of her reproductive life. Secondary amenorrhea is a disorder that physicians in other specialties are often asked to evaluate. Internists, family practitioners, and pediatricians are often approached about this problem.

The hormonal physiology that drives menstruation is complex, and as a result, unnecessary laboratory and radiologic studies are often ordered that do not uncover the source of the problem. Thus, an understanding of not only the physiology, but also of the appropriate studies and what information they elucidate is essential for effective and efficient treatment.

First and foremost, pregnancy, the most common cause of secondary amenorrhea, must be ruled out with a serum β-hCG test. If negative, 3 separate tests are usually ordered: TSH (thyroid stimulating hormone), FSH (follicle-stimulating hormone), and serum prolactin. Though an appropriate history and physical examination should dictate a logical sequence of these tests, many gynecologists will order all three tests simultaneously as a matter of patient convenience. Test results along with a thorough history and physical are the key to guiding your thought process towards the correct diagnosis and proper therapy.

The following exercise will help you consolidate your thoughts regarding the evaluation of secondary amenorrhea. In the yellow diamonds you will see the four most commonly ordered tests which help in the evaluation of secondary amenorrhea. The six purple rectangles contain the most likely diagnoses. Place the diamonds and rectangles into the algorithm appropriately, then check your work on the following page.

Place the four tests and six diagnoses where they make sense within the algorithm described for evaluation of secondary amenorrhea.

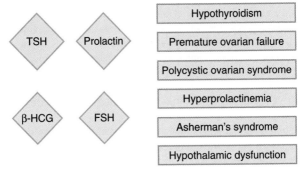

TSH   Prolactin

β-HCG   FSH

Hypothyroidism

Premature ovarian failure

Polycystic ovarian syndrome

Hyperprolactinemia

Asherman's syndrome

Hypothalamic dysfunction

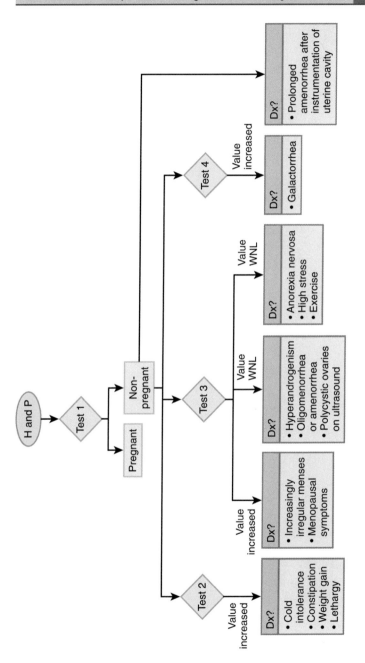

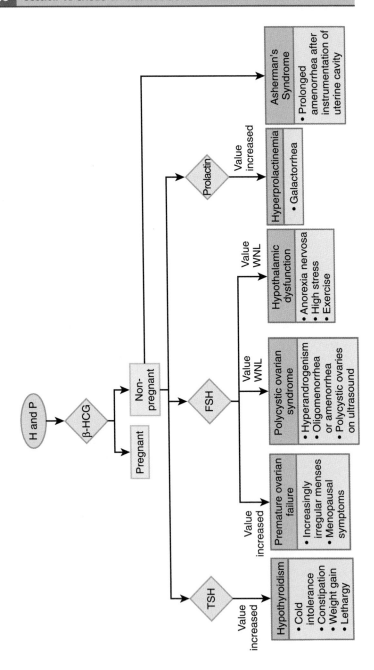

Professor's Pearls: Cases in Reproductive Endocrinology

Consider the following clinical problems and questions posed. Then refer to the professor's discussion of these issues.

1. A 33-year-old G0P0 presents to your office with her husband. She believes she has primary infertility. Her menstrual cycles over the last 18 months are 45 to 90 days apart. She reports that she is unable to lose weight and has gained 40 pounds over the last 2 years. On physical examination her body mass index (BMI) is 30, indicating obesity. She also notes hirsutism of the abdomen and chin. Her serum testosterone is 84 ng/dL (normal range, 20 to 70 ng/dL) and her prolactin and thyroid-stimulating hormone (TSH) levels are within normal limits.

2. A 29-year-old G0P0 reports a 3-year history of infertility with her male partner. You note that her history includes an episode of pelvic inflammatory disease at age 25 years. Her menses are regular. Her partner fathered a child, now 7 years old, during a previous relationship.

3. A 38-year-old comes to your office because she has not been able to achieve pregnancy. She tells you that despite painful intercourse, she has had unprotected sexual activity during the last 3 years. Her periods occur every 28 to 31 days, with severe pain 3 days before and during her menses. Her husband's sperm analysis is normal. You perform a laparoscopy and find severe adhesive disease, stage 3 endometriosis, and bilateral tubal occlusion. Discuss the possible therapeutic options.

4. A 31-year-old G1P1 complains of 4 months of amenorrhea and has been unable to conceive after 14 months of trying. She reports a history of regular menstrual cycles until 3 years ago, soon after her first child. Her history is otherwise uncomplicated and a normal physical examination is noted. A day 3 follicle-stimulating hormone (FSH) level is 46 ng/mL, and prolactin is 7 ng/mL. On further questioning, you discover that she had no difficulty conceiving her first child, and she delivered by cesarean section but "had to stay a few extra days in the hospital and take antibiotics."

Discussion by Dr. William Pfeffer, Main Line Fertility, Bryn Mawr, Pennsylvania

Answer 1: Clinical Considerations: Oligo-ovulation and Infertility
This vignette almost certainly describes a patient with polycystic ovaries and the metabolic syndrome. For the sake of completeness, a 17-OH progesterone level should be obtained in the follicular phase of her menstrual cycle to rule out congenital adrenal hyperplasia or

Cushing syndrome. The first step in addressing this patient's problem is to encourage lifestyle changes, including increased physical activity and low-carbohydrate diet. Although not firmly established in the literature, my preference is to simultaneously pursue issues of insulin resistance. Specifically, I would measure the patient's sex hormone–binding globulin and insulin levels. If any suggestion of insulin resistance is encountered, I would begin her on metformin (simultaneous with her attempts to improve her lifestyle activities).

I would allow 4 to 8 weeks of this program and reevaluate the patient. Has she begun to ovulate spontaneously on her own? How thick is her endometrial lining? Do we need to induce a withdrawal flow?

Unless the patient makes a remarkable improvement on metformin (ovulates spontaneously), after 8 weeks I would add clomiphene (Clomid) and begin to monitor her ovulations. I would also be sure to check that her partner has an appropriate semen analysis, and eventually check her fallopian tubes for patency with a hysterosalpingogram. I would look for her to become pregnant through this treatment.

Answer 2: Clinical Considerations: Infertility Caused by Pelvic Inflammatory Disease and Tubal Factor
The history invites the diagnosis of chronic tubal disease. Before we jump to that conclusion, despite his previous fathering of a child, the husband should undergo a semen analysis.

The first step in evaluating the patient's fallopian tubes is a sonogram. If hydrosalpinges are evident, we would skip the hysterosalpingogram and proceed to laparoscopy. If the patient has no hydrosalpinx evident on ultrasonography, she should have a hysterosalpingogram as her next step.

If we encounter tubal disease, this may be suitable for surgical treatment (for example, lysis of peritubal adhesions). If we encounter hydrosalpinges, the alternatives are removal of the fallopian tubes (with a future plan for in vitro fertilization) or lysis of adhesions with attempted salpineostomy with an attempt at surgical correction. The patient's inclinations regarding surgery and advanced reproductive technologies as well as insurance limitations might direct our choice of treatment. In any case, it is helpful to know whether we are likely to encounter a hydrosalpinx at the time of laparoscopy in order to make a preoperative decision regarding how we plan to treat the problem.

Answer 3: Clinical Considerations: The Treatment of Infertility Caused by Endometriosis
Similar to case no. 2, this patient has tubal disease. The damage to her tubes is likely to have been caused by her relatively severe endometriosis. Treatment alternatives include surgical resection of

endometriosis with tubal repair, followed by attempts to conceive "naturally" versus in vitro fertilization. If in vitro fertilization is an option, hydrosalpinges should be divided or removed to increase the patient's pregnancy rate. Therefore, a preoperative hysterosalpingogram anticipating the hydrosalpinges would have been helpful in deciding how to proceed at surgery.

The presence of endometriosis, in my experience, does not significantly affect the patient's prognosis for conception by in vitro fertilization. We have been careful not to aspirate endometriomas during oocyte retrieval because we have encountered some ovarian infections due to "seeding" of these endometriomas by vaginal bacteria introduced through the ovum retrieval procedure.

Answer 4: Clinical Considerations: Premature Ovarian Failure

Unfortunately for this patient, the diagnosis is most likely premature ovarian failure. When younger patients present with this condition, we are more interested in the karyotype to rule out variants of Turner syndrome. Similarly, evaluation of the fragile X status of the patient has implications for her existing child and potential future conceptions.

I often treat a patient such as this with low-dose unopposed estrogen (for example, 0.025-mg skin patch). On occasion, the estrogen therapy facilitates the return of ovulation. In any case, when estrogen is given unopposed by progesterone, one must keep track of the thickness of the patient's endometrial lining.

In situations like this (despite the patient's prior good pregnancy outcome), conception with the patient's own eggs is unlikely. Donor eggs remain an option. In the presence of low estrogen, one also should discuss bone health and sexual function with the patient.

Section VII
CASES IN GYNECOLOGIC ONCOLOGY

Section Editor
Mitchell Edelson MD

Chapter 51
Cervical Cancer (Case 35)

Kristen M. McCullen MD and
Norman G. Rosenblum MD, PhD

Case: A 40-year-old woman presents to a gynecologist with a 6-month history of ongoing spotting and postcoital bleeding. She has not been to a gynecologist since the birth of her son, 10 years ago. On several occasions she has also had a watery vaginal discharge.

Differential Diagnosis

Cervical cancer	Cervical polyp
Cervical myoma	Endometrial hyperplasia or endometrial cancer

Speaking Intelligently

When I encounter a patient with postcoital bleeding, my first questions are always directed to gynecologic history. Does she have normal menses? Women with anatomic causes of abnormal vaginal bleeding usually have regular menstrual cycles in addition to irregular bleeding. Is she having intermenstrual bleeding as well as postcoital bleeding? If the abnormal bleeding is limited to postcoital bleeding only, one can eliminate the upper genital tract causes of abnormal bleeding. Such upper tract uterine pathology includes uterine fibroids, endometrial hyperplasia, and endometrial cancer. Postcoital bleeding is almost always caused by a lower genital tract lesion of the cervix, vagina, or vulva. In the face of postcoital bleeding, the physical examination can shed much light on the situation. A speculum examination allows the physician to visualize any anatomic abnormalities or lesions immediately.

PATIENT CARE

Clinical Thinking
- Consider the most serious problem you may be facing: cancer of the lower genital tract.
- A thorough history and physical examination can allow for an accurate diagnosis.

- A physical examination should include a biopsy of any suspect lesion. The pathology diagnosis is the key to management.

History

- Menstrual history is critical. LMP, age of menarche, frequency and duration of menstrual cycles, and history of irregular bleeding must be ascertained to determine if and when the patient's menstrual cycle changed.
- Past history of human papillomavirus (HPV) infection, abnormal Pap tests or colposcopic examinations, or cervical dysplasia raises the strong possibility of cervical cancer.
- Epidemiologic risk factors for the development of carcinoma of the cervix include young age at first coitus, multiple sexual partners, high parity, and cigarette smoking. Smoking cessation should *always* be encouraged!
- Past history of uterine myomas, myomectomy, or uterine artery embolization raises the possibility of a prolapsed uterine fibroid or cervical fibroid.
- Past history of sexually transmitted infections (STIs), multiple sexual partners, or a new sexual partner suggests possible infectious causes of cervicitis or vaginitis.
- History of contraceptive use, especially an intrauterine device (IUD), is important. IUDs can cause abnormal uterine bleeding.
- Review of systems should focus on vaginal discharge, pelvic pain, pressure symptoms, and difficulty passing urine or stool.

Physical Examination

- **General appearance:** Usually within normal limits. Advanced cancer may cause wasting or cachectic appearance.
- **Lungs:** Should be clear bilaterally.
- **Abdominal examination:** Should include attempt to palpate the uterus because the uterus can be enlarged in the case of fibroids. The abdominal examination should also include palpation of the liver as well as examination for ascites.
- **Lymph nodes:** Palpation of the supraclavicular and groin nodes should be done to exclude the possibility of metastatic disease.
- **Pelvic examination:** Speculum examination provides direct visualization of the cervix and vagina. Gross lesions (tumor, ulceration) of the cervix/vagina/vulva should be sampled for biopsy. Colposcopy with endocervical curettage should be performed to evaluate cytologic abnormalities. Cervical cytology (Pap test) as well as genital cultures should be performed. An endometrial biopsy or endocervical curettage can also be performed in the absence of gross lesions. On bimanual examination, palpate the cervix for size and consistency.
- **Rectal examination:** A very effective method for determining size of the cervix and ovaries. Also necessary to detect extension of cervical disease into the parametrium.

Tests for Consideration

- **CBC with platelets:** Evaluates hemoglobin and white
  blood cell count. $38
- **Liver function tests:** Test for the possibility of metastatic
  disease to the liver. $56
- **Blood urea nitrogen (BUN)/creatinine:** Can detect possibility
  of renal dysfunction as a result of ureteral blockage. $28
- **Cervical cytology (Pap test):** Evaluates cells of the cervix. $315
- **Colposcopy with or without biopsy:** Cervical or cone
  biopsy as indicated by pathology. $423
- **Endometrial biopsy:** Evaluates endometrial pathology. $366
- **Endocervical curettage:** Evaluates for the possibility of a
  lesion that cannot be seen in the endocervical canal. $350
- **Cystoscopy:** Evaluates for tumor invasion into bladder. $570
- **Lower gastrointestinal endoscopy:** Looks for spread of
  disease into the rectum. $670

IMAGING CONSIDERATIONS

If the cervical biopsy is positive for carcinoma, proceed to imaging
to evaluate for metastatic disease:

→**Intravenous pyelogram (IVP):** To evaluate for
ureteral blockage. $300
→**Chest radiography:** To look for distant disease. $125
→**MRI of the pelvis:** Useful to distinguish tissue
densities of pelvic masses. $1500
→**Positron emission tomography (PET)/CT scan:** to
look for diffuse disease and metastases. $1800
→**Pelvic ultrasonography:** Evaluates uterine
abnormality such as myomas. $225
→**Barium enema:** Evaluates for spread to rectum. $550

Clinical Entities   Medical Knowledge

Cervical Cancer

Pφ Molecular biology has established a causal relationship between
persistent infection with high-risk HPV genotypes and cervical
cancer. Cervical cancer progresses from preinvasive cervical
intraepithelial neoplasia to invasive cancer.

TP Cervical cancer is often asymptomatic until quite advanced.
Vaginal bleeding is the most common presenting symptom of
invasive cancer of the cervix. In sexually active women, this

usually includes postcoital bleeding; however, many women present with intermenstrual or postmenopausal bleeding. Large tumors may become infected and women can also present with malodorous vaginal discharge. Pelvic pain and pressure symptoms secondary to size may be the chief complaint. Locally advanced disease can also present as renal failure secondary to ureteral obstruction.

Dx Diagnosis and staging is based on clinical examination, pathologic evaluation of the biopsy specimen, and imaging modalities to evaluate for metastasis. **See Katz 29, Hacker 38.**

Tx See Table 51-1.

Table 51-1 FIGO Staging Classification: Cervical Carcinoma

Stage	Classification	Diagnosis	Treatment
0	Carcinoma in situ	Cone biopsy	Cervical conization
IA1	Invasive carcinoma, confined to cervix, diagnosed only by microscopy. Stromal invasion ≤3 mm in depth and ≤7 mm in horizontal spread	Cone biopsy by cold-knife conization or loop electrosurgical excision procedure	Simple hysterectomy *or* Cone biopsy with negative margins if patient desires fertility
IA2	Invasive carcinoma, confined to cervix, diagnosed only by microscopy. Stromal invasion >3 mm and ≤5 mm in depth and ≤7 mm in horizontal spread	Cone biopsy with pelvic lymph node assessment by pelvic MRI or PET CT	Modified radical hysterectomy and pelvic lymph node dissection* *or* Pelvic radiation therapy *or* Radical trachelectomy and lymph node dissection for fertility preservation

Stage	Classification	Diagnosis	Treatment
IB1	Invasive carcinoma, confined to cervix. Microscopic lesion >IA2 or clinically visible lesion ≤4 cm in greatest dimension	Physical examination in case of gross lesion *or* cone biopsy by cold-knife conization or loop electrosurgical excision procedure	Radical hysterectomy with pelvic lymph node dissection* *or* Pelvic radiation therapy
IB2	Invasive carcinoma, confined to cervix, clinically visible lesion >4 cm in greatest dimension	Physical examination with IVP/CXR/ MRI/PET CT to evaluate for metastasis	Combination radiation therapy and cisplatin-containing chemotherapy
IIA	Tumor extension beyond cervix to vagina but not to lower third of vagina. No parametrial invasion	Physical examination with IVP/CXR/ MRI/PET CT to evaluate for metastasis	Radiation therapy with cisplatin-containing chemotherapy†
IIB	Tumor invasion beyond cervix. Parametrial invasion but not to pelvic sidewall and not to lower third of vagina	Physical examination with IVP/CXR/ MRI/PET CT to evaluate for metastasis	Radiation therapy with cisplatin-containing chemotherapy
IIIA	Tumor extension to lower third of vagina but not to pelvic sidewall	Physical examination with IVP/CXR/ MRI/PET CT to evaluate for metastasis	Radiation therapy with cisplatin-containing chemotherapy
IIIB	Tumor extension to pelvic sidewall or causing hydronephrosis or nonfunctioning kidney	Physical examination with IVP/CXR/ MRI/PET CT to evaluate for metastasis	Radiation therapy with cisplatin-containing chemotherapy

Table 51-1 caption: **FIGO Staging Classification: Cervical Carcinoma—cont'd**

Table continues

Table 51-1   FIGO Staging Classification: Cervical Carcinoma—cont'd

Stage	Classification	Diagnosis	Treatment
IVA	Tumor invasion into bladder or rectum	Physical examination with IVP/CXR/MRI/PET CT to evaluate for metastasis	Radiation therapy with cisplatin-containing chemotherapy
IVB	Distant metastasis	Physical examination with IVP/CXR/MRI/PET CT to evaluate for metastasis	Palliative radiation therapy for control of symptoms with cisplatin-containing chemotherapy (i.e., cisplatin and topotecan or taxol)

*If positive pelvic nodes, positive surgical margin, or positive parametrium, patients should be treated with postoperative pelvic radiation with concurrent chemotherapy.
†If small stage IIA cancer (<4 cm), may treat with surgical excision (radical hysterectomy and pelvic lymph node dissection).

Cervical Polyp

Pφ Most common benign neoplastic growth of the cervix. It is hypothesized that polyp growth is secondary to local inflammation or abnormal focal responsiveness to hormonal stimulation. May be endocervical or cervical.

TP Classic symptom is intermenstrual bleeding, most often after intercourse or physical examination. Occasionally, vaginal discharge can be associated if polyp becomes infected.

Dx Established on physical examination. Polyps may be single or multiple; soft; reddish-purple, red, or grayish-white in color. Cervical polyps are often pedunculated, and variable in length and size.

Tx Removal of the polyp by grasping base with clamp and avulsion at the base. This can typically be performed in the office setting, without anesthesia. Larger polyps on occasion require removal in the operating room. The polyp must then be sent to pathology for definitive diagnosis. **See Katz 18, Hacker 19.**

Cervical Myoma

Pφ Benign growth of smooth muscle fibers of the stroma of the cervix. May arise from the isthmus of the uterus.

TP Usually small and asymptomatic. Symptoms caused by size of myoma secondary to mechanical pressure of adjacent organs, including dysuria, urinary urgency and frequency, and dyspareunia. If myoma prolapses through the external os, ulceration and infection can cause abnormal bleeding or discharge.

Dx Physical examination allows for inspection and palpation. Usually identical to myomas originating from the corpus.

Tx Small myomas managed expectantly if agreeable to the patient. Enlarging myomas may be managed medically with a gonadotropin-releasing hormone agonist; surgically with a myomectomy or hysterectomy; or by uterine artery embolization. **See Katz 18.**

Endometrial Hyperplasia or Endometrial Cancer

Pφ Endometrial hyperplasia and cancer are two of the more common causes of abnormal bleeding from the female genital tract. See Chapter 52, Endometrial Cancer, for a more thorough explanation.

TP Variable. Most common complaint is irregular menstrual bleeding. Symptoms may range from prolonged, heavy vaginal bleeding to amenorrhea with infrequent light vaginal bleeding.

Dx Exclusion of anatomic causes of abnormal uterine bleeding, including uterine fibroids, inflammation of the genital tract, or cervical/vaginal lesions. Clinicians should have a low threshold to perform an endometrial biopsy to exclude carcinoma of the endometrium. Biopsy can often reveal proliferative or benign hyperplasia in states of unopposed estrogen stimulation.

Tx Goal of treatment is to address the underlying lesion. A D&C followed by medical therapy with progesterone is permissible for almost all types of hyperplasia. Endometrial cancer will require a complete surgical staging. **See Katz 32, Hacker 19, 41.**

ZEBRA ZONE

a. **Vaginal carcinoma:** Very rare, but give consideration to this malignancy, especially if the patient's history is significant for diethylstilbestrol (DES) exposure.

b. **Vulvar carcinoma:** More common in the elderly and immunocompromised. (See Zebra Zone box in Chapter 44, Human Papillomavirus–Related Vulvar Disease.)

c. **Foreign body:** Pessaries or retained tampons can on occasion present with vaginal bleeding.

d. **Vaginal trauma:** An unusual cause of vaginal bleeding that nevertheless must be addressed.

Practice-Based Learning and Improvement: Evidence-Based Medicine

Title
Randomised study of radical surgery versus radiotherapy for stage Ib-IIa cervical cancer

Authors
Landoni F, Maneo A, Colombo A, et al.

Institution
III Clinica Ostetrico Ginecologica, University of Milan, Milan, Italy

Reference
Lancet 1997;350:535–540

Intervention
Use of radiotherapy to cure stage Ib-IIa cervical cancer.

Quality of evidence
Level I: Evidence obtained form properly designed, prospective, randomized, controlled trial.

Outcome/effect
Noninvasive treatment of early-stage cervical cancer.

Historical significance/comments
First randomized trial to establish radiation therapy to be as effective as radical surgery for the treatment of early-stage cervical cancer. Allows an alternative treatment option for poor surgical candidates as well as allowing patients to avoid the major morbidity associated with surgery plus radiation therapy in cases of positive surgical margins.

Interpersonal and Communication Skills

Planning ahead for Complex Discussions

Most evidence-based literature suggests that radical hysterectomy and pelvic radiation therapy are equally effective in the treatment of early stage cervical cancer. In the absence of surgical contraindications, one must advise all patients about the advantages and disadvantages of, and alternatives to, all treatments. Beyond explaining diagnosis, prognosis, treatment options, and their potential complications, this discussion is complex. For example, one must inform younger women that the advantages of surgery include preservation of ovarian and sexual function, yet convey an understanding that if postoperative radiation is subsequently deemed necessary by the pathologic findings, then these advantages are obviously eliminated.

This type of discussion is one that will undoubtedly require time for patients and their supports to absorb. In this regard, at the outset, I often plan for both an initial discussion and a follow-up visit. It is helpful to acknowledge to the patient that the ideas you are discussing are complex and that most patients need time to think them through. I ask that, in the interim, my patient write down her questions so that she can remember to ask everything, and I can be sure to respond. In the follow-up visit it is easy to diverge from the patient's requests, so a list serves both patient and clinician well.

Professionalism

Principle: Commitment to Improving Access to Care

Invasive cancer of the cervix is a major cause of death worldwide. The reported incidence of cervical cancer in the developing world is much higher than the incidence reported in developed nations. Because cervical cancer can be diagnosed easily in its early, preinvasive, curable stages by effective screening, it is incumbent on physicians worldwide to foster such screening and to facilitate the development of screening mechanisms worldwide. Because of lack of awareness and deficiencies in patient education, many women present with invasive cancer that could have been detected at earlier and curable stages. Screening for cervical cancer is a clear example of an intervention that will prevent disease and eliminate suffering. We as physicians should support programs to improve access to care worldwide.

Systems-Based Practice

Vaccinations and the Cost of Inventory

For many years, the association between sexual behaviors and cervical cancer suggested a sexually transmissible agent as a causative factor, and now it is believed that HPV is involved in virtually all cases of cervical cancer. Until recently, the Papanicolaou screening test (the Pap smear) served as the greatest weapon in the reduction of cervical cancer mortality. However, with the recent development of the HPV vaccine, there is now an opportunity for *primary* prevention as well. In June 2006, the Centers for Disease Control and Prevention's Advisory Committee on Immunization Practices voted to recommend the use of **human papillomavirus vaccine (recombinant)**, the first vaccine to prevent cervical cancers caused by HPV. The vaccine, which was developed and marketed by Merck, protects against HPV types 16 and 18, which cause 70% of cervical cancers. The U.S. Food and Drug Administration licensed the vaccine for use in female patients 9 to 26 years of age. Ideally, the vaccine, which is given as a series of three shots over a 6-month period, should be administered before the patient becomes sexually active. The vaccine does not prevent all cervical cancers, and therefore women should continue routine screening with Pap smears.

Because this vaccine is administered in the outpatient setting, an issue to be considered is called the *cost of inventory*. At a price tag of $120 per dose—or $360 per full treatment—the cost of holding these drugs in the office is not an insignificant factor. Although one may expect eventually to be reimbursed for the cost of these drugs, holding 100 doses in your office means that at any given time $12,000 of cash—or what accountants refer to as "working capital"—is tied up in your drug cabinet. From an accounting perspective this is similar to your accounts receivable (A/R)—the money that you are owed for services you have delivered but for which you have not yet been paid. Just as having high A/R means you are losing interest or investment opportunity on the money you are owed, so does a high prepaid inventory. In addition, there is a certain inherent risk in holding inventory, such as the risk that you will never get paid for the drugs (e.g., if another drug comes out that is considered superior) and the risk that the drugs will expire before you have the chance to administer them. Although seldom the major determinant of a practice's financial bottom line, managing your inventory of drugs and supplies can help you keep your practice lean, efficient, and profitable, and ultimately contributes to the reduction of overall health care costs.

Chapter 52
Endometrial Cancer (Case 36)

Randolph Heinzel MD *and David Holtz* MD

Case: A 56-year-old white woman presents to her gynecologist's office with intermittent vaginal bleeding over the last 2 months. She underwent menopause at 50 years of age. An endometrial biopsy performed in the office reveals grade 2 endometrioid adenocarcinoma, with elements of complex endometrial hyperplasia with atypia seen as well.

Differential Diagnosis

Endometrial cancer, type I	Endometrial cancer, type II	Endometrial hyperplasia

Speaking Intelligently

When I see a patient with postmenopausal bleeding, my primary goal is to rule out malignancy. Approximately 15% of women experiencing postmenopausal bleeding have endometrial cancer. An endometrial biopsy performed in the office is a cost-effective, relatively convenient, and expeditious method to evaluate the endometrium of many patients. When the patient's endometrial lining cannot be easily sampled with an office biopsy, a D&C must be performed in the operating room. Transvaginal ultrasonography is another useful method in evaluating the endometrium of a patient with postmenopausal bleeding. Endometrial cancer is extremely unlikely if the endometrial stripe is no thicker than 4 to 5 mm. Endometrial cancer is not exclusively a disease of postmenopausal women, so premenopausal and perimenopausal women with abnormal uterine bleeding need to be evaluated as well.

PATIENT CARE

Clinical Thinking
- First determine if the patient has a malignancy. Endometrial cancer is the most common malignancy found in women with postmenopausal bleeding. Transvaginal ultrasonography, endometrial biopsy, or D&C

will often provide evidence to confirm or exclude endometrial cancer from the differential diagnosis.

- If malignancy is excluded, other possibilities on the differential diagnosis list for postmenopausal bleeding may be considered. (See Chapter 34, Abnormal Uterine Bleeding, for a comprehensive discussion of nonmalignant causes of such bleeding.)
- If a diagnosis of endometrial cancer is made, the patient's overall health status must be considered to determine if she is a candidate for surgical treatment.
- In postmenopausal patients with vaginal bleeding, I also consider the possibility of cervical cancer. There is a second rise in incidence for this cancer in certain women in the 50- to 60-year-old range. A Pap test or cervical biopsy is important in this setting.

History

- A thorough menstrual history, including the patient's age at menarche, age at menopause, and a previous history of abnormal uterine bleeding during the patient's menopausal years, is important. The amount of postmenopausal bleeding needs to be quantified, as well as associated symptoms such as nausea, vomiting, pain, and bowel or urinary changes.
- A history of hormone replacement therapy can sometimes cause postmenopausal bleeding, although malignancy needs to be excluded by more definitive measures. Unopposed estrogen exposure is a strong risk factor for endometrial cancer.
- A family history is always important when working up a patient for a potential malignancy.
- A history of obesity, chronic anovulation, diabetes mellitus, or tamoxifen use is significant because all are risk factors for endometrial cancer.
- Inquire if the patient has undergone age-appropriate screening tests such as colonoscopy and mammography.

Physical Examination

- Vital signs are usually within normal limits. Tachycardia or hypotension could be seen in patients with excessive blood loss.
- **Abdominal examination:** Large pelvic masses can be palpated on abdominal examination. Attention should be given to liver size.
- **Pelvic examination with bimanual and rectovaginal examination:** Try to evaluate the size of the uterus. Many patients with endometrial cancer will have an enlarged uterus. Evaluate the adnexa for size and tenderness. The vagina, inguinal lymph nodes, pelvic sidewall, bowel, and bladder should be assessed for possible tumor involvement.
- Consider the gastrointestinal and urinary systems as possible sources of the reported bleeding.

Tests for Consideration

- **Office endometrial biopsy:** Quick way to diagnose malignancy in the office. $220
- **D&C:** Operative procedure effective for diagnosis of malignancy. $760

IMAGING CONSIDERATIONS

→**Transvaginal pelvic ultrasonography:** Images the endometrial stripe; malignancy is very unlikely if stripe is less than 4 mm. $250

→**Saline infusion ultrasonography:** Particularly useful in making a diagnosis of uterine fibroids or endometrial polyps. $400

→**CT of the abdomen and pelvis:** Can evaluate other organs and structures for the possibility of metastases or advanced disease. $800

Clinical Entities	Medical Knowledge

Endometrial Cancer, Type I

Pφ Endometrial cancer is classified into two categories: type I and type II. Type I endometrial cancer accounts for nearly 80% of all endometrial cancer. Type I endometrial cancer is associated with chronic exposure of the endometrium to estrogen without exposure to progesterone. The most common histologic variety of type I endometrial cancer is *endometrioid*. Unopposed estrogen exposure can cause proliferation and hyperplasia of endometrial glands. Risk factors for this type of endometrial cancer include obesity, exogenous estrogen exposure, chronic anovulation, diabetes, and tamoxifen use. The degree of solid growth and glandular differentiation determines the grade of the tumor. Well-differentiated tumors are considered grade 1 and poorly differentiated tumors are considered grade 3. Intermediate tumors are grade 2.

TP Ninety percent of women with endometrial cancer present with abnormal uterine bleeding. Endometrial cells seen on a Pap smear in a woman older than 40 years of age can sometimes indicate an underlying malignancy.

Dx Diagnosis of endometrial cancer is made by histologic specimen. An endometrial biopsy performed in the office is often sufficient for diagnosis. A D&C may be used to obtain endometrial tissue for pathologic examination. Transvaginal ultrasonography is often useful for imaging the endometrial stripe, but it cannot replace a biopsy if you have a high level of suspicion. An endometrial stripe less than 4 to 5 mm is unlikely to be malignant in a postmenopausal woman with bleeding.

Tx Treatment for endometrial cancer is initially surgical. Abdominal exploration with collection of peritoneal fluid for cytology is performed. Hysterectomy and bilateral salpingo-oophorectomy, along with pelvic and para-aortic lymphadenectomy, are necessary for complete surgical staging. Women at low risk for recurrence require no further treatment. Women who have high-grade tumors, deep myometrial invasion, or cervical involvement often receive adjuvant radiation treatment in the form of vaginal brachytherapy to lower the risk of recurrence at the vaginal apex. Chemotherapy with or without radiation therapy is used for more advanced cases of endometrial cancer. Doxorubicin, paclitaxel, and cisplatin are the most commonly used chemotherapeutic agents for the treatment of endometrial cancer. In patients who have contraindications to surgery, radiation therapy or progestin therapy are alternatives to surgical treatment of endometrial cancer. **See Katz 32, Hacker 41.**

Endometrial Cancer, Type II

Pφ Type II endometrial cancers are those endometrial cancers not associated with excess estrogen exposure. Type II endometrial cancer is less common than type I and accounts for approximately 20% of all endometrial cancers. Type II cancers do not have the well-defined risk factors seen with type I endometrial cancer; however, women with type II cancers tend to be older. The most common histologic types of type II endometrial cancer are *papillary serous* and *clear cell*, which are higher-grade tumors, more aggressive than the *endometrioid* type, and carry a poorer prognosis.

TP As with type I endometrial cancer, type II endometrial cancer typically presents with abnormal uterine bleeding. Endometrial cells seen on a Pap smear of a woman older than 40 years of age must be evaluated to rule out malignancy. Type II endometrial cancers usually present at a more advanced stage than type I cancers because of their more aggressive nature.

Dx Diagnosis is by histologic sample. An endometrial biopsy or D&C is used to obtain endometrial tissue.

Tx Type II endometrial cancer is surgically staged. As in staging for type I endometrial cancer, peritoneal fluid is sent for cytology, hysterectomy and bilateral salpingo-oophorectomy are performed, and pelvic and para-aortic lymph nodes are removed. Because of the propensity for these tumors to spread intra-abdominally, like ovarian cancers, an omentectomy and peritoneal biopsies are also performed in this setting. Given the more aggressive nature of the type II endometrial cancer histologic types, chemotherapy is being used even in early-stage (I or II) disease. Adjuvant radiation therapy, such as vaginal cuff brachytherapy or whole pelvic radiation, may additionally be used to prevent pelvic recurrences. Chemotherapy is also used to treat type II endometrial cancers of a more advanced stage (III or IV). The choice of chemotherapeutic agents is controversial. Regimens with doxorubicin, cisplatin, and paclitaxel are commonly used. Carboplatin and paclitaxel, as used for chemotherapy in ovarian cancer, are also used for the adjuvant treatment of certain endometrial cancers, especially papillary serous tumors. **See Katz 32, Hacker 41.**

Endometrial Hyperplasia

Pφ Endometrial hyperplasia results when estrogen stimulates the proliferation of normal endometrium. Endometrial hyperplasia is categorized as simple or complex, depending on the degree of abnormality in glandular and stromal patterns. Simple and complex hyperplasias are further classified by whether nuclear atypia is present. Risk factors for endometrial hyperplasia are the same as those for type I endometrial cancer, namely, unopposed estrogen exposure. Endometrial hyperplasia can be a precursor for type I endometrial cancer. The risk of subsequent cancer after a diagnosis of endometrial hyperplasia has been made depends on the severity of the hyperplasia: simple hyperplasia, 1%; complex hyperplasia, 3%; simple hyperplasia without atypia, 8%; complex hyperplasia with atypia, 29%.

TP Endometrial hyperplasia often presents with abnormal uterine bleeding.

Dx Endometrial hyperplasia is a histologic diagnosis. Samples of endometrium obtained from biopsy or D&C are required for diagnosis. Endometrial hyperplasia must be suspected whenever a patient's endometrial stripe appears thickened on ultrasonography.

Tx The treatment of endometrial hyperplasia depends on the severity of the hyperplasia. Endometrial hyperplasia without atypia has a relatively low risk of progression to cancer. Oral progestins such as medroxyprogesterone, norethindrone, or megestrol, depot progestin, and levonorgestrel-releasing intrauterine devices may be used to treat endometrial hyperplasia without atypia. Hysterectomy is the preferred treatment for endometrial hyperplasia *with atypia* because of the increased risk of progression to malignancy that "atypia" adds to this disease. If a patient is a poor surgical candidate or desires preservation of fertility, progestin therapy may be used, but follow-up endometrial biopsies should be performed to monitor treatment results. Keep in mind that if you perform a hysterectomy for complex atypical hyperplasia, there is an up to 40% chance of finding endometrioid cancer in the hysterectomy specimen. **See Katz 32, Hacker 19.**

ZEBRA ZONE

a. Hereditary nonpolyposis colorectal cancer (HNPCC): Patients with HNPCC (Lynch syndrome II) are also at risk for extracolonic tumors. Endometrial carcinoma is the most common such tumor, affecting 40% of women with HNPCC by 70 years of age.

b. Uterine sarcomas: A much rarer form of uterine cancer. The most common histologic types of uterine sarcoma are leiomyosarcoma, endometrial stomal tumors, and carcinosarcoma (malignant mixed müllerian tumor). Uterine sarcomas tend to be more aggressive than uterine carcinomas and have a poorer prognosis. These cancers represent about 5% of all uterine malignancies.

Practice-Based Learning and Improvement: Evidence-Based Medicine

Title

Laparoscopy-assisted vaginal hysterectomy compared with abdominal hysterectomy in clinical stage I endometrial cancer: Safety, recurrence, and long-term outcome

Authors

Kalogiannidis I, Lambrechts S, Amant F, et al.

Institution
Division of Gynecologic Oncology, Department of Obstetrics and
Gynecology, University Hospitals Leuven, Katholieke Universiteit
Leuven, Leuven, Belgium

Reference
American Journal of Obstetrics and Gynecology 2007;196:248.e1–8

Problem
Surgical staging of endometrial cancer.

Intervention
Compares laparoscopy-assisted vaginal hysterectomy (LAVH) with
staging to abdominal hysterectomy with staging.

Quality of evidence
Level II-2.

Outcome/effect
This study shows that for patients with stage I endometrial cancer,
LAVH with lymphadenectomy compares favorably with total abdominal
hysterectomy and surgical staging.

Historical significance/comments
Confirms belief held by many that LAVH is a safe and effective
alternative to staging with total abdominal hysterectomy, bilateral
salpingo-oophorectomy, and lymphadenectomy. LAVH with staging is
characterized by slightly longer operating times, but with
significantly lower blood loss and time of hospitalization for the
patient.

Interpersonal and Communication Skills

Parceling the Delivery of News When Bad News Is Unexpected
You have just performed a hysterectomy on a patient for presumed
fibroids. The final pathology assessment reveals endometrial
carcinoma. Not only has the diagnosis been unexpected, but your
patient will require adjuvant therapy in the form of radiation,
chemotherapy, or both.

Delivering unexpected bad news is among the most difficult
situations the clinician encounters. You should consider the steps for
preparing the patient to hear the news, the need for the patient to
have support when receiving it, and the desirability of separating
the information into parcels that can be delivered when the patient
is adequately prepared to listen. First and foremost, careful
self-preparation is important. This involves ensuring that you have
all the information at hand that you might need, that you are
emotionally prepared, and that, wherever possible, you can provide
uninterrupted time with the patient. When seeing the patient, I
usually inform her that there has been an unexpected malignant

finding and I assure her as much as honestly possible that the ultimate outcome will be favorable. I suggest that we plan an initial discussion with her closest support(s) in attendance "as another set of ears." I try not to overwhelm my patient with too much information during the initial discussion. When I sense that the venue and time are right and that she is ready to absorb the information, I make sure she understands her condition and that her questions and concerns are answered. It is important to provide an avenue for further communication in any consultation and especially so in one where the news is unexpected.

Professionalism

Principle: Commitment to Honesty with Patients

Your patient is a 76-year-old Eastern European woman who speaks very little English and presents with abnormal uterine bleeding. Her son and daughter serve as your interpreters. You perform an endometrial biopsy that reveals endometrial carcinoma. At a follow-up visit, as you are about to discuss the findings and recommend hysterectomy, the patient's family entreats you not to mention the words "cancer" or "malignancy" and to suggest that hysterectomy is essential because of "fibroids."

Informed consent is both an ethical obligation and a legal requirement before any medical intervention and obviously mandates a discussion of the diagnosis. However, if the patient's family, motivated by cultural issues, is adamant that the patient not be told the diagnosis, there is a fine line that must be walked. The focus must be on what is best for the patient, yet the feelings of the entire family must be considered. When I have encountered this situation, I have generally recommended that the family not *infantilize* their elder by hiding the truth. Particularly in cases of malignancy, I explain that subsequent management will be more difficult if "we (the health care team and the family) are not dealing honestly with the patient." *I must admit that the preceding represents my own cultural bias*. In a few cases, when the family has persisted, I have gone to the patient and stated that the family wants all communication about the patient's diagnosis and treatment to be given to a specific family member who will then share it with the patient how and when the family member believes it would be best. This allows the patient the autonomy to decide her level of involvement in her care and gives her the opportunity to accept or reject her family's good intentions. Whatever is decided must be documented thoroughly in the patient's chart. This satisfies ethical obligations and legal requirements and treats the patient and family with respect.

Chapter 53
Teaching Visual: Ureteral Anatomy
Pinckney J. Maxwell IV MD *and Gerald A. Isenberg* MD

Objectives

- Map the course of the ureter through the pelvis.
- Identify the most common locations of surgical ureteral injury.
- Describe the principles of the most common ureteral repairs.
- Recognize that the possibility of ureteral injury should be included as part of informed consent for pelvic surgery.

Surgical injury to the ureter can occur in a variety of pelvic procedures; the majority of ureteral injuries (54%) occur as a result of hysterectomy.[1] Injuries also occur during colorectal surgery (14%), pelvic surgery (8%), and abdominal vascular surgery (6%). There is an overall ureteral injury rate of 0.5% to 1.5% in gynecologic surgery.

Medical Knowledge

Anatomy of Ureteral Injury

Ureteral anatomy lends itself to injury. The ureter appears similar to vascular structures, runs in close proximity to numerous structures throughout the retroperitoneum, and is closely adherent to the posterior peritoneum. The ureter lies near a number of structures that are commonly dissected during pelvic surgery: the uterine vessels, the inferior mesenteric artery and superior rectal artery, and the gonadal vessels. A consistent landmark in the pelvis for locating the ureter is at the bifurcation of the common iliac artery, where the ureter crosses over this structure. The most common site of injury in gynecologic surgery **is (1) the point where the distal ureter lies close to the uterine vessels. (2) The next most common site is at the pelvic brim, related to the peritoneal fold of the ovarian vessels, also known as the *infundibulopelvic ligament*. (3) A third vulnerable location is where the ureter lies close to the anterior vaginal fornix as it enters the bladder, more closely on the left than on the right (see Fig. 53-1 for corresponding locations).**

Mechanisms of Ureteral Injury

Factors predisposing to injury of the ureter include: increased uterine size, large adnexal or ovarian masses, endometriosis, pelvic inflammatory disease, prior pelvic procedures, radiation, advanced malignancy, and congenital or anatomic anomalies of the urinary tract. Significant inflammation, endometriosis, or malignant masses increase the risk of injury due to direct involvement or adjacent adhesions limiting visualization and exposure. Neoplastic conditions may necessitate partial resection and repair of the ureter.

The most common mechanisms of iatrogenic operative ureteral injury are the following:

1. Crushing the ureter by clamp application

2. Ligating the ureter with a suture

3. Partially or completely transecting the ureter

4. Causing ischemia from extensive ureteral dissection or electrocoagulation

5. Accidentally resecting a ureteral segment

6. Obstructing the ureter by angulation or extrinsic compression

Connect the dotted lines of the ureter's course. Identify and record below the three common sites of uretal injury. For reference, the common sites have been highlighted in Anatomy of Ureteral Injury on the preceding page.

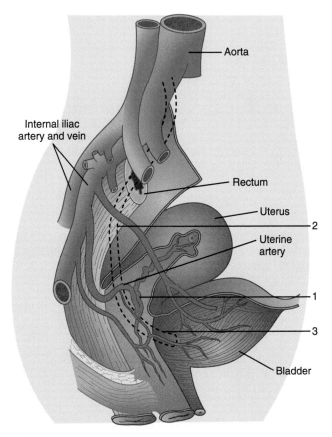

Figure 53-1

1. _____

2. _____

3. _____

Practice-Based Learning and Improvement: Avoidance of Ureteral Injury

Several techniques can be used to decrease the chance of ureteral injury, the most important of which are intimate knowledge of its location, adequate operative exposure, and meticulous hemostasis. Intraoperative hydration and diuresis can be used to enhance visualization. Preoperative stenting, especially with the use of fiberoptic catheters, has met with good success in high-risk procedures. Stents do not reduce the rate of injury to the ureter, but they do increase the chance of identifying an injury.[2-4]

Immediate intraoperative recognition of ureteral injuries occurs in approximately 33% of open procedures,[5] but less often in laparoscopic procedures.[6] Suspected intraoperative injuries can be diagnosed by dye extravasation within the operative field after administration of intravenous indigo carmine. Retrograde ureteropyelography and intravenous urography may be helpful intra-operatively. An intraoperative cystoscopy may be one of the easiest and safest ways to diagnose ureteral (or bladder) injuries.

Medical Knowledge

Clinical Presentation of Ureteral Injury

Recognizing a delayed or postoperative presentation of ureteral injury requires a high index of suspicion. Medina and colleagues have described a triad of fever, leukocytosis, and generalized peritonitis as being most diagnostic of ureteral injury.[7] Signs and symptoms of delayed injury include oliguria or anuria, urogenital fistula, fever, persistent generalized pain, flank pain from hydronephrosis, urinary leakage from the wound, hydronephrosis, hematuria, and uremia.[5] Serum creatinine levels may be elevated. Increased serous output from a surgical drain, wound, or suspected fistula should be checked for elevated creatinine. Leukocytosis may be evident with an infected urinoma, abscess, or infection of the urinary tract. Diagnostic imaging modalities include excretory urography, retrograde urography, and CT pyelography. Management strategies include either stent placement or open repair. Stent placement is successful only in 20%[5] to 50%[8] of cases. Open repair has been advocated by some authors publishing low complication rates,[5,9] and cautioned by others[10] citing 10% to 40% complication rates. Others suggest waiting 6 weeks to allow resolution of perioperative inflammation.[11] The correct approach depends on the status of the patient and the volume and character of any drainage.

PATIENT CARE

Treatment of Ureteral Injury

Minor-appearing injuries identified at the time of surgery, such as contusions or ligatures that have been removed, **may be observed.** *However, great caution must be exercised because underappreciated damage can lead to ischemia and necrosis with resultant early breakdown or late stricture.* Smaller ureteral contusions can be managed with simple **stent placement** and closed retroperitoneal drainage. With questionably viable tissue, the ureter should be débrided and a formal repair undertaken.

Primary repair may be used for partial transections or longitudinal lacerations, using the Heineke-Mikulicz procedure whereby a transverse closure is performed to avoid constriction of the lumen.

Ureteroureterostomy is most commonly used for injuries to the upper two thirds of the ureter. Principles of repair include (1) gentle mobilization of the ureter, conserving the adventitia widely to preserve the microvascularization; (2) liberal débridement to healthy, bleeding edges; (3) primary repair using an end-to-end, spatulated, watertight, interrupted or running anastomosis with 5-0 or 6-0 monofilament absorbable suture; (4) isolation of the repair with omentum when possible; and (5) ureteral stenting and closed drainage.

Ureteroneocystostomy can be used to repair injuries to the distal third of the ureter. This procedure involves reimplanting the distal ureter into the bladder. It is preferable to ureteroureterostomy in this location because of the more generous blood supply of the bladder. Technical considerations include forming a submucosal tunnel, usually three times the width of the ureter, to prevent urine reflux. The new orifice is completed by spatulating the ureter and performing a ureter-to-mucosa, interrupted, watertight, tension-free anastomosis with 5-0 or 6-0 monofilament absorbable sutures. The repair should be stented at the time of construction.

The **psoas hitch** is used to remove or reduce tension on a ureteroneocystostomy. It involves mobilization of the ipsilateral bladder and closing a transverse cystotomy longitudinally to add length to allow the bladder to be anchored above the iliac vessels. The bladder is secured to the tendinous portion of the psoas minor muscle and a ureteroneocystostomy constructed. Similarly, a Boari flap can be created by tubularizing a segment of bladder to manage injuries to the lower two thirds of the ureter with long defects.

A simple **skin-level ureterostomy**, possibly using an 8-Fr infant feeding tube, can be constructed. This may be useful for damage control surgery or in the unstable patient because it generally necessitates a more definitive future repair.

Transureteroureterostomy is a rarely used and somewhat controversial procedure. It involves mobilizing the injured ureter across the midline and performing an end-to-side anastomosis to the uninjured ureter. Although it is reported to have excellent success rates, there are a number of significant drawbacks. Most important, it carries the risk of converting a unilateral ureteral injury into a bilateral injury. It also limits access to the ureter cystoscopically, requiring a percutaneous nephrostomy tube for imaging or intubation. Consequently, this is a procedure for experienced hands and only if other repairs are not feasible or possible.

Resection and autotransplantation of the kidney may be required after significant ureteral loss or after failure of a number of attempts at repair. This is usually performed in consultation with a transplant surgeon.

Postoperative Care and Prognosis

Patients may be discharged when appropriate after surgery, with follow-up in the clinic in 14 to 21 days for stent removal. Some authors recommend leaving the stent for 6 weeks. If drains are not removed in the hospital, closer follow-up may be required for assessment and potential removal.

The Foley catheter is left in place for 7 to 10 days in patients requiring a cystotomy. Subsequently, a cystogram is performed. If no extravasation is observed, the Foley catheter can be removed. If there is no increase in drainage from external drains after removal of the Foley, these can also be removed. If extravasation is observed, the catheter and drain are left in place and studied again in 7 to 10 days.

Prognosis for ureteral injuries is excellent provided the diagnosis is made early and prompt correction is undertaken. Delayed recognition can worsen the prognosis owing to hydronephrosis, renal damage, infection or abscess, or fistula formation.

Interpersonal and Communication Skills

Informed Consent

Informed consent is a critical communication process that must occur between physician and patient prior to a specific medical intervention. This process is an ethical obligation as well as a legal requirement. Informed consent must contain the patient's dx (if known), the purpose of the proposed procedure, a description of the procedure, risks and benefits of the intervention, alternative tx with their risks and benefits, and finally the risks and benefits of no tx.

The intent is for the patient to use this information to generate questions before deciding to proceed with the intervention. Exceptions to informed consent include lack of decision-making capacity (lack of competence), emergencies, and therapeutic privilege (the physician feels that disclosure of medical information would harm the patient or affect the informed consent process).

Informed consent for a hysterectomy and other pelvic operations must include the risk of ureteral injury. Without unduly alarming patients, you must make them understand that while this severe complication may be infrequent, ureteral injury may result in additional surgical procedures.[12]

References

1. St Lezin MA, Stoller ML: Surgical ureteral injuries. Urology 1991;38:497–506.
2. Leff EI, Groff W, Rubin RJ, et al: Use of ureteral catheters in colonic and rectal surgery. Dis Colon Rectum 1982;25:457–460.
3. Bothwell WN, Bleicher RJ, Dent TL: Prophylactic ureteral catheterization in colon surgery: A five-year review. Dis Colon Rectum 1994;37:330–334.
4. Kuno K, Menzin A, Kauder HH, et al: Prophylactic ureteral catheterization in gynecologic surgery. Urology 1998;52:1004–1008.
5. Ghali AM, El Malik EM, Ibrahim AI, et al: Ureteric injuries: Diagnosis, management, and outcome. J Trauma 1999;46:150–158.
6. Grainger DA, Soderstrom RM, Schiff SF, et al: Ureteral injuries at laparoscopy: Insights into diagnosis, management, and prevention. Obstet Gynecol 1990;75:839–843.
7. Medina D, Lavery R, Ross SE, Livingston DH: Ureteral trauma: Preoperative studies neither predict injury nor prevent missed injuries. J Am Coll Surg 1998;186:641–644.
8. Cormio L, Battaglia M, Traficante A, Selvaggi FP: Endourological treatment of urologic injuries. Br J Urol 1993;72:165–168.
9. Witters S, Cornelissen M, Vereecken R: Iatrogenic ureteral injury: Aggressive or conservative treatment. Am J Obstet Gynecol 1986;155:582–584.
10. Campbell EW Jr, Filderman PS, Jacobs SC: Ureteral injury due to blunt and penetrating trauma. Urology 1992;40:216–220.
11. Cangiano TG, deKernion JB: Urologic complication of vascular surgery. AUA Update Ser 1988;17:306–312.
12. Mann BD: Surgery: A Competency-Based Companion, Elsevier, 2009, p. 70.

Chapter 54
Ovarian Cancer (Case 37)

Matthew Boente MD

Case: A 63-year-old G3P3 postmenopausal patient presents to you as a referral from her internist because of ongoing complaints of abdominal distention and early satiety. The internist ordered a CT scan that revealed ascites, a 6-cm complex right adnexal mass, and an omental mass.

Differential Diagnosis

Epithelial ovarian carcinoma	Germ cell tumor	Gonadal and stromal cell tumors
Serous/mucinous cystadenoma	Mature cystic teratoma	Krukenberg tumor

Speaking Intelligently

When I evaluate a patient with suspected ovarian cancer, I want to hear about the patient's concerns regarding subtle bowel or urinary tract symptoms, as well as other systemic complaints. I pay particular attention to specific physical examination findings, especially palpable pelvic masses, abdominal fluid waves, and cul-de-sac nodularity. I personally review CT scan or ultrasonographic findings (not just reading the reports) and the CA-125 value (if this is available). It is also important to inquire about any first-degree relatives who had breast, ovarian, endometrial, urinary tract, or colorectal cancers before the age of 50.

PATIENT CARE

Clinical Thinking

- Ask yourself when evaluating a patient with a pelvic mass or symptoms of a possible ovarian malignancy: what is the worst possible outcome? What important actions do I need to take to reassure myself and the patient that she doesn't have ovarian cancer?
- Are my decisions evidenced based, and can I support them with current standard-of-care studies?
- Is my thinking cost effective? Are my treatment recommendations likely to improve the long-term survival and the quality of life for the patient, and not just decisions based on what I as a surgeon can technically accomplish?

History

- Ovarian malignancies are difficult to diagnose and attention to subtle details may help raise your index of suspicion.
- Ask the patient about symptoms such as bloating, urinary urgency or frequency, difficulty eating, early satiety, and abdominal or pelvic pain.
- Ask about changes in bowel habits such as constipation, diarrhea, narrowing of stool caliber, or blood in the stool.

Physical Examination

- Pay attention to details of physical examination, including the possibility of pleural effusion (loss of breath sounds at the lung base), slight abdominal distention, or a fixed or nodular mass on pelvic examination.
- Specifically, a rectovaginal examination with one finger vaginally and one finger in the rectum is of vital importance on initial consultation (and on yearly follow-up exam) to evaluate the patient comprehensively. Be careful to sweep the middle (rectal finger) across the cul-de sac, looking for nodularity. If the patient is obese or cannot tolerate the examination, transvaginal ultrasonography should be performed when you have a high index of suspicion for a pelvic mass or malignancy.

Tests for Consideration

- **Serum CA-125:** Ideally, this test should be reserved for postmenopausal women with a pelvic mass or for premenopausal women with partially solid or complex (see later) pelvic masses. It should be noted that an elevated CA-125 and a pelvic mass in a postmenopausal woman is consistent with ovarian cancer in greater than 90% of cases. Unfortunately, about 50% of stage I ovarian cancers will have normal CA-125 values before surgery. In addition, about 20% of patients with advanced ovarian cancer will not have an elevated serum CA-125. Numerous benign conditions such as endometriosis, pelvic inflammatory disease, uterine fibroids, and pregnancy can elevate the CA-125 level in premenopausal women. However if ovarian cancer is suspected, a CA-125 should still be ordered in this age group. Most often, benign conditions will yield more moderate CA-125 elevations. Always remember that CA-125 is **not** a screening test, and should not be ordered as a matter of routine in asymptomatic patients. $100

- **Quantitative human chorionic gonadotropin (β-hCG):** Can be elevated with germ cell tumors. $35
- **Alpha-fetoprotein:** Can be elevated with germ cell tumors. $125
- **Inhibin B:** Can be elevated with granulosa cell tumor (sex cord stromal tumor). $215

IMAGING CONSIDERATIONS

→**Transvaginal ultrasonography:** The most sensitive test for adnexal masses and far superior to a bimanual examination. Pelvic/transvaginal sonograms should be ordered to investigate any symptoms or signs of a problem on physical examination. Sonographic findings such as mural nodules, papillary excrescences, or thick septations raise the suspicion for cancer. Transvaginal ultrasonography should be repeated in 3 to 4 months for equivocal cysts or masses, along with serial CA-125 levels. $225

→**Abdominal/pelvic CT:** A good test to evaluate the upper abdomen, especially the omentum, as well as to evaluate the retroperitoneal lymph nodes and look for the presence or absence of ascites. $800

→**MRI:** Rarely indicated before surgery. $1500

→**Positron emission tomography (PET) scan:** Rarely indicated before surgery. $2500

Clinical Entities	Medical Knowledge

Epithelial Ovarian Carcinoma

Pφ Epithelial ovarian carcinomas fall into four general categories. **Serous** cancers account for about 40% of tumors, **mucinous** cancers represent about 25% of tumors, **endometrioid** cancers account for about 20% of tumors, and **clear cell** cancers about 5%. Each tumor has different histologic characteristics. Serous tumors have the appearance of fallopian tube epithelium. Mucinous tumors resemble endocervical glands. Endometrioid tumors look like the endometrium, and clear cell tumors have an almost transparent appearance secondary to an abundance of clear, glycogen-rich cytoplasm.

TP Patients typically present with nonspecific complaints of bloating, pelvic or abdominal pain, urinary symptoms, change in eating and bowel habits, and occasional weight loss in the face of abdominal distention.

Dx Diagnosis is made at surgical staging. A total abdominal hysterectomy, bilateral salpingo-oophorectomy, pelvic washing, pelvic and periaortic lymphadenectomy, omentectomy, and peritoneal biopsies must be included.

Tx Therapy is by surgical staging with cytoreductive surgery to remove the primary tumor as well as any associated metastatic implants. Most patients will then receive combination chemotherapy with a platinum agent, typically carboplatin, and paclitaxel. **See Katz 33, Hacker 39.**

Germ Cell Tumors

Pφ Rare tumors that arise in ovarian oocytes. These tumors are typically characterized by their cell types and histologic appearance: dysgerminomas, immature teratomas, endodermal sinus tumors, and embryonal carcinomas.

TP Germ cell tumors typically present in younger, premenopausal patients and sometimes children.

Dx Diagnosis is made at laparotomy with appropriate surgical staging. In patients of reproductive age, this surgery should be fertility sparing if possible. Fertility-sparing surgery would include removal of the involved ovary, accompanied by pelvic washings, an omentectomy, pelvic and periaortic lymphadenectomy, and peritoneal biopsies.

Tx Therapy is achieved with removal of the primary tumor and appropriate staging, as described previously. Staging is followed with adjuvant chemotherapy consisting of bleomycin, etoposide, and cisplatin, except for women with stage IA dysgerminoma or grade 1 stage IA immature teratoma. **See Katz 33, Hacker 39.**

Gonadal and Stromal Cell Tumors

Pφ Gonadal and stromal cell tumors arise from the stromal cells that make up the endocrinologically functional tissue of the ovary, which surrounds the oocytes. In normal situations these cells produce hormones, and when the cells become cancerous they are capable of producing elevated levels of these hormones. **Granulosa** cell tumors produce estrogen, and **Sertoli-Leydig** cell tumors often produce testosterone.

TP Because these tumors often produce hormones, they often present with symptoms associated with increased hormone production. Granulosa cell tumors secrete estrogen, which can cause abnormal uterine bleeding in older patients or precocious puberty in prepubescent patients. Sertoli-Leydig cell tumors sometimes produce testosterone, which can be masculinizing.

Dx Diagnosis is made at staging laparotomy.

Tx Therapy is with tumor removal, and possibly fertility-sparing surgery for carefully selected patients. **See Katz 33, Hacker 39.**

Cystadenomas

Pφ The etiology of serous and mucinous cystadenomas is unknown. These benign tumors can have a complex appearance on radiologic studies, and often can cause a mild elevation of the serum CA-125 level, which can allow them to masquerade as malignancies. Serous cystadenomas are often multilocular and can have papillary components on the inner surface. Mucinous cystadenomas can grow quite large and usually have mucoid material within cystic loculations.

TP These cysts can arise at any age but typically are seen in adults. They can cause symptoms such as pain, pressure, bloating, or increasing abdominal girth. Occasionally they enlarge and cause early satiety or nausea and vomiting. Ultrasonography or CT scan typically reveals a unilocular cyst, occasionally with septations, but rarely with a significant solid component.

Dx The diagnosis of a mucinous or serous cystadenoma is made surgically with a frozen section. Gross examination cannot distinguish benign versus malignant neoplasm. The decision to perform a cystectomy instead of complete removal of the ovary is based on the clinical situation and the experience of a seasoned gynecologist or gynecologic oncologist. Younger physicians should always consult with a senior surgeon when malignancy is suspected or if there is sufficient doubt that the mass encountered in the operating room is likely to be benign. Surgical experience cannot be underestimated in these circumstances, and the failure to perform the correct surgery the first time, especially in the face of a potentially malignant gynecologic cancer, can have significant impact on the outcome for the patient.

Tx Treatment is either ovarian cystectomy or unilateral salpingo-oophorectomy. **See Katz 8, Hacker 20.**

Mature Cystic Teratomas

Pφ The etiology and pathophysiology of mature cystic teratomas are unknown. All germ cell layers are represented (ectoderm, mesoderm, endoderm). They are the most common cause of adnexal masses in premenopausal women.

TP The presentations of these benign cysts are quite variable. Presentation can range from pelvic pain and an acute abdomen when the cysts rupture or torse, or they can present as a completely asymptomatic mass. Transvaginal ultrasonography is quite characteristic, with sharp contrast noted radiologically between the various components of the cyst.

Dx The diagnosis is suspected radiologically, but made surgically. Although malignant transformation of a benign cystic teratoma is reported to occur in 1% to 3% of the tumors, there is no literature to document the safety of following a dermoid cyst expectantly.

Tx Unilateral cystectomy or salpingo-oophorectomy is the treatment of choice. Frozen section should be done to rule out carcinoma or immature teratoma. **See Katz 18, Hacker 20.**

Krukenberg Tumor

Pφ Krukenberg tumors are metastases that travel to the ovary from a primary **gastrointestinal** site. These tumors are characterized by mucin-secreting cells that have a "signet-ring" appearance. Interestingly, approximately 5% of all malignant ovarian tumors are metastatic from sites elsewhere in the body. Krukenberg tumors are an example of this phenomenon. The pathophysiology involved is tumor spread through lymphatics or blood. Breast, colon, and endometrial cancers are some of the other primary tumors that can metastasize to the ovary.

TP Patients with Krukenberg tumors have the same subtle symptoms as patients with ovarian primaries: nausea, vomiting, indigestion, and early satiety. Subtle pelvic pain and pressure are also common. Intermittent constipation and loose bowel movements are reported. Many patients have no symptoms and their tumors are discovered on routine CT scans that are performed for surveillance of their primary tumors.

Dx The diagnosis and treatment of these situations is usually with surgery.

Tx An exploratory laparotomy is often performed because a second "new" ovarian primary cannot be ruled out noninvasively. The surgeon needs to be prepared to debulk a new ovarian primary or simply remove the ovaries if metastatic carcinoma (Krukenberg tumor) can be confirmed on frozen section. **See Katz 33, Hacker 39.**

ZEBRA ZONE

a. **Pedunculated fibroid:** Can often be confused with an ovarian mass on radiologic studies.

b. **Ovarian fibroma with ascites and pleural effusion:** This entity is classically described as Meigs syndrome.

Practice-Based Learning and Improvement: Evidence-Based Medicine

Title
Surgical resection of tumor bulk in the primary treatment of ovarian carcinoma

Authors
Griffiths CT

Institution
Massachusetts General Hospital, Boston, Massachusetts

Reference
National Cancer Institution Monographs 1975;42:101–104

Problem
Advanced ovarian cancer.

Intervention
Debulking surgery.

Quality of evidence
Level II-3.

Outcome/effect
Improved survival with optimal surgical debulking (<2 cm residual disease).

Historical significance/comments
This study from 1975 was the first study to report the benefit of surgical debulking in ovarian cancer stratified by the volume of residual tumor. This paper was instrumental in describing the benefit of debulking surgery, which has become one of the mainstays of modern gynecologic oncology. The concept of debulking revolves around the principle that if you leave a patient with a minimum volume of cancer after surgical resection, then adjuvant chemotherapy will be more effective.

Practice-Based Learning and Improvement

Improvement Project
A resident works with a mentor to identify an aspect of his/her own practice that requires improvement.

Consider, for example, that early in the fall of final year of residency a senior resident accepts a job at a small rural community hospital where there is no "Gynecologic Oncology" back-up. The president of the hospital's medical staff informs her that she may, on occasion, be called upon to do full surgical staging for gynecologic cancer patients.

The resident proceeds to identify a mentor in the Gynecology Oncology Division at her training program and works to improve her surgical skills so that she can safely and reliably perform lymph-node dissections unassisted and safely. In such an instance, the department chair should be able to "sign-off" on credentialing documents that would permit the resident to perform such procedures in her new rural location when called upon to do so.

Interpersonal and Communication Skills

Choosing Hopeful Language and Attitude

Sometimes the imaging studies we obtain in patients with ovarian carcinoma show obvious metastatic disease, which can be very discouraging to patients who understand the implications of distant metastases. Accordingly, I always emphasize that whereas most metastatic solid tumors are incurable, *ovarian cancer is an unusual exception*. With proper debulking surgery and effective chemotherapy, patients with widely metastatic disease can, in some instances, be cured.

Just as we try to remain positive when discussing ovarian cancer with our patients, physicians and other health care providers should always try to emphasize whatever positives the particular clinical situation might offer. It is also helpful to reflect on the language that is used in consultations in which serious issues are discussed. Carefully consider the words you use in giving this message.

Professionalism

Principle: Commitment to Professional Competence

Gynecologic oncology is a rapidly changing field, driven for the most part by well-designed studies that have been devised by the Gynecologic Oncology Group (GOG), a nonprofit organization whose purpose is to promote excellence in the quality and integrity of clinical and basic scientific research in the field of gynecologic malignancies. In the design of its clinical trials, the GOG is committed to maintaining the highest standards in development, execution, analysis, and distribution of results.

Numerous studies have demonstrated that patients who are appropriately staged at their first exploration for ovarian carcinoma have a much higher likelihood of 5-year survival and better outcomes overall. Accordingly, it is advisable to have a gynecologic oncologist available to act as primary surgeon or first assistant when an ovarian neoplasm is suspected. The primary surgeon should have the most up-to-date surgical strategies and therapies available, and these are usually based on GOG studies.

Systems-Based Practice

Avoiding Unnecessary Studies

When a patient is referred with an abnormality discovered on pelvic ultrasonography and a CA-125 elevation, the question arises as to whether CT imaging is warranted prior to surgical exploration. Traditional consensus has been that it is cost effective to operate on patients without further imaging because a CT or PET/CT is unlikely to change the surgery required, and, once surgical access is established, the pathology is viewed directly. Others contend that CT or MRI may demonstrate sites of metastatic spread, which can be helpful in planning the optimal surgical procedure. Ponder the following: "Why not just order that CT scan, just to be safe?" In general, there are multiple reasons not to order unnecessary imaging studies. Cost is certainly a legitimate concern. More important, however, is avoidance of unnecessary risks for the patient. Iodinated contrast can cause both allergic and non-allergic complications and renal compromise, particularly in diabetic patients. Furthermore, abdominal CT scans expose patients to much higher levels of radiation than physicians realize: an abdominal CT scan exposes a patient to a 5.3-mSv effective dose of radiation (approximately 100 chest radiographs), a dose almost doubled by a chest-abdomen-pelvic CT.

Never hesitate to order an imaging study that is required, but always consider whether the study is going to change the course of care, and whether potential overall benefit outweighs the potential risks.

Reference

1. Brenner DJ, Hall EJ: Computed tomography: An increasing source of radiation exposure. N Engl J Med 2007;357:2277–2284.

Chapter 55
Gestational Trophoblastic Disease (Case 38)

Jonathan C. Cook MD *and Norman G. Rosenblum* MD, PhD

Case: A 21-year-old G3P0020 migrant worker presents at 16 weeks' gestation dated by her LMP, of which she is certain. She presents to your clinic for the first time with complaints of new-onset vaginal bleeding, and a dramatic increase in nausea and vomiting. Her vital signs are as follows: BP 158/96, HR 90, RR 20, Temp 98.8, and Sa_{O_2} 99% on room air. You observe 3+ proteinuria on an office urine dipstick test. The fetal heart rate cannot be auscultated with a hand-held Doppler, and her uterine fundal height measures 33 cm, suggesting a pregnancy at 33 weeks' gestation.

Differential Diagnosis

Gestational trophoblastic disease (molar pregnancy)	Gestational hypertension/ preeclampsia	Spontaneous abortion

Speaking Intelligently

"Chance favors the prepared mind."

—Louis Pasteur.

Although complete molar pregnancies are by all accounts uncommon, the cost of missing a potentially malignant disease can be devastating for a patient's life and future fertility. Most cases of molar pregnancy should be diagnosed early in a patient's prenatal care, especially when a "size versus dates" discrepancy necessitates a first-trimester sonogram, or when a patient may be interested in first-trimester screening. Nevertheless, there still exists a large population of patients in whom the diagnosis can be missed. Therefore, my index of suspicion must always be high when there is a possibility of molar pregnancy. For example, preeclampsia before 20 weeks in a properly dated pregnancy is rare, especially in the case of patients who have no history of preexisting hypertensive disorders. "Size greater than dates" with preliminary absence of fetal heart tones and intractable vomiting all should be setting off alarm bells! I have a high level of suspicion for gestational trophoblastic disease (GTD) when things don't "add up" from a clinical standpoint, and I use ultrasonography to figure things out. Complete molar pregnancies will be picked up readily once the patient is imaged, and earlier diagnosis leads to better prognosis with this disease process.

PATIENT CARE

Clinical Thinking

- How do I identify the most serious condition that might underlie this patient's presentation? More important, which one of these seriously threatening clinical entities will need rapid action rather than expectant management?
- What laboratory tests/imaging studies will be **essential** and guide treatment in the first few hours? Which tests are important, but can wait?
- What takes priority in treatment decisions? Fertility, overall morbidity, fetal morbidity versus maternal morbidity?
- Which additional services should I be consulting? Maternal-fetal medicine, gynecologic oncology, and medical endocrinology are all considerations.

- Should a generalist Ob/Gyn be working alone if he or she is faced with a clinical situation suggesting GTD?

History
- Correct dating of the pregnancy is essential. If a patient is truly 16 weeks by an accurate LMP but her uterine fundal height suggests 33 weeks, then there is something wrong. Fetal macrosomia does not normally present in this dramatic a fashion. A multiple gestation is still a possibility, but still this is a large discrepancy.
- Obstetric history: What were the circumstances involving her prior pregnancy losses? Elective terminations? Spontaneous first- or second-trimester miscarriages? Repeated molar pregnancies?
- What about vaginal bleeding? Is this a threatened abortion? Has there been a recent history of trauma, sexual intercourse, or drug abuse (i.e., cocaine/methamphetamine)? Is there any associated cramping or abdominal pain? How much bleeding can be accurately quantified (pad count)? Is the patient currently hemodynamically stable?
- Quantify the nature and frequency of the vomiting. Is there an imminent intravascular volume depletion or electrolyte imbalance developing? What is her current nutritional state? Could the nausea the patient is experiencing be a result of an infectious etiology or gastritis versus a more straightforward case of hyperemesis gravidarum? Don't forget to think about a potential diabetic ketoacidosis in a patient with diabetes mellitus or a past history of gestational diabetes.
- Does the patient have any history of thyroid disturbance before becoming pregnant? Is there a family history of endocrinopathies?
- Do we know anything about the patient's medical history that may suggest a predisposing factor to early-onset preeclampsia, such as chronic hypertension or renal disease?

Physical Examination
- **Vital signs:** Blood pressure elevations may suggest some form of gestational hypertension such as preeclampsia. Tachycardia may be suggestive of thyroid dysfunction or volume depletion. An increased respiratory rate, although nonspecific like most vital signs, can suggest pain, volume depletion, or primary pulmonary compromise.
- **HEENT:** Is exophthalmos present?
- **Chest:** Are the lungs clear or is there evidence of pulmonary edema? Again, most lung findings will be nonspecific with our differential diagnosis, but GTD can easily metastasize to the lungs if ignored.
- **Abdominal examination:** Fundal height, tenderness, etc.? Is this presenting as a normal intrauterine pregnancy? Are fetal parts palpable?

- **Pelvic examination:** Is the cervical os open or closed? Are there signs of bleeding, discharge, or cervical motion tenderness?
- **Extremities:** Does the patient have edema or hyperreflexia?

Tests for Consideration

- **Human chorionic gonadotropin (β-hCG):** Molar pregnancies produce very high amounts of this pregnancy hormone because of proliferating syncytiotrophoblastic tissue. Following the β-hCG levels of a patient with gestational trophoblastic neoplasia is crucial, and is done at very frequent intervals. $32
- **Chem7:** Prolonged vomiting will produce a hypochloremic metabolic alkalosis. Creatinine should not be elevated in a pregnant woman without prior renal compromise. $12
- **CBC:** Low platelet counts and signs of hemoconcentration (as evidenced by an increased hematocrit with normal hemoglobin) will be clues for possible preeclampsia. $12
- **Liver function tests:** Should always be checked in pregnant women with a preeclamptic-like presentation! Elevations in alkaline phosphatase are to be expected secondary to endogenous placental manufacture of this enzyme. But aspartate aminotransferase (AST) and alanine aminotransferase (ALT) should be normal in a normal pregnancy. $29
- **Thyroid function tests:** The elevated levels of β-hCG can cause significant disruption of thyroid metabolism seen in approximately 7% of molar pregnancies. This is thought to be due to cross-reactivity between thyroid-stimulating hormone (TSH) and β-hCG molecule. Get a TSH and free thyroxine (T_4) to make sure a thyroid storm is not imminent. $32

IMAGING CONSIDERATIONS

→**Ultrasonography:** The imaging modality of choice. The key finding in molar pregnancies will be the classic "snowstorm" appearance. Ultrasonography can also distinguish singleton from higher-order pregnancies. Obstetric ultrasonography will typically be able to distinguish between GTD and normal pregnancy early and effectively. $300

→**CT scan (pelvis, abdomen, chest, and head):** Can be used if you are faced with the possibility of metastatic disease. $800–$3200

Clinical Entities   **Medical Knowledge**

Gestational Trophoblastic Disease (Molar Pregnancy)

Pφ Gestational trophoblastic disease is a complex clinical entity that can be subdivided into three separate categories: **"complete" and "partial"** molar pregnancies (these are benign), **invasive** molar pregnancy (locally invasive within the uterus), and **choriocarcinoma** (malignant). It is reasonable to think of this disease process as the development of potentially malignant products of conception with a strictly **paternal** genetic complement within the endometrial cavity. There is no trophoblastic tissue containing maternal chromosomes.

- **Complete moles** are typically 46XX and **partial moles** are typically of triploid karyotype—(69XXY, 69XXX, or 69XYY). Triploid molar pregnancies can often develop with a concomitant fetus. Complete moles are generally considered "good prognosis" and do not exhibit malignant characteristics.
- **Invasive moles** invade into the wall of the uterus. Only rarely are invasive moles metastatic. The diagnosis of invasive mole is most commonly reached when a patient who is treated with chemotherapy for a persistently elevated β-hCG level ultimately undergoes hysterectomy.
- **Choriocarcinoma** is the malignant form of GTD. Choriocarcinoma is most likely to occur after a molar pregnancy, but it can occur after miscarriages, pregnancy terminations, ectopic pregnancies, or normal pregnancies as well. The tumor cells have a propensity to spread through the bloodstream. The lungs, liver, brain, kidney, gastrointestinal tract, and vagina are all potential sites of metastatic disease.

TP The most common presenting symptoms/findings for all subgroups of GTD are vaginal bleeding, uterine size greater than gestational size suggested by dates, cystic ovaries, preeclampsia, and hyperemesis.

Dx The correct diagnosis is made from tissue curettings after surgical evacuation of the uterus. However, a "snowstorm" appearance on ultrasonography is nearly always pathognomonic. The diagnosis of metastatic disease is presumptive, using radiologic studies, in cases of metastatic invasive molar pregnancy or choriocarcinoma. Usually by the time you are ordering radiologic studies you have some indication that the pregnancy involved GTD to begin with.

Tx Surgical evacuation of the uterus using suction curettage is the first line of therapy, and from that point further therapy can proceed. Understand that a D&E procedure in the face of GTD can put the patient at a high risk for hemorrhage, so be sure to have blood products, platelets, and clotting factors readily available, and expect that you may have to use them. Women who are Rh negative should receive RhoGAM. After the D&E, β-hCG levels are used to monitor the patient's progress. Chemotherapy is indicated if there is radiologic suspicion of distant spread, or if the β-hCG level does not fall as expected. **Methotrexate** is usually the first-line agent, but **actinomycin-D** can also be used. In some instances, GTD can be resistant to methotrexate or actinomycin-D, or considered "poor prognosis," with metastases to the brain or liver. For these patients, further treatment is given with combined agents such as **MAC** (methotrexate, actinomycin-D, and cyclophosphamide) or **EMA-CO** (etoposide, methotrexate, actinomycin-D, cyclophosphamide, and vincristine). Hysterectomy can be a consideration for persistent disease, or for selected women who have completed their childbearing. **See Katz 35, Hacker 42.**

Gestational Hypertension/Preeclampsia

Pφ In some instances it may be initially difficult to distinguish early-onset gestational hypertension or preeclampsia from GTD. Ultrasonographic dating and evaluation is invaluable in these instances. The exact pathophysiology of preeclampsia remains unclear. It is believed to be directly related to inadequate trophoblastic invasion into the spiral arterioles of the uterus during initial placental implantation.

TP Patients usually present with elevated blood pressure and proteinuria. Other signs and symptoms include headache, visual field changes, hyperreflexia, right upper quadrant pain, shortness of breath, and pulmonary congestion/edema.

Dx Typically, preeclampsia is considered to occur only after 20 weeks' gestation, but there may be exceptions to this rule. There are specific criteria regarding elevations in blood pressure (140/90 mm Hg [mild] vs. 160/110 mm Hg [severe]), with associated proteinuria (300 mg/24 hr [mild] vs. 5 g/24 hr [severe]). The patient must meet these criteria if you are considering the diagnosis of preeclampsia.

Tx The definitive treatment is delivery. Blood pressure can be managed with antihypertensives and magnesium sulfate can be used during labor and postpartum. See Chapter 21, Hypertensive Disorders in Pregnancy, for a more comprehensive explanation of illness associated with gestational hypertension. **See Gabbe 33, Hacker 14.**

Spontaneous Abortion

PФ	Thirty percent of women will complain of spotting in the first trimester and of those, about half will go on to lose the pregnancy. However, miscarriage can occur in any trimester, particularly in the third trimester in the face of poorly controlled gestational hypertension. Bleeding is typically due to separation of the developing placenta from the vascularized decidua basalis.
TP	Cramping and vaginal bleeding or spotting are the most common presenting symptoms/signs.
Dx	An open os with products extruding makes the diagnosis; often ultrasonography will be necessary to assess the viability of the pregnancy. Third-trimester miscarriages on many occasions present with labor.
Tx	Initial management can be expectant, medical, or surgical, with misoprostol being the most common medical therapy, and D&E the appropriate surgical therapy. **See Katz 16, Hacker 7.**

ZEBRA ZONE

a. **Hyperemesis gravidarum:** Poorly understood reaction to elevated levels of β-hCG. Seen especially in molar pregnancies because of the excessive levels of this pregnancy hormone. There is intractable nausea and vomiting, especially pronounced in the first trimester (between 4 and 8 weeks). Can be seen with electrolyte abnormalities (e.g., hypokalemia, hypochloremia, metabolic alkalosis), ketosis, and dehydration.

b. **Incorrect gestational dating:** An unlikely, but plausible explanation for certain cases when the uterine size is inconsistent with what you would expect based on the LMP. Women who have irregular menstrual cycles or poor recollection of their menstrual cycles, or who become pregnant while on hormonal birth control all have the potential of incorrectly dating their pregnancy.

Practice-Based Learning and Improvement: Evidence-Based Medicine

Title
Gestational trophoblastic disease

Authors
Garner EI, Goldstein DP, Feltmate CM, Berkowitz RS

Institution
Brigham and Women's Hospital, New England Trophoblastic Disease Center, Boston, Massachusetts

Reference
Clinical Obstetrics and Gynecology 2007;50:112–122

Problem
Gestational trophoblastic disease.

Intervention
Describes various surgical and chemotherapeutic options.

Quality of evidence
Review article; level III.

Outcome/effect
Describes strategies to optimize good outcomes for this typically treatable gynecologic malignancy.

Historical significance/comments
A recent review article describing advances in diagnosis and treatment of GTD with special mention of possible familial syndromes of hydatidiform moles.

Interpersonal and Communication Skills

Anticipating the Conversation
Although it is a rare complication of pregnancy, GTD is a potentially fatal malignancy. The word "cancer" will undoubtedly stimulate fear, and it is essential, therefore, that compassion and concern be demonstrated. Try to anticipate the conversation and be prepared to:

- Counsel your patient on prognosis and future fertility.
- Deal with your patient's fear and confusion about this seemingly paradoxical entity. Your patient will undoubtedly be stunned to learn that for the last several months she was carrying a nonviable and potentially dangerous pregnancy.
- Offer reassurance that this cancer is one of the few malignancies that can be cured (some solace in the face of such a tragic revelation).
- Discuss chemotherapy, if the clinical situation dictates.
- Discuss the relatively low probability of having the same events recur with subsequent pregnancies (approximately 1/100).

In this scenario, you are the bearer of bad news and there is much evidence that patients remember very clearly what happens at such times. With thought and consideration, it is possible to make a difficult situation bearable and even positive. It is not unusual for patients to "shut down" while being given bad news. This is when the patient appears to stop listening. She may change the subject and avoid eye contact. There are several things to do at this time. Acknowledge that the patient may not wish to hear any more information. Encourage her expression of emotions ("How are you feeling now?") and respond empathetically ("I can see this is very difficult for you."). Silence can also be helpful in simply giving the patient time to process the information you have delivered.

Professionalism

Principle: Commitment to Improving Quality of Care: Administrative Follow-up
Women who have been treated with a D&E for gestational trophoblastic neoplasm need close follow-up of their β-hCG levels for 6 months to be certain that there is no recurrence of tumor. This type of long-term follow-up can be difficult for private medical offices to coordinate logistically, and it is even more difficult for such careful follow-up to take place in clinics for the underinsured. In these instances there is great potential for patients to slip through the cracks. Obviously, missing the recurrence of an invasive gestational trophoblastic neoplasm may lead to a worse outcome for the patient. In general, the medical community needs to be committed to improving the administrative aspects of health care to prevent medical errors and to improve outcomes.

Systems-Based Practice

Malpractice Insurance
Because of the inherent risks of the profession, an obstetrician/gynecologist needs to be concerned about malpractice insurance. On an annual basis (coverage period), the obstetrician/gynecologist will be required to purchase malpractice coverage, and this cost will probably range from 4% to 20% of the expenses for the entire practice. There are principally two major types of coverage, "occurrence" and "claims made." Occurrence malpractice covers you for a claim during the entire 1-year coverage period, and for any subsequent claims that may arise from a patient encounter during the coverage period. In contrast, claims-made coverage is limited to any claims that need to be paid during the coverage period. To the

physician, both forms of coverage work the same way if you stay with the same insurance carrier during your entire career. However, occurrence coverage, which generally costs more initially but covers you regardless of when a claim arises, allows you to change malpractice carriers (especially likely if you relocate because not every malpractice carrier will offer coverage in every state, or even in every city within a state). A physician may change malpractice carriers with claims-made coverage, but the physician would be required to pay what is called a "tail," which is additional malpractice insurance for any claims that may arise after the coverage period. Tail coverage typically costs two to three times the annual cost of claims-made coverage, a significant cost for any obstetrician/gynecologist. Thus, the physician's ability to relocate or shop around for malpractice coverage to obtain the best price is severely limited with claims-made coverage. Many large physician employers, such as hospital systems or physician groups, may self-insure, taking on the malpractice risk themselves, rather than paying a malpractice carrier for coverage.

Professor's Pearls: Cases in Gynecologic Oncology

Consider the following clinical problems and questions posed. Then refer to the professor's discussion of these issues.

1. A 35-year-old G1P0, status post molar pregnancy, presents for preconception counseling at the request of her obstetrician. She inquires about the recurrence rate of this disease for a woman like her, as well as the likelihood that it could progress to gestational trophoblastic disease.

2. A 25-year-old G0 presents at the request of her family physician, who has been managing her Pap tests for several years. Two years before, this patient had a low-grade squamous intraepithelial lesion (LGSIL) Pap test result, but did not have a colposcopy done at that time because she was about to travel overseas to perform missionary work. Recently, she describes some abnormal vaginal bleeding and bleeding after intercourse. She wants to know what her next step should be.

3. A 57-year-old G2P2 presents with the likely diagnosis of ovarian cancer. She has been evaluated by her gynecologist, who took seriously her complaints of diminished appetite and abdominal bloating. A CT scan of the abdomen and pelvis revealed ascites, complex bilateral ovarian masses, and an omental mass. She has mild hypertension, for which she takes an angiotensin-converting enzyme inhibitor. How should she be evaluated before proceeding to surgical staging?

4. A very elderly and debilitated woman was noted to have postmenopausal bleeding in the hospital, where she is currently admitted for treatment of urosepsis. An examination at the beside is unrevealing, and her family compels you to take her for an examination under anesthesia with a D&C. Three days later the pathology report returns: FIGO grade 1 endometrioid adenocarcinoma. The patient's family wants to know what you recommend for the patient.

Discussion by Dr. Donald Gallup, Professor and Chair, Department of Obstetrics and Gynecology, Mercer University School of Medicine, Savannah, Georgia

Answer 1: Clinical Considerations: Counseling Regarding Pregnancy after Molar Pregnancy

Our gynecologic oncology service would ensure that she had adequate initial follow-up with serum β-hCG titers every 2 weeks until she has two consecutive negative values, and then bimonthly negative values for at least 6 months after her prior pregnancy. We usually recommend a 6- to 12-month delay before attempting a new conception. During this time, the patient should have contraception provided. We prefer oral contraceptives. Pelvic examinations should be done every 2 to 3 months while titers are dropping to normal. We would advise her that molar pregnancy can occur in about 1% to 2% of subsequent pregnancies. About 20% of molar pregnancies progress to gestational trophoblastic disease and require chemotherapy. A molar pregnancy may recur regardless of whether the prior mole was partial or complete. We would stress that most patients with a prior molar pregnancy will have a normal subsequent pregnancy.

Answer 2: Clinical Considerations: Management of Abnormal Cervical Screening

The first step we would take is to obtain the records and slides from her prior abnormal Pap test. The slides would be reviewed by one of our attendings with our pathologist. A careful intake interview would be obtained regarding sexually transmitted infection history, history of genital warts, cigarette smoking history, age at onset of coitus, number of sexual partners, etc. She needs a physical examination, pelvic examination, and Pap test. Our office uses the ThinPrep for Pap test preparation, and the liquid can be saved for possible later human papillomavirus determination. Obviously, if a gross lesion is seen on speculum examination, an immediate biopsy should be done. She should be informed before the examination and sign appropriate consents for a cervical biopsy. Because of a 2-year delay and the postcoital bleeding, we would advise her she needs a colposcopic examination, even if the Pap smear is normal. Our practice is to request human immunodeficiency virus (HIV) testing in patients with significant cervical intraepithelial neoplasia on biopsies. Depending on where she did her missionary work, HIV testing may also be indicated.

Answer 3: Clinical Considerations: Preoperative Evaluation in a Patient with Likely Ovarian Cancer

We would agree that this patient most likely has an advanced ovarian malignancy. However, a careful history, particularly related to the gastrointestinal tract, should be obtained. Is there a family history of malignancy? A woman with bilateral adnexal masses could have metastatic carcinoma to the ovaries. Before any operative intervention, she needs a complete gastrointestinal evaluation, including a serum carcinoembryonic antigen (CEA), colonoscopy, and possible upper tract endoscopy. A baseline serum CA-125 should be obtained for later monitoring during chemotherapy and postchemotherapy surveillance. A mammogram should be obtained, along with a chest radiograph to evaluate for cardiomegaly, metastatic disease, or significant pleural effusion. If significant pleural fluid is present, a preoperative thoracentesis should be done for staging and to improve possible impaired postoperative ventilation. We would also obtain preoperative "clearance" from her internist, who will obtain an electrocardiogram and possibly further cardiac studies as indicated. Patients with ascites are at risk for significant intraoperative and postoperative fluid shifts, which can lead to pulmonary edema and congestive heart failure in inappropriately managed patients.

Answer 4: Clinical Considerations: Treatment of Endometrial Cancer in a Very Elderly Patient

Such patients are occasionally managed by our gynecologic oncology service. The family should be informed that her urosepsis must be stabilized. A nutrition consult should be obtained and parameters, such as serum prealbumin, assessed for possible intervention with enteral alimentation. A CT (or MRI) of the abdomen and pelvis should be obtained to rule out ureteral obstruction or extrauterine malignancy. We would review our own operative findings from the D&C. How large was the uterus on examination under anesthesia and by sounding? Was the cervix involved? These data would help in *clinical* staging and further treatment plans. She should be placed on low–molecular-weight heparin, until fully ambulatory, to avoid deep vein thrombosis and pulmonary embolism. Physical therapy should be consulted. If the clinical stage is I, we would place her on high-dose oral megestrol acetate (unless contraindicated). If she cannot undergo a major operation after these interventions, we would perform another endometrial biopsy or repeat D&C (depending on the size of the uterus) about 2 to 3 months later. If persistent invasive cancer is found, radiation should be considered. Either brachytherapy alone or with the addition of external-beam irradiation is possible. The family can be told that in this scenario, the 5-year survival rate drops about 10% for stage I disease to around 80%, compared with operative management. If there is no cancer found on repeat D&C, consideration for continued oral megestrol acetate should be given.

Section VIII
THE COMPETENCIES: CHALLENGES AND PATIENT PERSPECTIVES

Section Editor
Linnea S. Hauge PhD *and Sara N. Mann*

Section Contents

Chapter 56
Issues in Primary Care for the Obstetrician/Gynecologist

Kirsten Jacobson MD and Ernest Enzien MD

Primary care is the foundation of good medicine. Family physicians attend to episodic health needs, coordinate services from other providers, and help patients negotiate an often-mystifying world of referrals and third-party payers. Along with knowledge of a patient's physical condition, the primary care physician is attuned to the patient's overall well-being, including the context (family, work, community) in which she functions. Evidence shows that a long-term relationship with a primary care physician results in better health.[1]

The U.S. health care system has grown increasingly bureaucratized and fragmented over the past decade. On the one hand, many patients have unprecedented access to specialists and high-tech interventions. On the other hand, nearly half of all patients do not receive basic preventive care. This occurs even when these services would be covered by insurance, mostly because of the discouraging complexities of health care delivery. Also, because of a dwindling supply of primary care practitioners in many communities, too many patients have either limited access to their overburdened regular medical provider or no access to primary care at all. This results in a confusing fragmentation of specialty medical care with increased possibilities of negative consequences and poor outcomes. In such a climate, communication among providers is more essential than ever.

The medical care of a single patient is often delivered by more than one provider, at multiple outpatient and inpatient facilities. The greater the number of medical professionals involved in a woman's care, the more likely it is that tests and treatments will be inappropriately duplicated or omitted. It becomes possible to make (sometimes incorrect) assumptions about who is responsible for various aspects of the patient's health care. For example, a gynecologist may believe incorrectly that a patient's family physician will arrange for follow-up of an abnormal mammogram, whereas the family physician believes the opposite, conceivably resulting in harm to the patient.

Obstetrician/gynecologists have a long history of providing exceptional primary care to their patients. With most HMOs allowing female patients direct access to obstetrician/gynecologists without referral, there are many women whose only contact with a physician is at the annual gynecologic examination. Young women without comorbidities are especially likely to obtain much of their general medical care and counseling from their gynecologist. Still, it is important to determine how much contact these patients have with their actual primary care physicians, especially in areas where health insurance regulations restrict obstetrician/gynecologists from delivering primary care. If a patient presents to her family physician only for acute minor illness and sees her gynecologist for continuity care, important preventive interventions may be neglected.

Because obstetricians are unique in simultaneously extending both specialty and primary care to their patients, a woman will often disappear from her usual primary care practice during pregnancy. During pregnancy, it is not uncommon for a patient to direct most of her health care concerns, obstetric and otherwise, to her obstetrician. Often there is scant communication between a woman's family physician and her obstetrician during this transfer of care, before, during, and after pregnancy. Most pregnancies are admittedly uncomplicated and involve young, healthy women with no serious medical concerns. Still, the presence of conditions with the potential to become serious or chronic at some point after the pregnancy, such as depression, gestational diabetes, and pregnancy-induced hypertension, necessitates a note or telephone call between physicians.

The postpartum period is rife with change. A new mother is learning not just how to care for her new child but how to manage her new role within the context of a changed family unit. An ideal time for the family physician to touch base with the mother is at her newborn's first doctor's visit. Her physical condition, emotional state, and social supports can be assessed, and interventions delivered as needed. This valuable contact may never be established, however, if the baby's doctor is not also the mother's doctor. It becomes essential to know who will assume care of the mother and her child.

In the case of gynecologic cancer, the patient is often referred by the primary care doctor or the general obstetrician/gynecologist to a gynecologic oncologist. Surgery, with the possibility of both chemotherapy and radiation, follow. Weeks later, the primary physician may be called on to treat chemotherapy-related pain, immunosuppression, or electrolyte abnormalities. This can be disconcerting for a physician who has not been kept informed about the treatment plan and may not even know which chemotherapeutic agents have been administered. Again, the importance of communication among treating physicians cannot be overemphasized.

As the organization and delivery of medical care continue to evolve, the quality and safety of that care depend on organized and efficient interaction among the collaborators in the health care system. Ideally, physicians, nurses, institutions, and communities are all players united in a single mission: the best possible care for patients.

Reference

1. Phillips RL Jr, Starfield B: Why does a U.S. primary care physician workforce crisis matter? Am Fam Physician 2003;68:1494, 1496–1498, 1500.

Chapter 57
The Importance of Screening for Violence in the Teen Population

Michelle Vichnin MD

One of my patients confided to me, "My daughter's boyfriend pushed her through a glass door. The door shattered, and shards of glass cut her all over her hands and face. She needed stitches. My daughter is so terrified now that we had to get a restraining order."

The statistics on abuse in teenage girls are shocking: one in five teen girls has suffered sexual or physical abuse from a boyfriend. In addition to being more likely to smoke, use cocaine, acquire eating disorders, and have unsafe sex, high school–aged girls who have been abused by their boyfriends are four to six times more likely to become pregnant than teens who are not abused, and teen girls who are in abusive relationships are eight to nine times as likely to make a serious suicide attempt.

Unfortunately, amid all of the things we need to do for our patients in the short time allotted for gynecologic visits—check vital signs, review the chief complaint, obtain past medical, surgical, and family histories, and perform thorough physical examinations—screening for violence is sometimes overlooked. Given that violence in the teen population has a prevalence of 20%—greater than some of the most common STIs, such as chlamydial infection—it is essential that any physician who provides medical services to teens include routine screening for domestic and sexual abuse.

Obstetrician/gynecologists can play a critical role in identifying teens who are at risk for abuse. First, many girls and women are comfortable discussing intimate issues with their gynecologists. If the doctor asks about abuse as part of each visit and it is routine, teens will often feel free to open up to have a frank discussion. Also, gynecologists have many opportunities to see teens for ongoing care, such as contraceptive management and treatment of dysmenorrhea and menorrhagia. Each visit provides an opportunity to screen for abuse. Because we often treat mothers of teens, we have the opportunity to educate them about abuse and other issues their daughters may face.

The following are some tips for screening for violence in teens:

- Ask a teen how she is doing—overall, in school, and in activities. Poor grades or lack of interest in her favorite activities may be signs of depression or abuse.
- Ask about her relationships. Is anybody hitting or hurting her?
- Remain nonjudgmental, but remind patients that no means no, no matter what!
- Remind teens that their answers are confidential (and then maintain confidentiality).
- Let girls know that they deserve to be treated well.
- Let girls know that you screen everyone in your practice for violence at every visit.
- Be yourself. Teens know when you are sincere.
- Have literature on violence, along with hotline numbers, available in the restrooms.

Chapter 58
Obesity and Obstetrics:
Using Systems and Early Intervention

Kelly C. Allison PhD, *Chad O. Edwards* MS, RD,
and Thomas A. Wadden PhD

Obesity increases the risk of gestational diabetes, preeclampsia, infection, macrosomia, shoulder dystocia, cesarean delivery, stillbirth, and other complications.[1,2] Evidence is mounting that excess weight gain during pregnancy is linked to overweight status among offspring as early as 3 years of age.[3] The impact of both pregravid obesity and excess weight gain during pregnancy should be addressed by physicians, medical assistants, registered dietitians, and other health professionals on the health care team. This approach includes discussing weight loss with overweight and obese gynecologic patients during routine visits if they are considering pregnancy. During pregnancy, weight gain guidelines should be explained and weight gain throughout the pregnancy should be carefully monitored.

In 1990, an expert panel of the Institute of Medicine (IOM) issued guidelines for weight gain during pregnancy to decrease the number of small-for-gestational-age births.[4] The panel recommended that during the course of pregnancy, underweight women (body mass index [BMI] <19.9 kg/m^2) gain 12.3 to 18 kg; average-weight women (BMI 19.9 to 26.0 kg/m^2) increase approximately 11.5 to 16 kg; overweight women (BMI 26.1 to 29.0 kg/m^2) gain 7 to 11.5 kg; and obese women (BMI >29 kg/m^2) gain no more than 7 kg. These guidelines have recently been updated. While the weight gain ranges for the average-weight and overweight groups remained the same, the recommended weight gain range for obese women decreased to 5 to 9 kg.[5]

It has proven difficult to limit women to the current recommended ranges. Typically, about half of all pregnant women gain in excess of the amount recommended by the IOM.[1,2] Efforts of multiple health care providers are likely needed to control weight gain to subsequently reduce the incidence of negative birth outcomes for obese women. Care providers should start by calculating the BMI of patients considering pregnancy and informing them of the reductions in risks to both mother and baby that result from a pregravid weight loss. Small losses of 5% to 10% of initial body weight (e.g., 4.5 to 9 kg for a 90-kg woman) improve blood pressure, glucose and cholesterol levels, and fertility.[6] Modest weight losses can also be expected to have a positive impact on pregnancy outcomes, although more data are needed in this area. Intake of approximately 3500 calories above an individual's energy requirements can lead to a gain of 2.2 kg of body weight; similarly, a deficit of 3500 calories can lead to the loss of 2.2 kg of body weight (e.g., a deficit of 500 calories per day, equivalent to one cookie and one bagel a day, would lead to a 2.2-kg weight loss each week). Physical activity can also contribute to a calorie deficit.

Appropriate communication and empathy are important in achieving a patient's trust and compliance. When discussing weight issues with patients, the words "obese" and "fat" are perceived in an extremely negative fashion and should be avoided. The most preferred terms are simply "weight" or "excess weight."[7]

Overweight or obese patients who are considering pregnancy should be referred to a dietitian whenever possible. Teaching patients the healthy methods of preparing and choosing foods, using recommended portion sizes, and eating regularly throughout the day can promote weight loss. Lower-calorie foods with higher nutritional value are encouraged. Education about these principles will help to ensure that patients consume an appropriate level of calories and key nutrients (folate, calcium, iron, protein) that are recommended for healthy pregnancy outcomes. By developing healthy eating habits before conception, obstetric patients will have the foundation to make appropriate diet choices, achieve proper weight gain goals, and consume recommended supplements during pregnancy.

After conception, the health care provider should provide weight gain criteria appropriate for each stage of pregnancy. If this rate is exceeded, the care provider should caution that precipitous weight gain can increase the risk of negative birth outcomes. Capitalizing on the "teachable moment" that pregnancy often represents for women, small, simple behavioral weight control strategies, continued physical activity, and clear nutritional counseling should be used to minimize weight gain or to maintain weight status among overweight and obese patients. Weight loss during pregnancy is not recommended. Dietitians are useful for controlling weight gain, and psychologists and social workers also may be enlisted to help patients control eating in response to stress and negative emotions. Disordered eating patterns seen more frequently among the overweight and obese population, such as binge eating disorder and night eating syndrome, should be assessed, along with the belief that patients are "eating for two," instead of only consuming approximately 300 extra calories per day in the second and third trimesters. In summary, consistent, straightforward information about weight gain recommendations combined with nutritional or psychological counseling will likely limit negative pregnancy outcomes that health care professionals increasingly are required to manage.

References

1. Catalano PM: Management of obesity in pregnancy. Obstet Gynecol 2007;109:419–433.
2. Sarwer DB, Allison KC, Gibbons LM, et al: Pregnancy and obesity: A review and agenda for future research. J Womens Health 2006;15:720–733.
3. Oken E, Taveras EM, Kleinman KP, et al: Gestational weight gain and child adiposity at age 3 years. Am J Obstet Gynecol 2007;196:322e1–322e8.
4. Institute of Medicine: Nutrition during Pregnancy: Part I: Weight Gain, Part II: Nutrient Supplements. Washington, DC, National Academy Press, 1990.
5. Institute of Medicine: Weight gain during pregnancy: Reexamining the guidelines. Washington, DC, National Academies Press, 2009.
6. Vidal J: Updated review of the benefits of weight loss. Int J Obes Relat Metab Disord 2002;26:525–528.
7. Wadden TA, Didie E: What's in a name? Patients' preferred terms for describing obesity. Obes Res 2003;11:1140–1146.

Chapter 59
Pregnancy Termination and the Competencies

Richard D. Kaplan MD and Frank White MD

Editor's Note: On January 22, 1973, in his majority opinion on the legality of abortion in the case *Roe v. Wade*, Supreme Court Justice Harry Blackmun wrote,

This right of privacy, whether it be founded in the Fourteenth Amendment's concept of personal liberty and restrictions upon state action, as

we feel it is, or, as the District Court determined, in the Ninth Amendment's reservation of rights to the people, is broad enough to encompass a woman's decision whether or not to terminate her pregnancy. The detriment that the State would impose upon the pregnant woman by denying this choice altogether is apparent.[1]

About 50% of the 4.5 million pregnancies in the United States each year are unintended. Of those unintended pregnancies, 50% are electively terminated. Since 1973, an estimated 46 million legal abortions have been performed. But the national debate on abortion continues, both publicly and privately.

In 1998, an international study found that some of the most common reasons women chose to terminate pregnancies were:

- Desire to delay or end childbearing.
- Concern over the interruption of work or education.
- Issues of financial or relationship stability.
- Their own perceived immaturity.[2]

A 2004 study in which American women at abortion clinics answered a questionnaire yielded similar results.[3]

In the United States, most abortions are performed by an obstetrician/gynecologist. Of the approximately 28,000 board-certified obstetrician/gynecologists in the country, about 23% perform pregnancy terminations. Some of the most common rationales among the 77% who do *not* perform abortions are

- Lack of proper training or proper facilities.
- Ethical, moral, or religious beliefs.
- Health risk to the mother.
- Pressure from antiabortion activist groups.

In the following, Dr. Richard D. Kaplan of Greensboro, North Carolina and Dr. Frank White of Philadelphia, Pennsylvania offer their thoughts on abortion as practicing obstetrician/gynecologists.

WHY I OFFER TERMINATIONS OF PREGNANCY TO MY PATIENTS

Richard D. Kaplan MD

In 1991, my home was picketed by demonstrators who threatened my life and brandished signs that called me a murderer. In order to protect my wife, my children, and my own safety, I sued for an injunction against residential picketing. During my deposition, the protesters' attorney demanded accusingly, "What do you feel when you perform abortions?" I thought about it and replied, "I feel satisfaction." I feel the satisfaction of knowing that I provide an important service to my patients in a caring, professional, and safe environment.

As I reflect on my having been raised in a principled, ethical, and caring family, I am reminded that providing abortion care to my patients falls completely within my personal moral framework and belief system. I grew up in New York, and I can recall my parents' positive reaction when the New York State legislature, by a single vote majority, legalized unrestricted abortion of a pre-viable fetus. "No more bloody coat hangers or women dying from septic shock," they said. "No more need for a woman to convince a psychiatrist or gynecologist that her life or her psychiatric health are threatened by her pregnancy. No more need for a woman who has taken thalidomide to fly to Sweden for a legal abortion of her deformed fetus."

In 1973, when I was in medical school, the Supreme Court affirmed many patients' needs by ruling that a woman has a constitutional right to choose to abort her pre-viable fetus. Many argued that legalized abortion on demand would cause psychological harm to women. Studies have failed to confirm this claim.[3] Others argued that, despite the Supreme Court's analysis, a fetus is a person from the moment of fertilization and has a right to life whether it is in a woman's womb or a freezer in an infertility clinic. My rational upbringing and my scientific and medical training have led me to conclude that a pre-viable fetus is biologically incapable at conception and experientially deficient at any point thereafter of having thoughts or feelings. I accept the *Roe v. Wade* decision as just because I believe that a fetus is not a person. I choose to use my Ob/Gyn training to help my patients either carry or terminate their pregnancy according to their informed wishes.

Working directly with my patients gives me another perspective in addition to my scientific one on my decision to perform abortions. Since 1979, when I entered private practice, I have worked 4 to 8 hours per week in an abortion clinic. One of the forms that each of my patients completes before undergoing the procedure allows her space to state why she is having the abortion. Many patients choose not to comment, but others share their situation. "I had a baby 3 months ago," one woman wrote. "Raped," another said. "Forty-five years old and have grandchildren," "Single, going to college," "My boyfriend beats me," "I have three children and cannot afford another," "I'm thirteen years old and not ready to be a mother," others said. Whatever their situation, I do not believe that any of these women should be forced by law or the lack of trained and willing physicians to carry an unwanted pregnancy to term.

WHY I DO NOT PERFORM TERMINATIONS OF PREGNANCY

Frank White, MD

I do not perform abortions. My decision is founded on two principles: the right to life of all human beings, and the professionalism principle of social justice.

My upbringing is rooted in Catholicism, and studies have shown that religious affiliation is a strong predictor of one's opinion on this issue. Traditionally, many practicing Catholics have adopted a pro-life stance.[4] Catholics are not alone on this issue, though. Other groups, including many Muslims, Orthodox Jews, and Fundamentalist Christians, feel similarly.

I agree with the Catholic Church's position that "Human life must be respected and protected absolutely from the moment of conception. From the first moment of existence, a human being must be recognized as having the rights of a person—the foremost of which is the inviolable right of every innocent being to life." In my opinion, Pope John Paul II has summarized it best:

It is impossible to further the common good without acknowledging and defending the right to life, upon which all the other inalienable rights of individuals are founded and from which they develop. A society lacks solid foundations when, on the one hand, it asserts values such as the dignity of the person, justice and peace, but then, on the other hand, radically acts to the contrary by allowing or tolerating a variety of ways in which human life is devalued and violated, especially where it is weak or marginalized. Only respect for life can be the foundation and guarantee of the most precious and essential goods of society, such as democracy and peace.[5]

Other reasons for my position are not necessarily grounded in Catholic teaching, but in the principles of social justice. Abortion terminates what I believe to be an innocent life. The aborted fetus is voiceless and vulnerable, and abortion makes the fetus party to a procedure for which it cannot give informed consent.

For me, however, the debate over whether or not abortion is acceptable is not always clear. There are certain circumstances in which abortion is an appropriate decision. For example, I have no objection to terminating a pregnancy conceived after an assault, molestation, or rape. Other instances require more consideration. For example, consider the shock of discovering, at a 16-week ultrasonography or amniocentesis, that a fetus has anencephaly, Down syndrome, or an anatomic abnormality incompatible with life. In such instances, my commitment to professionalism and patient care requires me to encourage my patient to seek a second opinion, similar to a referral I might recommend for a complex procedure such as a tubal reanastamosis or surgical staging that I am not experienced at performing. I recognize that some would consider me a hypocrite for referring women in these situations to doctors who may agree to end their pregnancies. We are fortunate that the preceding scenarios are rare and recognize that these types of situations account for only a small fraction of the abortions performed.

References

1. *Roe v. Wade*, 410 U.S. 113 (1973).
2. Aiyer AN, Ruiz G, Steinman A, Ho GY: Influence of physician attitudes on willingness to perform abortion. Obstet Gynecol 1999;93:576–580.
3. Major B, et al: Report of the APA task force on mental health and abortion, Washington, DC: American Psychological Association, 2008, p 68.
4. Eastwood KL, Kacmar JE, Steinauer J, et al: Abortion training in United States obstetrics and gynecology residency programs. Obstet Gynecol 2006;108:303–308.
5. John Paul II: Evangelium Vitae (Encyclical Letter). Presented in Rome, March 25, 1995. Available at http://www.vatican.va/holy_father/john_paul_ii/encyclicals/.

Chapter 60
On Birthing Plans and Birthing Outcomes
Perspectives from a Physician-Patient

Cynthia D. Smith MD

As doctors, constantly surrounded by a scientific community, it is often difficult for us to understand patients' decisions to explore alternative medicine, especially during pregnancy. When I was pregnant with my first child, I began to understand one patient mindset that had often confounded me before my own pregnancy. I found myself reading nonscientific books written by people other than doctors for lighthearted advice, and I even tried yoga and contemplated the benefits of giving birth at home rather than at a hospital. Although I was an internist in a full-time private practice, it took my husband, an infectious disease physician, to help me remember that there is nothing shameful about delivering a baby in a hospital in a safe, well-monitored environment.

I found myself avoiding obstetrical scientific literature when I was pregnant with my first child. The last thing I wanted to read about was everything that could possibly go wrong in my pregnancy and delivery. I wanted to read something that would make me laugh and make me feel that everything would be all right. I read the *Girlfriends' Guide to Pregnancy* and would quote it repeatedly to anybody who would listen. This embarrassed my husband, who would ask me, "How on earth can you quote a former *Penthouse* model on the risks of pregnancy and not pay attention to what the real doctors are telling you?" The book made me laugh. It made me less anxious.

Not only did my husband put up with passages read aloud from the *Girlfriends' Guide*, he supported the maternity yoga class I did three times a week. When the yoga instructor offered a special weekend natural childbirth class, he agreed to give up a Saturday and come with me. During the first part of the class, which a diverse array of couples attended, we went around in a circle explaining our individual birth plans to the group. Nearly half the class had chosen to have natural childbirth in water tanks at home. I had planned to have my child at the hospital, a decision that was expected among my colleagues at work. But when it came to my turn to explain I felt so nervous and exposed. "I plan to have my child at the hospital," I stuttered.

The other parents seemed horrified. "Won't that be awfully invasive and impersonal?" one of the women in the group asked, tapping into my deepest fears.

"I hope not," I said. Then, I burst into tears.

I was able to pull myself together and spent the remainder of the day practicing breathing and contractions on the birthing ball, learning about the joys of labor in the shower, and putting my swollen body into a variety of labor positions. In the car on the way home my husband and I talked about our birthing decision and decided we were doing the right thing for us.

In my mind, my delivery would take place in the hospital, but would be a perfect combination of science and new-age magic. I would have mood lighting, massage, a birthing ball, and, of course, the shower that I was now convinced was the panacea for labor pain. I would be in control at all times, and I would smile lovingly at my husband. I would not poison my baby with unnecessary medicine or invasive procedures, and I would give birth naturally.

Two weeks before my due date, I was seeing patients in my office when I noticed a trickle of fluid running down my leg. I excused myself from the room and locked myself in the bathroom to try and figure out whether or not I had broken my water. I asked the secretary to cancel my remaining patients, changed into scrubs and drove myself home to do a maneuver I had read about to help identify if I had actually broken my water. I was terrified about going to the hospital unless something real had happened. I was more concerned about a false alarm and bothering the doctors unnecessarily than I was with my own health and the health of the baby. The "maneuver" was positive and my husband came home to drive me to the hospital.

My water was broken and my doctors induced my labor after I failed to progress. Despite the fact that I now had an IV and Pitocin was running into my veins, I was feeling optimistic: I could hear the shower and the birthing ball call my name. But moments later I felt the real thing, a stabbing pain so penetrating it took my breath away. Worse than the pain itself was the anticipation of the next contraction. I was no longer smiling at my husband. I grabbed his hand and told him to call the anesthesiologist. He placed his hand on my head and said he would take care of it. I withdrew my hand from his and screamed "Now!" My epidural went in quickly and painlessly, but with it came numbness in my legs, difficulty urinating on my own, and the shower and birthing ball were out of the question.

When the fetal monitor alarmed, I glanced up at the tracing. My medical student obstetrics rotation was a distant memory, but my baby's heart rate tracing looked worrisome to me. Naively, until that moment, I had not entertained the possibility of danger to my baby. Suddenly, I was surrounded by nurses, doctors, medical students, and residents. I could no longer see my husband's face. They worked quickly and efficiently turning the Pitocin drip down, moving me into a variety of positions, and placing a fetal scalp monitor on my baby. I was terrified, and I was no longer in control of anything. Suddenly my labor and delivery was no longer about me, no longer about my birth plan, and no longer about my relationship with my husband—it was all about getting my baby out safely. At that moment there was no place that I would have rather been than in the teaching hospital where I trained, surrounded by a competent and caring team of students, doctors, and nurses. At 2:00 AM on July 1, 1999, I gave birth to a healthy baby boy named Christopher.

As I recall my first pregnancy now, I laugh at how unrealistic my birth plan turned out to be for me. My colleagues and I routinely hear far-fetched birthing plans from our patients. Pregnancy can be scary, and the medical environment often provides less comfort than alternative medicine and lay press books. It is important to remain nonjudgmental and to keep in mind that the traditional, scientific perspective may not always be the most comforting while talking to patients about their pregnancies. Having had the experience of being such a patient myself has helped me better relate to my patients and provide them the explanations that they need to understand the joy and risks of the birthing process.

Chapter 61
A Defense Attorney's Perspective

Mary Grady Walsh Esq.

It is the very rare physician who survives a career practicing medicine and is not the subject of a malpractice lawsuit. In many jurisdictions, plaintiffs often name a host of treating doctors as defendants. This can result in an inordinate amount of time determining which doctors belong in the lawsuit. Although most medical malpractice cases do not ultimately end in a verdict against the physician, the experience is nonetheless disconcerting and consumes valuable time and attention that otherwise could be spent treating patients.

The truth is there is no advice that will render a physician "lawsuit-proof." However, there are some practical guidelines you can follow to reduce the likelihood of being sued. Physician defendants often lament that they have been forced to resort to practicing "defensive medicine." The important principle is to practice smart medicine.

In a lawsuit, the medical record is sacrosanct. It is a road map of both the treatment provided and the recommended treatment. For an attorney who defends physicians, a medical record that supports the physician-client's version of events is of paramount importance. It stands to reason, then, that the record must be an unadulterated document. Unfortunately, it is not uncommon to be faced with a case in which the course of treatment is otherwise defensible, and then have it rendered indefensible by an altered record. I learned first-hand some years ago the lengths to which plaintiffs will go to verify the accuracy of a record. In this particular instance, I was required to present a client's original chart to a laboratory for forensic testing to determine if all the ink on a record was written at the same time. If a portion of a handwritten record is added later, the technology exists to conclusively identify such discrepancies. Creating a comprehensive contemporaneous record bolsters not only the physician's ability to treat patients, but also provides a foundation for the physician's testimony if a suit is filed.

What I tell my clients, and what is universally true, is that a defense attorney can defend most actions except a changed record. Although defendants who do attempt to add to or change a medical record believe it will protect them in a lawsuit, in reality, it does just the opposite. Importantly, an attorney is not permitted by the Code of Professional Ethics to use a record that is known to be false at trial. I have never seen a record change where the alteration was to the physician's advantage. Once you lose your credibility with the jury, your chances of victory at trial diminish exponentially. Likewise, all of the various Physician Codes of Medical Ethics would suggest that dishonesty and fraud cannot be tolerated. The take-away point here is to not change or alter a medical record in any way after an event has occurred. Keep in mind, however, that late addendums or additions, dated as such, which may help clarify how care was provided are allowable, and may help in the long run if there are issues or events you feel justify clarification.

It is often difficult to predict which patients are likely to sue if an adverse outcome occurs. However, there are strategies that can be used from the beginning of a physician–patient relationship that can reduce the likelihood of a lawsuit and ensure a better outcome from a legal standpoint should a suit be filed. If a patient is noncompliant, it is critical to record that behavior in the patient's chart. If a specialist or testing is recommended and your patient ignores or refuses your advice, document it each time. Live by the adage "if it wasn't noted, it wasn't done." That way, you are not later faced with a contest over whose memory is most accurate. If a patient comes to trial ill or maimed, you can ameliorate much of the sympathy a jury may feel for your patient if it is clear that you recommended the appropriate treatment all along. The extra few moments it takes to accurately record an encounter in the medical record will pay dividends if you are ever named in a lawsuit. Document, document, document.

Patients are less likely to sue physicians whom they like or whom they believe are truly interested in their well-being. Unfortunately, as many of us practice today, doctors have less time to spend with each patient, and this can make patients feel as though they are just one of an assembly line of patients who need to be seen in a given day. Try to find a balance between running a cost-effective practice and giving patients the time and attention they invariably expect and deserve. Patients are likely to communicate better with a doctor who actively listens, invites patient questions, and demonstrates empathy. Open communication often leads to a better opportunity to diagnose and treat the patient. Although you may only have mere minutes to spend with each patient, spend that time wisely.

Never disregard your common sense when treating patients or when deciding whom to treat. I once deposed a middle-aged woman who had undergone numerous cosmetic surgery procedures. She suffered a cardiac arrest during breast enhancement surgery. Her medical record contained a nurse's note that indicated that she was distraught, not from almost losing her life, but because she looked "puffy" as a result of the fluids given to her during the effort to revive her. Her records were, in fact, replete with notations indicating that she had a distorted body image. This was not a patient that the surgeon was required to operate on. The surgery was clearly elective. The bottom line is, try to show good sense and judgment when you are treating and caring for patients. When performing elective surgery, put yourself in the best position possible to obtain a good outcome: sometimes this means showing good judgment by choosing *not* to operate on people.

In a busy practice, it is not easy to maintain a protocol for ensuring that test results are communicated to a patient, but this is a crucial element in preventing a disaster. It only takes one suspect mammogram, off-kilter INR, or abnormal blood sugar to fall through the cracks to initiate a difficult-to-defend lawsuit. Take some time to establish practice protocols to ensure patients are promptly and accurately advised of their test results in person, over the phone, or in writing. Imagine the feeling of the family physician who attempted to call her patient with a worrisome mammogram report but had difficulty reaching the patient and left it to her office staff to pursue the matter. The chart was inadvertently re-filed before the contact was made, compounding the communication failure. Thirteen months later, the patient returned for a routine visit when the doctor realized the cancer had been growing since the mammogram first identified it without the patient's knowledge, and with no intervention—all because there was no protocol to ensure the test results were reported.

The law dictates that a mere mistake in judgment or poor outcome does not constitute medical negligence. But patients who feel wronged or injured may seek legal counsel and file lawsuits. It is important not to take it personally if you are named as a defendant. Instead, maintain the sanctity of your records, stay in contact with your attorney, and understand that even the finest physicians find themselves as defendants in lawsuits.

Chapter 62
Coping with the Malpractice Insurance Crisis and Rising Costs: The Advantages of a Physician-Organized System

Stephen P. Krell MD

This chapter gives a brief background on the principles by which the United States' malpractice insurance system operates, and explains why consolidated practices present a promising way to cope with the current malpractice insurance crisis that is currently affecting obstetricians and gynecologists.

The cost and availability of medical malpractice insurance for physicians are cyclical. Malpractice insurance premiums charged to physicians are directly related to an insurance carrier's financial performance. The investment returns of the malpractice carrier and the efficiency of the carrier's management can directly affect the cost to the physician when it comes to establishing the true cost for a policy. Other important determining costs relevant to the carrier include the frequency of claims against physicians and tort laws, which vary greatly from state to state. When malpractice carriers experience a financial downturn, they usually compensate for their poor performance by increasing the insurance premiums of their insured physicians. Simply stated, they pass on their increasing cost of doing business to the physicians they insure.

In Pennsylvania in 2003, a severe medical malpractice insurance crisis began, and has not yet ended. The crisis reflects a larger national trend in the dramatically rising costs of malpractice insurance. Especially hard hit in Pennsylvania were high-risk specialties such as neurosurgery, orthopedics, general surgery, and obstetrics/gynecology. There was no legislative relief on the horizon, and because the cost of malpractice insurance was so high (if a physician could get it at all), physician incomes plummeted. Many well-established physicians opted to leave the state to practice in more physician-friendly environments. For many patients, especially those in urban and rural communities, access to health care was in jeopardy.

An alternative to legislated tort reform was for the physicians to find ways to reduce practice costs while increasing revenues. One solution to this problem was to create a physician-organized system based on the principle of practice consolidation. By consolidating practices, certain "economies of scale" could be better implemented. Consolidation allows for better and more efficient analysis of outcomes and risk, more efficient control of costs, and, most important, enhanced ability to approach payers for more fair and equitable reimbursement for services.

The Women's Healthcare Group of Pennsylvania (WHCGPA) was incorporated and began to operate on January 1, 2005. This organization was the first successful attempt in the southeastern Pennsylvania region to consolidate obstetric and gynecologic practices to take advantage of the benefits of consolidation. WHCGPA originally included 39 obstetrician/gynecologists in 6 hospitals in suburban Philadelphia. Now, in its third year, it comprises 56 physicians who deliver over 6000 babies annually, perform thousands of surgical procedures, and treat well over 200,000 patients every year. This business model is by no means unique. It has been used elsewhere in the United States with great success in many different specialties.

There are many advantages for physicians who consolidate their practices. Some of the major benefits of such a system include the following:

- Group purchase of supplies and equipment.
- The purchase of health insurance benefits for all physicians and their employees at favorable rates.
- Contracting for an efficient billing and practice management service.
- The establishment of common and fair human resource policies.
- Joint accounting and legal services.
- The establishment of a high-quality retirement plan.
- Ease of instituting an electronic medical records program.
- The ability to do meaningful clinical research as a group.
- Increased negotiating power with third-party payers.

In a consolidated practice, **negotiation power** for service and supplies is improved. The group can negotiate with health insurance payers to obtain **improved reimbursement** for provider services. This is a reasonable expectation provided the group demonstrates its ability to become more efficient and provide high-quality care. Being attentive to formulary prescription drugs, avoiding overutilization of testing, and performing procedures safely in the office rather than in the more expensive hospital or surgical center settings are a few ways to demonstrate savings to the payers. The group also must be able to demonstrate a higher quality of medical care and better outcomes for patients. Many physician-organized groups have been successful in establishing *Pay for Performance* programs with the payers in their respective communities.

Another extremely important advantage of consolidation is the establishment of a **risk management program** within the larger group. Physician-organized practices must be very serious about improving patient safety, reducing medical errors, and providing the highest quality of care for patients. Less-than-optimal patient outcomes should be reviewed by a risk management committee and steps for improvement should be identified and implemented. Well-managed groups often establish a partnership with a medical malpractice insurance carrier to reduce claims and improve patient outcomes. Many groups have been successful in this regard and have obtained substantial discounts on malpractice premiums and the establishment of a risk-sharing deductible program.

Although physicians are widely regarded to be independent thinkers who are often inclined to "go it alone," sometimes there is no choice but to collaborate. In hostile practice environments where costs continue to rise and reimbursements often remain static, it is often advantageous for physicians to band together in physician-organized, physician-run systems. These collaborative business models enable us to continue to provide care to the patients we are trained to treat.

Section IX
OPERATIVE DELIVERY AND GYNECOLOGIC PROCEDURES

OPERATIVE DELIVERY PROCEDURES
Section Editor: Michael Belden MD

GYNECOLOGIC PROCEDURES
Section Editor: Mark Finnegan MD

Operative Delivery Procedure 1: Vacuum-Assisted Vaginal Delivery

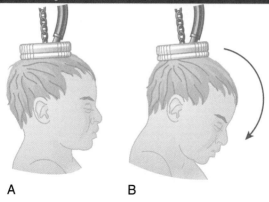

A   B

Application of vacuum extractor. The application shown in **A** is incorrect. The application shown in **B** is correct; the vacuum is properly placed over the posterior fontanelle.

Indications

- Prolonged second stage of labor
- Maternal exhaustion
- Fetal distress

Medical Knowledge—You Need to Know

- Fetal heart rate tracings that would dictate delivery
- ACOG recommendations regarding appropriate length of second stage of labor
- Perineal anatomy and blood supply
- The specifics of the vacuum extractor you have selected

Major Steps

1. Establish that the fetus needs to be delivered expeditiously
2. Ascertain that cervix is fully dilated
3. Drain bladder
4. Confirm adequacy of anesthesia
5. Examine the patient and estimate fetal station and position
6. Apply vacuum to fetal vertex
7. Pull gently during contractions as the patient pushes
8. Be prepared to discontinue if the fetus does not make successive progression with each push
9. Be prepared to abandon procedure if baby not delivered after three pushes with vacuum applied to the vertex

Anticipating Potential Complications

- Failure to establish fetal movement → Abandon procedure
- Maternal trauma → Prepare for thorough postdelivery examination and be prepared to do repair
- Fetal cephalohematoma → Do not pull too hard if there is no progress

Issues for Discussion

- How does one determine when it is appropriate to abandon procedure and perform an cesarean delivery?

| Vacuum-Assisted Vaginal Delivery | Dx V22.2 | CPT code 43280 | $3000 |

Operative Delivery Procedure 2: Forceps-Assisted Vaginal Delivery

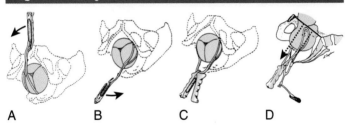

A   B   C   D

Proper application of obstetric forceps. **A,** Application of the left branch; **B,** movement of the left branch so that it lays appropriately adjacent to the parietal bone; **C,** addition of the right branch; **D,** correct axis of traction.

Indications

- Prolonged second stage of labor
- Maternal exhaustion
- Fetal distress

Medical Knowledge—You Need to Know

- Fetal heart rate tracings that would dictate delivery
- ACOG recommendations regarding appropriate length of second stage of labor
- Perineal anatomy and blood supply
- The different types of forceps available
- The clinical situations that dictate the use of specific types of forceps

Major Steps

1. Establish that the fetus needs to be delivered
2. Confirm adequacy of anesthesia
3. Examine the patient and estimate fetal station and confirm fetal position
4. Confirm that the bladder is drained
5. Between contractions, carefully apply the branches of the forceps
6. Make sure the application is correct
7. Pull gently during contractions as the patient pushes
8. Be prepared to abandon procedure if the fetus does not make progression during each push

Anticipating Potential Complications

- Failure to establish successive movement with each pull
- Maternal trauma

- Fetal trauma

→ Abandon procedure

→ Prepare for a thorough postdelivery examination, including an examination of the upper vagina and cervix, be prepared to repair
→ Do not pull too hard if there is no progress

Issues for Discussion

- Given the controversy associated with obstetric forceps, how does one best reassure patients when their use is indicated?

Forceps-Assisted Vaginal Delivery   Dx V22.3   CPT code 43280 $3000

Operative Delivery Procedure 3: Episiotomy Repair

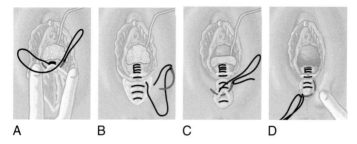

A   B   C   D

Episiotomy repair. **A,** Anchoring stitch placed at apex of defect; **B,** repair of posterior vaginal wall; **C,** repair of deeper tissue of the perineum; **D,** repair of perineal skin.

Indications

- Need to create larger pelvic outlet
- High likelihood of difficult-to-repair perineal tear
- Certain instrumental deliveries
- Shoulder dystocia

Medical Knowledge—You Need to Know

- Advantages and disadvantages of midline versus mediolateral approach
- Pelvic floor anatomy, including perianal anatomy
- Pelvic blood supply
- Properties of the various sutures used for repair
- Proper use of instruments and assistants

Major Steps

1. Establish adequacy of vaginal/pelvic outlet during second stage of labor
2. Assess possibility of a third- or fourth-degree tear (for which episiotomy is indicated)
3. Prep the perineum
4. As the fetal head is crowning, use a scissors to surgically increase vaginal outlet
5. Use absorbable suture; begin above apex of episiotomy
6. Carefully reapproximate

Anticipating Potential Complications

- Third- and fourth-degree extensions
- Inadequate repair
- Bleeding and hematoma

→ Pay particular attention to supporting the perineum at the time of delivery, as well as controlling the delivery of the head and shoulders
→ Meticulously dissect out the capsule of the external anal sphincter, if damaged
→ Know the blood supply of perineum, and apply best techniques for hemostasis

Issues for Discussion

- Are episiotomies really required?

| Episiotomy Repair | Dx V22.2 | CPT code 43280 | $275 |

Operative Delivery Procedure 4: Cesarean Section

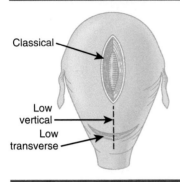

Classical

Low vertical

Low transverse

Types of uterine incisions for cesarean section.

Indications

- Arrest of dilation
- Arrest of descent
- Breech presentation
- Fetal distress with no opportunity for vaginal delivery
- Placenta previa
- Elective repeat cesarean
- Elective primary cesarean at patient's request
- Medical conditions precluding trial of labor

Medical Knowledge—You Need to Know

- Types of cesarean: low transverse, low vertical, classical
- Blood supply to the uterus
- Innervation and blood supply of other pelvic organs
- Properties of sutures
- Proper use of instruments and assistants

Major Steps

1. Make skin incision: Pfannenstiel or vertical
2. Open rectus fascia
3. Enter peritoneal cavity and reflect bladder off lower uterine segment
4. Incise uterus and deliver fetus
5. Remove placenta and begin uterine repair
6. Reapproximate rectus fascia
7. Reapproximate skin incision

Anticipating Potential Complications

- Difficult cesarean → Have assistants available; use meticulous technique
- Infection → Provide antibiotics; use best surgical technique
- Hemorrhage → Obtain blood products and be prepared to transfuse; be prepared to perform hysterectomy, if required

Issues for Discussion

- The rate of cesarean section in the United States now approaches 30% (up from around 5% in 1970). Why has there been no demonstrable improvement in neonatal outcomes attributable to this change in practice?

| Cesarean Delivery | Dx V22.2 | CPT code 43280 | $3100 |

Gynecologic Procedure 1: Dilation and Curettage/Hysteroscopy

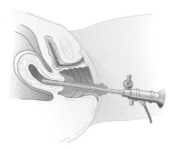

Proper placement of hysteroscope before curettage.

Indications

- Abnormal uterine bleeding
- Submucous uterine fibroids
- Postmenopausal bleeding
- Endometrial polyps

Medical Knowledge—You Need to Know

- Blood supply of cervix and uterus
- Endometrial physiology
- Causes of abnormal uterine bleeding and postmenopausal bleeding

Major Steps

1. Empty bladder, perform bimanual pelvic examination
2. Sound uterus
3. Insert hysteroscope
4. Examine endometrial cavity
5. Use polyp forceps as indicated
6. Use sharp curettage

Anticipating Potential Complications

- Cervical stenosis   → Consider use of preoperative misoprostol (prostaglandin E_1)
- Uterine perforation   → Exercise care in curettage

Issues for Discussion

- Can the procedure be performed in the office setting?
- What is the value of hysteroscopy?

Dilation and Curettage/Hysteroscopy   Dx: 626.a   CPT code 58558 $425

Gynecologic Procedure 2: Endometrial Ablation

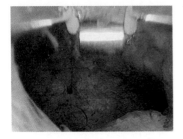

Endometrial cavity before beginning ablation.

Indications

- Endometrial polyps
- Submucosal uterine fibroids
- Abnormal uterine bleeding

Medical Knowledge—You Need to Know

- Blood supply of cervix and uterus
- Anatomy of endometrial cavity
- Resectoscope assembly and use
- Management of intraoperative fluids, especially uterine distention medium

Major Steps

1. Empty bladder, perform bimanual pelvic examination
2. Sound uterus for depth of endometrial cavity
3. Examine endometrial cavity with hysteroscope
4. Resect myoma or polyps as indicated
5. Perform ablation

Anticipating Potential Complications

- Cervical stenosis → Preoperative misoprostol (prostaglandin E_1) for cervical softening
- Uterine perforation → Use meticulous technique; consider diagnostic laparoscopy if perforation results in heavy bleeding
- Postoperative bleeding → Oral contraceptives, leuprolide, progestins

Issues for Discussion

- Does endometrial ablation have a high enough success rate to make it a viable option for the correctly chosen patient, and is it cost effective?
- What is the next step if the endometrial ablation is a failure?

| Endometrial Ablation | Dx 218.1 | CPT code 58563 | $466 |

Gynecologic Procedure 3: Cone Biopsy and Loop Electrocautery Excision Procedure (LEEP)

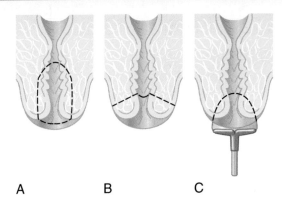

A   B   C

Three different strategies for performing a cone biopsy. **A,** A deep cone; **B,** a more superficial cone biopsy; **C,** a standard LEEP procedure.

Indications

- Cervical dysplasia (typically cervical intraepithelial neoplasia [CIN] grade 2 or greater)
- Discordant Pap test and colposcopy findings

Medical Knowledge—You Need to Know

- Blood supply of uterus and cervix
- Bethesda System for evaluating Pap test abnormalities
- Pathologic nomenclature for describing cervical dysplasia
- Cervical cancer staging
- Properties of local anesthetic agents

Major Steps

1. Empty bladder, perform bimanual pelvic examination
2. Place sutures at 3 and 9 o'clock (for "cold knife" cone biopsy only)
3. Perform cone biopsy
4. Cauterize cone bed
5. Apply Monsel solution if required

Anticipating Potential Complications

- Bleeding   → Sutures, electrocautery, Monsel solution

Issues for Discussion

- How does one choose between cone biopsy and LEEP?
- What is the rationale for expectant management of CIN2?

Cone Biopsy of cervix/LEEP procedure	Dx 622.10	CPT code 43280	$317

Gynecologic Procedure 4: Marsupialization of Bartholin's Cyst

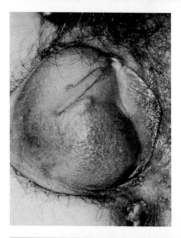

A large Bartholin's cyst before surgical excision and marsupialization.

Indications

- Bartholin's gland cyst
- Pain, cellulitis, fever associated with Bartholin's gland cyst

Medical Knowledge—You Need to Know

- Vulvar anatomy
- Location of Bartholin's glands

Major Steps

1. Provide intravenous sedation or local anesthesia, or both
2. Incise gland on its medial aspect
3. Drain and culture fluid
4. Suture epithelium to cyst wall (outside to inside)

Anticipating Potential Complications

- Cellulitis   → Antibiotics
- Bleeding   → Local anesthesia with epinephrine

Issues for Discussion

- What are the indications for complete excision (removing cyst wall) versus incision and drainage?

Marsupialization of Bartholin's Cyst   Dx 616.3   CPT code 56440 $367

Gynecologic Procedure 5: Laparoscopy

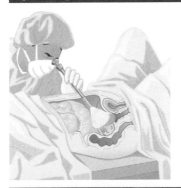

Diagnostic laparoscopy with proper placement of laparoscope.

Indications

- Complex adnexal mass
- Symptomatic ovarian cysts associated with pain
- Tubo-ovarian abscess
- Evaluation of pelvic pain
- Ectopic pregnancy

Medical Knowledge—You Need to Know

- Interpretation of sonograms, CT scans, and MRIs
- Etiologies of chronic pelvic pain
- Anatomy of pelvis and pelvic sidewall
- Differential diagnosis of ovarian masses

Major Steps

1. Empty bladder, perform bimanual pelvic examination
2. Insert Harris-Kronner uterine manipulator injector (HUMI uterine elevator)
3. Insert Veress needle
4. Insufflate abdomen with carbon dioxide gas
5. Insert primary port
6. Evaluate pelvis
7. Insert secondary ports
8. Identify ureters; follow these steps to remove an ovary, if required:
   a. Coagulate and cut ovarian vessels
   b. Coagulate and cut utero-ovarian anastomosis
   c. Cut any remaining peritoneal attachments
   d. Insert Endo-Bag (need 12-mm port)
   e. Remove specimen, send for frozen section
   f. Irrigate and check for bleeding
   g. Close fascia at 12-mm port sites
9. Drain CO_2 gas and remove ports
10. Close skin
11. Remove HUMI uterine elevator

Anticipating Potential Complications

- Bleeding
- Bladder, bowel or vessel injury
- Ureteral Injury
- Possible malignancy

→ Adequate cautery; use clips and endoloops as needed
→ Insert ports under direct vision; use meticulous dissection
→ Know course of ureter at all times
→ Gynecologic oncology consultation

Issues for Discussion

- When is it appropriate to convert to open laparotomy?
- When is it appropriate to manage pelvic malignancy with laparoscopy?

Laparoscopy: Diagnostic or Operative   Dx 625.9   CPT code 49320 or 58661 $910

Gynecologic Procedure 6: Fulguration of Endometriosis

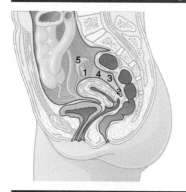

Likely locations of pelvic endometrial implants. 1, Ovaries; 2, cul-de-sac of Douglas; 3, bowel serosa; 4, uterine serosa; 5, fallopian tubes.

Indications

- Pelvic pain
- Infertility
- Dyspareunia

Medical Knowledge—You Need to Know

- Pelvic anatomy
- Location of ureters
- Diagnosis of endometriosis
- Staging of endometriosis
- Types of endometrial implants

Major Steps

1. Empty bladder, perform bimanual pelvic examination
2. Perform laparoscopy (or laparotomy if required)
3. Examine pelvis
4. Identify pathology
5. Cauterize or excise endometrial implants
6. Send excised implants to pathology

Anticipating Potential Complications

- Bowel, bladder, ureteral injury → Identify anatomy and use caution

Issues for Discussion

- Recurrence rates of endometriosis
- Etiology of chronic pelvic pain
- Hormonal suppression of endometriosis
- Use of leuprolide to suppress endometriosis

| Fulguration of Endometriosis | Dx 617.3 | CPT code 58662 | $662 |

Gynecologic Procedure 7: Abdominal Hysterectomy

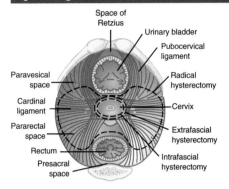

Space of Retzius
Urinary bladder
Pubocervical ligament
Paravesical space
Radical hysterectomy
Cardinal ligament
Cervix
Pararectal space
Extrafascial hysterectomy
Rectum
Intrafascial hysterectomy
Presacral space

Types of hysterectomy: extrafascial, intrafascial, and radical.

Indications

- Uterine fibroids
- Menorrhagia
- Pelvic pain
- Endometriosis

Medical Knowledge—You Need to Know

- Abdominal wall and pelvic anatomy
- Path of ureter
- Evaluation of pelvic pathology using ultrasonography, CT scan, and MRI

Major Steps

1. Prep vagina and insert Foley
2. Prep and drape abdomen
3. Enter abdomen through vertical or transverse incision
4. Use an appropriate retractor
5. Grasp cornua of uterus with Kelly clamps
6. Clamp, cut, and ligate round ligaments
7. Incise vesicouterine peritoneum and develop bladder flap
8. Clamp, cut, and ligate tube and utero-ovarian anastomosis
9. Clamp, cut, and ligate uterine arteries
10. Clamp, cut, and ligate cardinal ligaments
11. Clamp, cut, and ligate uterosacral ligaments
12. Enter vagina anteriorly
13. Excise cervix circumferentially
14. Close vagina with continuous or interrupted suture

Anticipating Potential Complications

- Bowel or bladder injury
- Bleeding
- → Careful dissection
- → Identify vessels clearly; secure ties

Issues for Discussion

- When is an abdominal hysterectomy indicated?
- Can the operation be done as a laparoscopy-assisted vaginal hysterectomy?
- Is there a role for supracervical hysterectomy?
- When should you leave the ovaries, and when should you remove them?

Total Abdominal Hysterectomy with or without removal of tubes, with or without removal of ovaries	Dx 218.1 (uterine fibroids)	CPT code 58150	$920

Gynecologic Procedure 8: Vaginal Hysterectomy

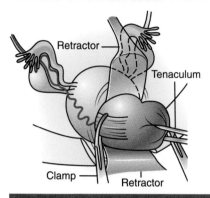

General technique used for vaginal hysterectomy.

Indications

- Uterine prolapse
- Menorrhagia
- Uterine fibroids
- Pelvic pain

Medical Knowledge—You Need to Know

- The degrees of uterine prolapse
- Pelvic anatomy from vaginal viewpoint
- Path of ureters

Major Steps

1. Empty bladder
2. Grasp cervix with tenaculum
3. Inject cervix with local anesthesia and epinephrine
4. Incise vaginal mucosa around cervix
5. Dissect vaginal mucosa in cephalic direction
6. Identify and enter posterior peritoneum
7. Identify and incise vesicouterine peritoneum
8. Clamp, cut, and ligate uterosacral ligaments
9. Clamp, cut, and ligate cardinal ligaments
10. Clamp, cut, and ligate uterine arteries
11. Clamp, cut, and ligate utero-ovarian anastomosis
12. Clamp, cut, and ligate uterotubal anastomosis
13. Close peritoneum using pursestring suture
14. Close vaginal cuff with interrupted suture

Anticipating Potential Complications

- Bleeding → Inject cervix with local anesthesia containing epinephrine
- Bladder injury → Identify vesicouterine peritoneum
- Ureteral injury → Maintain traction on cervix; keep dissection close to uterus

Issues for Discussion

- When is it appropriate to convert to laparotomy?
- Is the patient's anatomy appropriate to perform the procedure from a vaginal approach?
- Is it vital to remove the ovaries?

| Vaginal Hysterectomy | Dx 618.1 | CPT code 58260 | $1256 |

Gynecologic Procedure 9: Surgical Staging for Endometrial and Ovarian Cancers

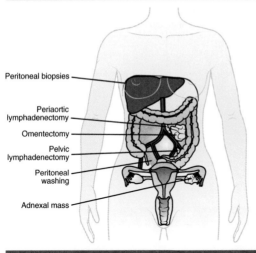

Anatomy that should be addressed at surgical staging for endometrial or ovarian cancer.

- Peritoneal biopsies
- Periaortic lymphadenectomy
- Omentectomy
- Pelvic lymphadenectomy
- Peritoneal washing
- Adnexal mass

Indications

- Endometrial cancer
- Ovarian cancer

Medical Knowledge—You Need to Know

- Natural history of endometrial and ovarian cancer
- FIGO surgical staging for endometrial and ovarian cancer
- Survival associated with each stage
- Likely locations of metastatic spread
- Pelvic anatomy, including blood supply and lymphatic drainage
- Path of ureters
- Appropriate preoperative evaluation
- How to manage difficult postoperative complications

Major Steps

1. Perform total abdominal hysterectomy and bilateral salpingo-oophorectomy
2. Obtain pelvic washings
3. Perform pelvic lymphadenectomy
4. Perform periaortic lymphadenectomy
5. Perform omentectomy (ovarian cancer only)
6. Obtain peritoneal biopsies (ovarian cancer only)

Anticipating Potential Complications

- Metastases to small → Be prepared to perform bowel resection or large bowel
- Pelvic hemorrhage → Anticipate the need for blood products
- Ureteral damage → Stent ureters before surgery if necessary, be prepared for ureteral reanastomosis or reimplantation to bladder as required

Issues for Discussion

- What is the role of consultants in this surgery?
- Should preoperative chemotherapy be given?

| Total Abdominal Hysterectomy with bilateral salpingo-oophorectomy and surgical staging | Dx 182.0 (endometrial cancer) 183.0 (ovarian cancer) | CPT code 58951 | $1975 |

Gynecologic Procedure 10: Pfannenstiel Incision

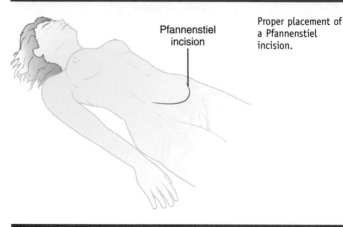

Pfannenstiel incision

Proper placement of a Pfannenstiel incision.

Indications

- Abdominal hysterectomy
- Abdominal myomectomy
- Cesarean section
- Exploratory laparotomy

Medical Knowledge—You Need to Know

- Abdominal wall anatomy

Major Steps

1. Make transverse skin incision with scalpel approximately two fingerbreadths above pubic symphysis
2. Incise subcutaneous tissue with Bovie electrocautery
3. Make transverse incision in anterior sheath of rectus fascia
4. Extend fascial incision past lateral edge of rectus muscles
5. Separate fascia from underlying rectus muscles
6. Separate rectus muscles in the midline
7. Separate preperitoneal fat
8. Grasp and incise peritoneum
9. Extend peritoneal incision in cephalic and caudal directions

Anticipating Potential Complications

- Bleeding from subcutaneous veins and subfascial vessels
- Intraperitoneal adhesions

→ Identify likely "bleeders" before you cut

→ Anticipate adhesions and dissect meticulously

Issues for Discussion

- When is a Pfannenstiel incision contraindicated?

| Pfannenstiel Incision | Dx 218.1 | CPT code 58150 | $980 |

Credits

Text

Definition of interpersonal and communication skills competency: Used with permission of Accreditation Counsel for Graduate Medical Education ©ACGME 2007. Please see the ACGME website: www.acgme.org for the most current version.

Communication behaviors and skills in Table 4-1 from *Successfully Navigating the First Year of Surgical Residency: Essentials for Medical Students and PGY-1 Residents* in Table 4-1: From *Successfully Navigating the First Year of Surgical Residency: Essentials for Medical Students and PGY-1 Residents,* p. 20, Division of Education, American College of Surgeons ©2005.

Definition of professionalism competency in text and Table 5-1: Used with permission of Accreditation Counsel for Graduate Medical Education ©ACGME 2007. Please see the ACGME website: www.acgme.org for the most current version.

Principles of the American Medical Association Code of Ethics: Principles of Medical Ethics, Adopted by the American Medical Association House of Delegates, June 2001. Accessed at http://www.ama-assn.org/ama/pub/category/2512.html on 2/13/08.

Physician's Charter principles and commitments: From ABIM Foundation, ACP Foundation, European Federation of Internal Medicine. Medical Professionalism in the New Millennium: A physician charter. Annals of Internal Medicine, 2002; 136:243-246.

Definition of systems-based practice competency: Used with permission of Accreditation Counsel for Graduate Medical Education ©ACGME 2007. Please see the ACGME website: www.acgme.org for the most current version.

Section I Appendix 1

ACGME Competency definitions: Used with permission of Accreditation Counsel for Graduate Medical Education ©ACGME 2007. Please see the ACGME website: www. acgme.org for the most current version.

Table 46-1: From the American College of Radiology (ACR) Breast Imaging Reporting and Data System Atlas (BI-RADS® Atlas). Reston, Virginia: ©American College of Radiology; 2003. All rights reserved.

Figures

Figures 10-1, 14-1, 14-2, 14-3, 14-4, 16-1, 19-1, 19-2, 19-3, figure in Operative Delivery Procedure 2: From Gabbe SG, et al.: Obstetrics: Normal and Problem Pregnancies, 5th edition. Copyright 2007, Elsevier.

Index

Note: Page numbers followed by f indicate figures; those followed by t indicate tables.